Fetal Echocardiography

Fetal Echocardiography
A Practical Guide

By

Lindsey D. Allan

Andrew C. Cook

and

Ian C. Huggon

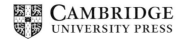

CAMBRIDGE UNIVERSITY PRESS
Cambridge, New York, Melbourne, Madrid, Cape Town, Singapore, São Paulo, Delhi, Dubai, Tokyo, Mexico City

Cambridge University Press
The Edinburgh Building, Cambridge CB2 8RU, UK

Published in the United States of America by Cambridge University Press, New York

www.cambridge.org
Information on this title: www.cambridge.org/9780521695206

First published 2009
3rd printing 2010

Printed in the United Kingdom at the University Press, Cambridge

A catalog record for this publication is available from the British Library

Library of Congress Cataloging in Publication data
Allan, Lindsey D. (Lindsey Dorothy)
  Fetal echocardiography : a practical guide / Lindsey D. Allan, Andrew C. Cook, Ian C. Huggon.
      p. ; cm.
  Includes bibliographical references.
  ISBN 978-0-521-69520-6 (hardback)
  1. Fetal heart–Ultrasonic imaging. I. Cook, A. C. (Andrew C.) II. Huggon, Ian C. III. Title.
  [DNLM: 1. Fetal Heart–anatomy & histology. 2. Fetal Heart–ultrasonography. 3. Echocardiography.
  4. Heart Defects, Congenital–ultrasonography. 5. Ultrasonography, Prenatal. WQ 210.5 A417f 2009]
  RG628.3.E34A453 2009
  618.3′26107543–dc22   2008052569

ISBN 978-0-521-69520-6 Hardback

I would like to dedicate the book to my friend and co-editor, Ian Huggon, who sadly died during the preparation of this book. Despite that, his input was considerable. He contributed a great deal to my knowledge and understanding of cardiac malformations, not to mention the computer skills I learnt from him during the 6 years we worked together, especially in obtaining clips and stills from the stored ultrasound images. I sorely missed his constructive criticism of the work latterly, and am sure there would have been a better book had he survived. With his agreement, I decided to use his recent teaching DVD as an enclosure to support and complement the text, as the moving image is so important to understanding and recognizing the heart and its malformations.

Contents

Preface

The term "congenital heart disease" refers mainly to anatomical malformations of the heart, which, in general, arise during cardiac formation prior to 8 weeks' post-conception. An accurate definition of any anatomical abnormality of the heart, to a large extent, predicts function and therefore postnatal symptomatology. An organized approach to defining the anatomy of the heart is therefore essential. The anatomy of the heart is evaluated in a sequential fashion, beginning below the diaphragm in the abdomen, and ending at the inlet of the thorax. In addition to the prediction of likely physiology, the anatomical definition allows any potential surgery or intervention to be planned, the results of which will correlate with the functional outcome for the child.

Fetal cardiac diagnosis depends first on the technical ability to obtain standard cardiac views. Technical skill is achieved both from understanding the relationships of the intrathoracic structures and from practice in obtaining cardiac views. Diagnosis depends second on the ability to distinguish normal from abnormal and third, on the ability to recognize and describe accurately the difference between the normal and the abnormal. Once the abnormality has been defined, giving it an accurate diagnostic label, and being able to predict the prognosis from the anatomical features of the diagnosis, are relatively easy steps. The book is aimed at anyone involved in fetal scanning who wants to learn each of these steps; how to obtain views, how to recognize the normal, how to distinguish and describe the abnormal and, from this last step, reach a diagnosis. The implications of a particular diagnosis are then described in the Outcome chapter.

There is no ideal way to construct a book on this topic. I have tried different approaches in previous books, but none is perfect. I have elected this time to concentrate on the standard views in separate chapters and how they may manifest abnormalities, but this means that the composite picture of a malformation, which may show abnormal features in various views, is rather lost, which is a pity. I have also separated the material on the implications of a defect into the chapter on outcome, which has its advantages, but also its disadvantages. However, I would hope that this book can be kept in the scan room and used as a quick and handy reference guide, to answer questions such as "is what I see within normal?" or "I think I see such and such in this fetal heart, what are the possible diagnoses?" or "I think the diagnosis is x, what could that mean for the child's future?"

We acquired a new machine near the end of the preparation of the book. This inevitably produced better images and new ways of illustrating the heart, which made it tempting to throw out all the old images and wait for another 10 years of new material. However, I resisted this temptation and have been able to distribute many of our new images throughout the text. It is just the way of things, of course, that one has lots of really good images of one type of malformation and none of another. I hope that the images of anatomy specimens prove helpful in understanding the echocardiography. I learnt so much from the anatomical dissections in my early years when correlative pathological specimens were readily obtained. It is a tragedy that this valuable teaching resource has been largely taken from us, but I hope the pathological images go some way towards reversing this loss.

I was not going to provide a bibliography at all initially, but decided in the end to include some of what I considered the most relevant ones, but grouped together in a separate chapter. I apologize if I have missed some important ones, but the ease of using resources such as PubMed, more or less make references obsolete in my opinion. Every statement can be checked or further explored in a minute, far more thoroughly than any reference list can do.

I have specialized in this subject for nearly 30 years now and have tried to communicate a distillate of that knowledge in this book. I make no apology for my individual approach, which is perhaps different from others, but has worked pretty well for me for a long time. I have illustrated examples of almost everything I have ever seen, and have been lucky in having had access to a huge volume of cases over the years.

I hope there is material here which will add to the understanding of the complete beginner, as well as to the knowledge of the fairly experienced practitioner, and that it is presented in a manner which is accessible for everyone.

Acknowledgments

I would like to thank my current colleague, Vita Zidere for her support and help with the project, allowing me quiet time and space to complete it, as well as help with obtaining images. Also, I would like to thank Sven-Erik Sonesson for his help with the chapter on arrhythmias, which Ian had not been able to finish. Sven-Erik's images were much better than ours and he was generous in contributing them.

Technique of obtaining cardiac views

Successful ultrasound diagnosis in any context depends first, on obtaining a series of defined cross-sectional images and, second, on the correct interpretation of those images. The plane of cross-section is modified according to the structures identified, in order to demonstrate the structure of the three-dimensional whole in an optimum fashion. The relationship between movements of the transducer, and alteration in the image obtained by those movements, is a complex one. Practice and intuition play a large part in the skilled manipulation of a transducer to obtain the desired views. However, a methodical and deliberate approach may improve the initial rate of learning and of continuing skill development, and also help in teaching those skills to others. There is no universal terminology to describe the axes of the transducer, or the different movements that the transducer can make relative to the abdomen. Figure 1.1 shows the three axes of an ultrasound transducer, which we have labeled X, Y, and Z. The following scheme may be helpful in directing others to scan and also in disciplining oneself into a methodical approach to scanning. Every transducer images in a plane or sector, which is usually evident from its shape or markings, and corresponds to the plane that includes the X- and Y-axes in Fig. 1.1. There are six possible movements of a transducer each in two possible directions. Three of these movements conserve the imaging plane, whilst viewing that plane from a different aspect, whereas the other three alter the imaging plane itself (Figs. 1.2 and 1.3)

In-plane slide

In-plane slide describes the movement of the transducer across the abdomen in line with the initial plane of imaging, or movement in its X-axis. As the transducer slides, new structures will appear on the side of the image corresponding to the leading edge of the transducer and others will disappear from the trailing edge side. Structures in the image will appear to move laterally relative to the sector margins (and eventually

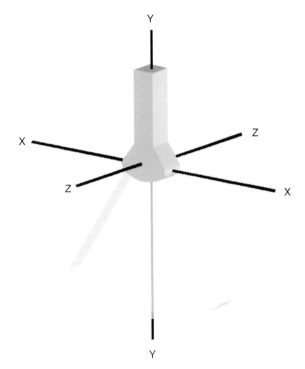

Fig. 1.1. The three axes of an ultrasound transducer, labeled to help with the description of the transducer movements that follows.

disappear from the edge), but their appearance remains otherwise unaltered.

Rocking

Rocking the transducer describes the movement in which the sector remains in the same plane and the point of contact with the maternal abdomen is unchanged but the angle between the transducer and the abdomen is altered. This is movement in the X- and Z-axes of the transducer. In the image, new structures will appear on the side of the image corresponding to the leading edge of the transducer and others will disappear from the trailing edge side, as with an in-plane slide. The difference between the in-plane slide and rock is best appreciated when the two are used

(a)

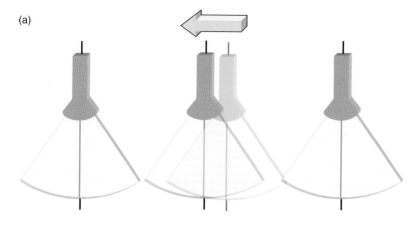

Fig. 1.2. The three types of transducer movements that keep the plane of imaging the same but alter the view within that plane are shown. In each diagram, the left-sided drawing is where the transducer starts, the middle panel represents the movement of the transducer and the right-hand panel is where the transducer ends up after the movement. **(a).** In-plane slide. The transducer slides over the maternal skin in the line of its X-axis. The angles made with the skin by all three axes remain unchanged.

(b)

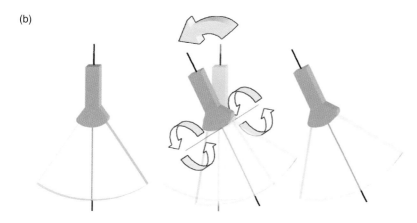

Fig. 1.2.(b). Rock. The point of contact of the transducer with the maternal abdomen remains unchanged. The angles that both the X- and Y-axes of the transducer make with the skin change, but the angle that the Z-axis makes with the skin remains the same.

(c)

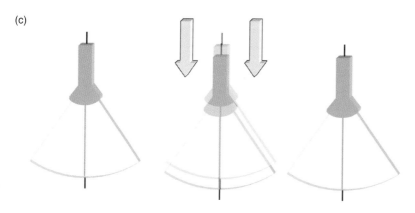

Fig. 1.2.(c). Change in pressure. Both the point of contact of the transducer with the skin and the angle of contact with the skin in all three axes remain unchanged, but the transducer moves up or down in its Y-axis. The transducer moves nearer or further away from a given point in the fetus because of compression displacement or release of intervening tissue.

(a)

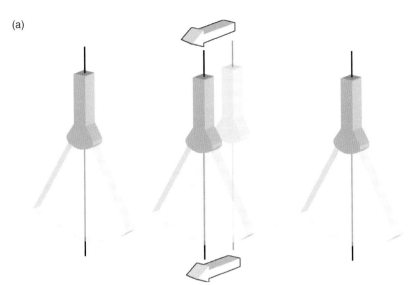

Fig. 1.3. The three types of transducer movement that alter the imaging plane as well as the view. **(a).** Out-of plane slide. The transducer is moved along the line of its Z-axis. The angles that all three axes make with the skin are unchanged but the point of contact with the skin moves.

(b)

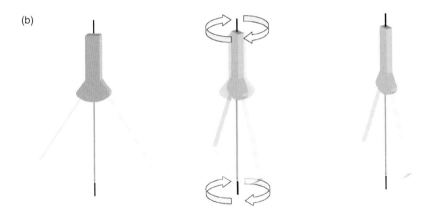

Fig. 1.3.(b). Rotation. The transducer rotates or spins around its Y-axis. The angles that all three axes make with the skin are unchanged as is the point of contact with the skin.

(c)

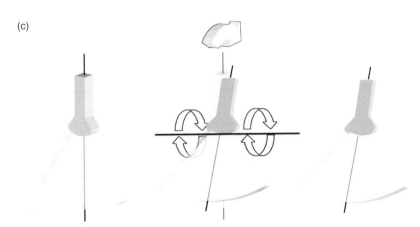

Fig. 1.3.(c). Angulation. The point of contact with the skin remains unchanged, but the angle that the Y- and Z-axes makes with the skin alters. The angle between the X-axis and the skin remains constant.

together in combination (Fig. 1.4). An initial in-plane slide moves a central area of interest towards the edge of the image, but a subsequent rock of the transducer in the appropriate direction will bring the area of interest back to the center of the image. The difference between images before and after this combination of movements is that the path of ultrasound to the structure of interest is altered, so that shadows due to intervening structures may be avoided. Also, the angle with which the ultrasound beam strikes the structure of interest is altered, affecting the quality and appearance of the image.

Change of pressure

Change of pressure on the transducer allows a limited amount of vertical movement within the imaging plane. This movement is in the Y-axis of the transducer. Increasing pressure moves the transducer nearer to a distant area of interest, by displacing intervening fluid and soft tissue. Structures will appear to move up within the image. The quality of the image also changes. Within limits, image quality generally improves as the transducer moves nearer to the area of interest, but this may be counteracted by the displacement of amniotic fluid from between the transducer and the area of interest, a modest amount of which generally enhances image quality. Excessive pressure may be counterproductive, may cause discomfort to the patient, and can nearly always be avoided.

Out-of-plane slide

Out-of-plane slide describes the movement of the transducer across the maternal abdomen parallel to the initial imaging plane. This is movement in the Z-axis of the transducer. The images obtained are therefore parallel planes to the initial imaging plane. As the transducer moves, the images show new structures appearing within the body of the image, rather than appearing to slide in from the edge, as with an in-plane slide.

Rotation

Rotation of the transducer describes the movement whereby the central point of the transducer surface remains in a fixed position on the abdomen, but the transducer is spun about this point (around the Y-axis or the axis of the transducer cable). As the transducer rotates, structures in the center of the image remain in view but are cut in a different plane. Structures more peripheral in the image will disappear from view as the transducer rotates.

Angulation

Angulation of the transducer is when the point of contact of the transducer with the abdomen remains constant, but the angle that the transducer makes with the initial imaging plane is varied. This produces a similar change in the image to the out-of-plane slide, except that in the out-of-plane slide, near and far structures pass through the image at the same rate, whereas angulation has a greater effect on the appearance of distant structures than it does on near ones. This is movement in the Y- and Z-axes of the transducer.

Transducer movements in practice

Although the possible movements of a transducer have been described individually, they will often be used in combination. Indeed, a slide in any direction across the curved, rather than flat, surface of the maternal abdomen will inevitably involve an element of rock or angulation. The combination of an in-plane slide of the transducer with a rock in the "opposite" direction has already been described.

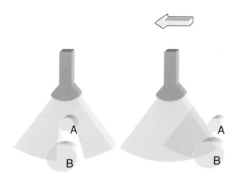
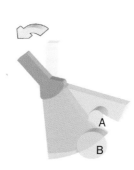

Fig. 1.4. Use of a combination of movements. A structure in the near-field casts an ultrasound shadow obscuring the deeper structure B of interest. An in-plane slide of the transducer removes structure A from the near field, but leaves the structure B at the periphery of the image. A subsequent rock of the transducer brings structure B to the centre of the image, without interference from structure A.

This is a useful method of obtaining clearer views of a structure, already in view in the desired plane, but partially obscured by intervening structures, such as a limb (Fig. 1.4).

Although the terms "view" and "plane" tend to be used interchangeably, an important distinction can be made between them. Any defined plane can be imaged from different directions to obtain different views. The actual structures within a given plane are fixed, but their appearance may vary considerably in different views (or approaches to the plane). This is because ultrasound, and therefore the image obtained using it, has a directional quality. The axial resolution of an ultrasound image is always greater than the lateral resolution. Structures consisting of reflective surfaces perpendicular to the ultrasound beam are generally demonstrated more clearly than those oriented parallel to the beam. Ultrasound shadows from dense structures interposed between the transducer and areas of interest may also detract from the image quality of some views within a plane. Usually more than one view of a particular plane will be required to demonstrate all of the anatomical features within that plane to best effect. Subtle adjustments to the angle of view within a plane explain at least in part the ability of an experienced echocardiographer to obtain clearer views than a less experienced pupil scanning the same patient. Methodical scanning dictates that the operator should understand how different movements of the transducer will alter the plane of section of the fetus and the effect of this relationship on the position and size of the fetus and its distance from the imaging probe. If the echocardiographer has already achieved the appropriate plane of section, but needs to change the view within that plane in order to optimize imaging of a particular structure, then this can be achieved by a combination of in-plane slide, rock, and change in pressure. These are the three movements that conserve the initial plane of imaging, whilst altering the view. If the desired plane of imaging has yet to be obtained, then a combination of out-of-plane slide, angle, and rotation will be required to move to the required plane. Once the desired plane has been obtained, further manipulation by in-plane slide, rock, and pressure will demonstrate the optimum view within that plane. Most of these movements are performed instinctively with experience, but understanding how they operate can accelerate the learning curve.

The combination of movements required to move from one plane to another depends not only on the initial and final planes, but also the aspect from which the initial plane is being viewed. For example, consider the movements of a transducer required to move from a standard transverse four-chamber plane to the left ventricular outflow plane, passing through the right shoulder. With the fetus prone relative to the transducer, this change in plane can be achieved by an almost pure clockwise rotation of the transducer (Fig. 1.5(a)). However, if the same initial plane is viewed with the fetal right side uppermost, a combination of an out-of-plane slide towards the fetal head, combined with an angulation towards the abdomen, is required to achieve the same change in plane (Fig. 1.5(b)).

Sweeps through the fetus to provide a series of approximately parallel image slices are an important element of fetal echocardiography. For a small fetus, some distance from the transducer, this can be achieved entirely by angulation of the transducer from a fixed point on the maternal abdomen. In contrast, for a larger fetus, or for one closer to the transducer, an out-of-plane sliding motion of the transducer is required to produce a similar series of image slices (Fig. 1.6). Those whose prior experience is with pediatric echocardiography need to adjust their technique to the fact that fine movements of the transducer can produce large alterations in the plane of section of the small heart of the fetus. As a practical point, it is helpful in fetal cardiac scanning to support the hand and arm by maintaining direct contact between the hand and the maternal abdomen as well as with the probe, or by leaning or resting the hand and arm on the mother's thigh or abdomen, in order to facilitate the fine controlled movement which is necessary.

Left–right orientation

Determination of the fetal position and establishing the left and right, anterior and posterior, and superior and inferior aspects of the fetus is vital. It is important at the outset to ascertain the right–left orientation in the fetus, as this is indefinite in a cross-sectional image. In order to establish this, the operator must be aware of the relationship between the sector on the screen and the transducer in their hand and also that between the transducer on the abdomen and the fetus beneath. On most ultrasound systems, a marker on the side of the transducer corresponds to a symbol on the corresponding side of the sector image on the screen. Correct orientation of the transducer can also

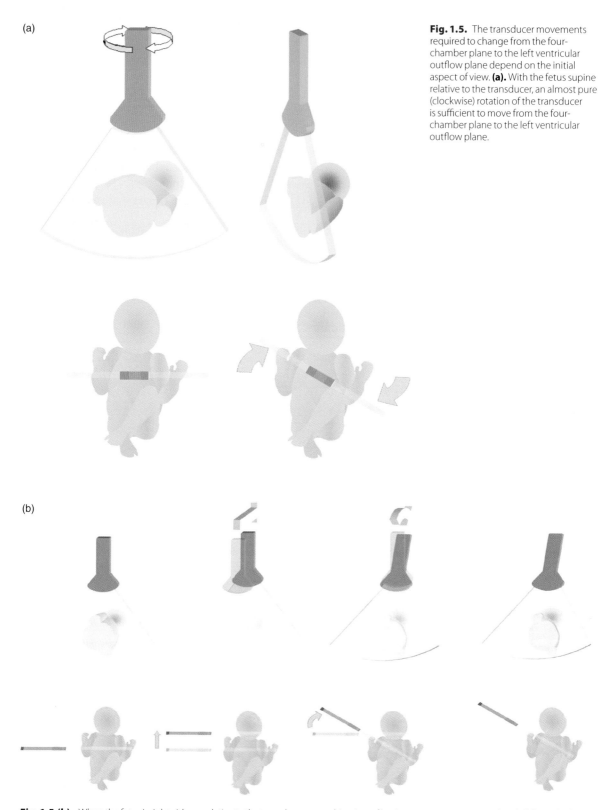

Fig. 1.5. The transducer movements required to change from the four-chamber plane to the left ventricular outflow plane depend on the initial aspect of view. **(a).** With the fetus supine relative to the transducer, an almost pure (clockwise) rotation of the transducer is sufficient to move from the four-chamber plane to the left ventricular outflow plane.

Fig. 1.5.(b). When the fetus is right-side up relative to the transducer, a combination of basic movements is required to shift from the four-chamber plane to the left ventricular outflow plane. Initially an out-of-plane slide towards the head gives a transverse imaging plane parallel to the four-chamber plane but close to the head. Subsequent angulation of the transducer to point back towards the heart gives an imaging plane passing through the right shoulder and demonstrating the left ventricular outflow. Note that the amount of initial out-of plane slide required will depend on the distance of the fetus from the transducer and the size of the fetus.

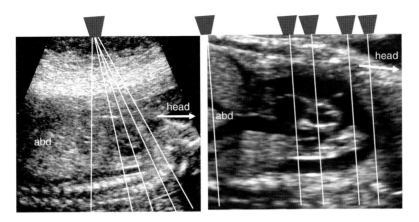

Fig. 1.6. The beam is positioned in a transverse section about the level of the diaphragm. The beam is then swept or angled, down to image the stomach in the abdomen (abd) and then up towards the head end of the baby, to the inlet of the thorax. It can be seen that, in a small fetus, some distance from the transducer as in the left-hand panel, this is achieved by angulation of the beam but in a larger fetus, closer to the transducer (right-hand panel), by an out-of-plane slide. Usually an element of both movements are involved. Note that the five important planes to be examined are not equidistant from each other.

be confirmed by the effect of transducer movements on the image. Viewing the fetus in transverse section and keeping the transducer in the same plane of section, as the operator slides the transducer laterally (in-plane) to his or her left, the image on the screen moves appropriately, with "new" structures being revealed on the left of the screen and others disappearing from the right. (Should this not be the case then the transducer

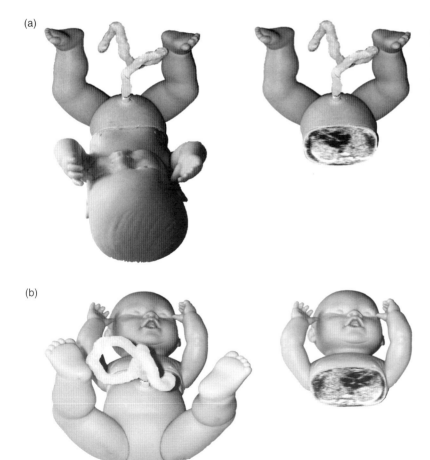

Figs. 1.7 and 1.8 Establishing right–left orientation. The operator has already confirmed that the right side of the image as displayed on the screen is generated by the right side of the transducer as viewed by the operator. Subsequent small movements of the transducer, parallel to the four-chamber plane, will then allow the operator to decide if the image displayed corresponds to a section of the thorax viewed as though looking from above (Fig. 1.7(a) and 1.8(a)) or from below (Fig. 1.7(b) and 1.8(b)), whether the fetus is in a supine (Fig. 1.7) or prone position (Fig. 1.8). In Fig. 1.7(a) and 1.8(a), therefore, the head is in front of the screen (HF), whereas in Figs. 1.7(b) and 1.8(b), the head is behind the screen (HB). Many four-chamber views in the book will be labelled HF or HB to stress the understanding of this point. Look out for disorders of heart position.

(a)

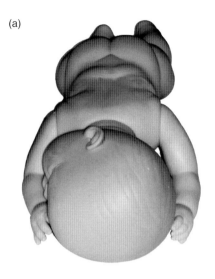
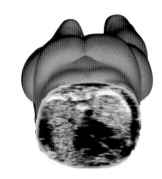

Fig. 1.7 and 1.8 Continued

(b)

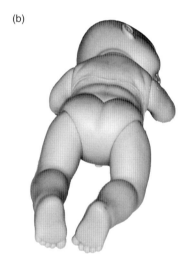
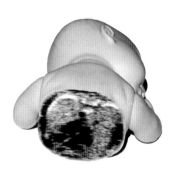

should be rotated 180° about the axis of its cable, to ensure that it is.) Alternatively, touching the edge of the transducer or adjacent abdominal skin should demonstrate distortion of the image at the corresponding side of the screen. This confirms the "correct" orientation of the transducer relative to the screen image. Then the transducer is moved parallel to the imaging plane (out-of-plane-slide), away from the operator. From the change in the structures seen, the operator should then be able to determine whether the transducer is moving up or down the fetus. If the appearance is consistent with the transducer moving down the

fetus (caudad) as it moves away from the operator, then the section of the fetus will be as though viewing a cut section from above (Fig. 1.7(a) and 1.8(a)). Conversely, if the image moves up the fetus (cephalad) as the transducer is pushed away from the operator, then the section of the fetus will be as though viewing a cut section from below (Fig. 1.7(b) and 1.8(b)). If one imagines the whole fetus viewed from either above or below as in Fig. 1.7(a) and (b) and 1.8(a) and (b), there should be no difficulty in ascertaining left and right, regardless of whether the fetus is supine or prone. Various other specific methods of establishing orientation have been described, including that from Cordes as follows. In the long axis of the fetus, the head is positioned to the right on the screen (whichever side it truly lies). The transducer is turned 90° clockwise from this position to the four-chamber view. This effectively positions the head behind the screen. Thus, in the normal fetus, if he/she lies face up, this will display the liver on the left and the heart on the right of the screen, the reverse if face down. Each operator will have their own preferred method for establishing orientation with which they feel most secure. One cannot, however, establish the right–left orientation of the fetus on the basis of the position of internal organs, such as the stomach or heart, since their position may vary from the normal. Moreover, abnormalities of laterality often affect both the stomach and the heart. Thus, the appearance of the stomach and cardiac apex on the same side of the fetus as each other in no way guarantees that both are normally positioned on the left. Fig. 1.9 demonstrates how an abnormality of position of the heart may be evident

only if the operator ascertains right and left independently of the supposed position of the internal organs. However, once the left–right orientation is determined and a normal (or otherwise) position of the stomach and cardiac apex is established, these structures are then useful points of reference to maintain appreciation of right and left throughout the rest of the scan, during which the fetus may move from its original position.

After the first step on ultrasound examination of the maternal abdomen – identifying the position of the fetus relative to the maternal pelvis, breech, cephalic or transverse lie, which will allow the correct identification of left and right in the fetus – the transducer should then be lined up in a transverse section of the fetal trunk, approximately at the level of the diaphragm. Maintaining a more or less horizontal cut, the ultrasound beam is then swept from the level of the stomach, in a cranial direction, through the cardiac structures to the inlet of the thorax. This is achieved

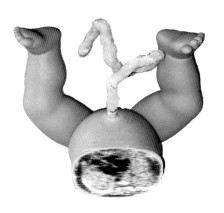 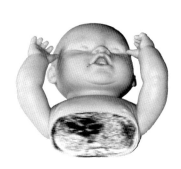

Fig. 1.9. The two ultrasound images are identical. It is only by understanding the relationship of the image slice to the whole baby that the operator can know if he or she is viewing a normally positioned heart as though from above (left-hand image), or mirror-image dextrocardia viewed as though from below (right-hand image). Instead of the right-hand fetus lying HF as would be expected, it is HB.

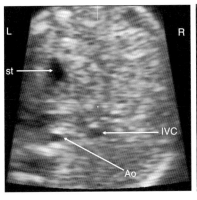 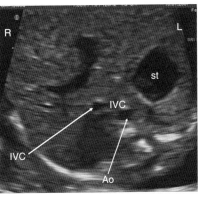

Fig. 1.10. On the left-hand panel, the fetus lies with the head in front of the screen (HF). The stomach is seen in a cross-section of the abdomen lying on the left of the fetus in the usual position relative to the other abdominal structures. The abdominal aorta lies anterior and slightly to the left of the spine with the inferior vena cava anterior and to the right of the aorta. Note these normal spatial relationships. On the right-hand panel, the fetus lies with the head behind the screen (HB). The same positional relationships of the aorta, inferior vena cava and stomach are seen.

9

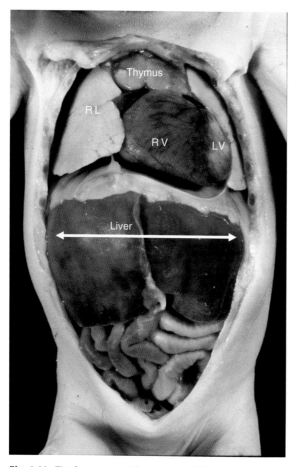

Fig. 1.11. This fetus is viewed from the front following removal of the anterior chest and abdominal walls to show the heart lying in the left chest with its apex pointing leftward. As a result of the large fetal liver extending to the left abdominal wall, the apex is pushed cranially. This renders the right heart structures anterior. The left atrium and ventricle lie posteriorly, so are hidden from view from the front. The arterial trunks in the upper thorax are covered by the thymus. Note that there is a good portion of right lung (RL) between the right atrium and right thoracic wall.

mainly by angulation in the first half of pregnancy or by out-of-plane slide in the larger fetus (Fig. 1.6). This "sweep" shows all the cardiac structures that are necessary to check during a fetal echocardiogram and, from the correct starting point, can be accomplished in seconds.

The cross-section of the abdomen (Fig. 1.10) shows the stomach on the left. As the beam is swept up to the heart, the inferior vena cava can be followed to its connection to the right atrium. The stomach is noted to be on the same side as the cardiac apex. The four-chamber plane is seen in a completely transverse section of the thorax just above the diaphragm. This is because the large fetal liver, extending to the left abdominal wall, tilts the apex cranially so that the base of the heart almost lies flat on the diaphragm (Fig. 1.11). Note that this is in contrast to the situation in postnatal life and especially in the adult, where the apex points caudally and the four-chamber plane does not correspond to an orthogonal transverse plane. The correct technique of obtaining the four-chamber plane is vital, as the ultrasound beam must be positioned in the correct orthogonal plane at the right level in the heart, in order to analyze it accurately. Confirmation that the plane obtained is indeed a standard four-chamber plane should precede any attempt at detailed analysis. The correct plane is a completely transverse section, as evidenced by a round shape to the thorax and at least one complete rib in the image. When multiple ribs are seen, this indicates that the section is oblique, either laterally or antero-posteriorly (Fig. 1.12). The correct level within the heart for assessment of the four-chamber plane shows the crux or center of the heart and is a precise point in the heart, which in the early fetus is quite small. If the level is too low in the heart, the

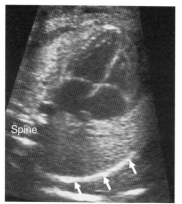

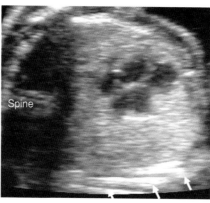

Fig. 1.12. In the left-hand panel, the ultrasound beam is positioned correctly across the thorax in order to image the four-chamber view. The thorax has a round shape and one almost complete rib is seen. In the right-hand panel, the transducer beam cuts obliquely across the thorax, as can be seen by multiple ribs on one side of the image. Something of the four-chamber view is seen in the heart, but this is not adequate for either analysis of the view, nor is it the correct starting point to initiate a sweep to the great artery views (HF).

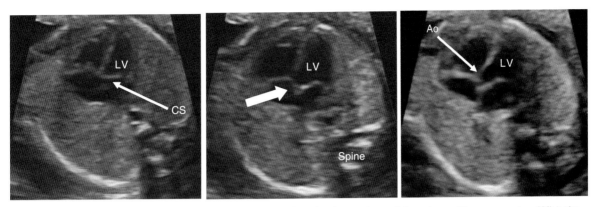

Fig. 1.13. In the left-hand panel, the beam cuts just below the true four-chamber section and shows instead the coronary sinus (CS). In the right-hand panel, the beam is too high in the heart and shows the origin of the aorta. In the center panel, the beam is at the right level cutting through the crux of the heart (broad arrow). In a small fetus, the distance between these planes is a matter of millimetres and fetal movement or maternal breathing can readily displace the beam from the crux. It is important to be aware of this and make sure the true crux is seen (HB).

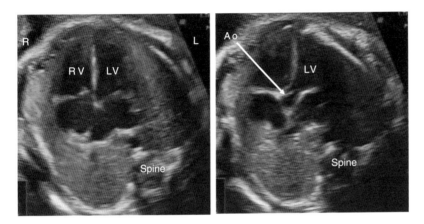

Fig. 1.14. In the left-hand panel, the beam is correctly positioned on the four-chamber view both for analysis and for initiating a sweep. In the right-hand panel, the ultrasound beam has been tilted, or slid, slightly cranially to image the view immediately cranial to the four-chamber view, of a great artery arising from the left ventricle. In the normal heart, this should be the aorta but until the other great artery is seen, or a longer course of the artery is seen, this may not be the case. Note that the posterior wall of the artery is continuous with the anterior leaflet of the mitral valve and the anterior wall is continuous with the septum. This view is very close to the four-chamber view, especially so in the small fetus (HB).

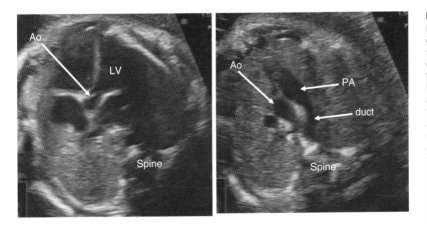

Fig. 1.15. The view obtained in the right-hand panel is just above the level of the section on the left-hand panel and shows the origin of the other great artery, close to the anterior chest wall as it arises from the right ventricle. In the normal heart, this should be the pulmonary artery. Seeing the artery, which arises from the right ventricle, crossing over the great artery arising from the left as shown here (almost always), indicates that the great arteries are normally connected. Thus, the artery seen on the left panel arising from the left ventricle is the aorta and the artery on the right panel arising from the right ventricle is the pulmonary artery. Note that the direction of the outflow tracts at their origin is at right angles to each other, with the aorta initially directed rightwards, whereas the pulmonary artery is directed straight back towards the spine.

coronary sinus is seen instead of the crux; if it is too high, the aortic origin is seen in the center of the heart instead of the true crux (Fig. 1.13). Immediately above the level of the four-chamber plane lies the aortic outflow tract plane, with the aorta "wedged" between the two atrioventricular valves (Fig. 1.14). At its origin, the aorta sweeps out towards the right shoulder. Scanning more cranially, the right ventricular outflow tract and pulmonary artery lie above the aorta. The main pulmonary artery "crosses over" the aortic origin and, in its continuation with the arterial duct, is directed straight posteriorly (Fig. 1.15). Thus, the two great arteries are at right angles to each other at their origin. Moving further cranially the transverse aortic arch is seen just below the inlet of the thorax (Fig. 1.16). The anatomical specimen is shown to improve understanding of the position and direction of the standard sections of the heart used in fetal echocardiography and their relationship to cardiac structures (Fig. 1.17(a) and (b)).

The great arteries are distinguished from each other by their morphological features rather than by

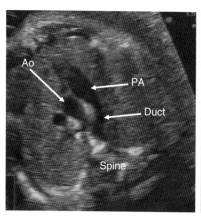 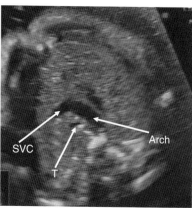

Fig. 1.16. The right-hand panel shows the final section of the same fetus imaged in Figs. 1.14 and 1.15. A small portion of the duct is still seen as well as the transverse arch, which is the most superior (or cranial) arterial vessel. Note that the aortic arch crosses the midline from right to left in front of the trachea (T). The superior vena cava (SVC) lies at the right-hand end of the aorta as it turns towards the left.

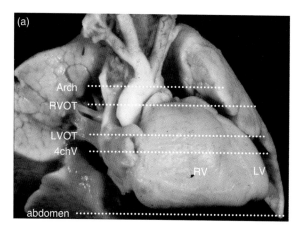

Fig. 1.17.(a). The unopened heart specimen is viewed from the front. The successive cuts across the specimen in order to achieve standard planes are shown. Note that there are five standard planes from the abdomen to the transverse arch and they are not equidistant from each other.

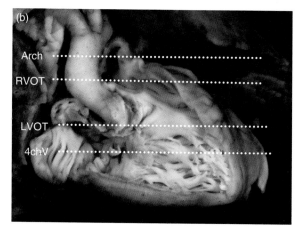

Fig. 1.17.(b). The transverse sections are shown in relation to the opened cardiac specimen as viewed from the right ventricular side of the septum. The four-chamber view (4chV) cuts through the middle of the tricuspid valve. The mitral valve lies in the same plane behind the septum. The origin of the left ventricular outflow tract (LVOT) is just above the four-chamber plane. Note that the right ventricular outflow tract (RVOT) is much further from the four-chamber view than the left ventricular outflow tract.

their connections to the heart, as the latter can vary in heart malformations. The immutable morphological characteristics of the aorta are that the first branches seen echocardiographically arise in a superior direction some distance from the arterial valve. (To be more precise, the aorta first gives off the coronary arteries from the aortic sinuses just above the valve, but these are usually too small to be seen on fetal echocardiography.) In contrast, the pulmonary artery branches after a short distance from the arterial valve and branches laterally into three, the left and right pulmonary arteries, with the arterial duct in the middle. In addition, the

aorta forms the most superior arch, whereas the ductal arch lies below the level of the aortic arch.

During the transverse sweep, a slight rotation, or combination of out of plane slide and angulation of the transducer from the four-chamber plane (depending on the initial aspect of view, Fig. 1.5) images a left ventricular outflow plane, which passes between the right shoulder and left iliac crest of the fetus. This plane will open out the aortic origin, allowing it to be identified more positively as the aorta by virtue of its lack of early branching (Fig. 1.18(a) and (b)). In contrast, slight adjustment of the transducer beam will show that

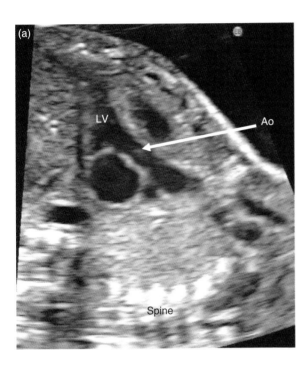

(a)

LV — Ao

Spine

Fig. 1.18.(a). By rotating the transducer on the origin of the vessel arising from the left ventricle, it can be imaged in a long axis view, which allows a longer length of vessel to be seen. The lack of visible early branching and the sweeping course towards the right shoulder designates it the aorta. This view often demonstrates more clearly than the view of the aorta seen in Fig. 1.14, that the aorta is wholly committed to the left ventricle, an essential normal feature.

Arch views

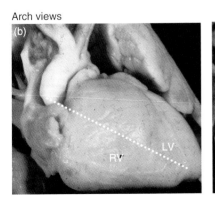

(b)

RV — LV

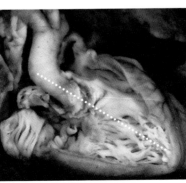

Fig. 1.18.(b). The orientation of the transducer necessary to produce the long-axis view of the left ventricular outflow tract is shown in relation to the unopened and opened anatomical specimens.

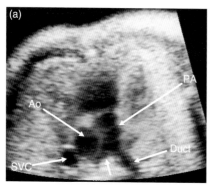
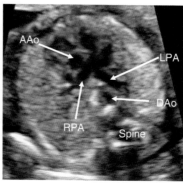

Fig. 1.19.(a). When the pulmonary artery and duct are imaged in a transverse section (the three-vessel view) the origin of the right pulmonary artery just above the level of the pulmonary valve, is often seen (HB). It arises from the pulmonary artery after only a short part of the main pulmonary artery and travels behind the ascending aorta to the right lung. By slightly tilting the transducer from the view on the left-hand panel, the right and left pulmonary arteries can be seen, as on the right-hand panel. Note that the duct cannot usually be seen in the same cut as both branch pulmonary arteries as it really lies slightly above the level of the branches. The right pulmonary artery lies between the ascending (AAo) and descending (DAo) aorta.

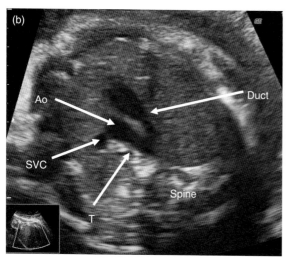
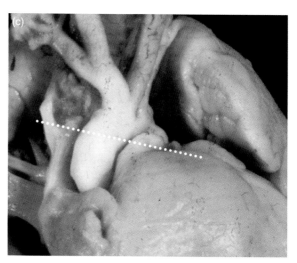

Fig. 1.19.(b). Slight angulation of the transducer from the truly transverse plane in the upper thorax allows the transverse aortic arch and arterial duct to be seen in the same section. They can be compared in relative size and position. Usually the duct is the same size or slightly smaller than the transverse arch. The two vessels in this view lie close together before they join just in front of the spine. The aorta crosses the midline in front of the trachea (T).

Fig. 1.19.(c). The anatomical specimen is seen from the front. The orientation of the ultrasound beam necessary to produce an image of the arch and duct simultaneously is indicated. It only needs to be slightly tilted from the truly transverse plane.

the artery arising from the right ventricle does branch soon after its origin, identifying it as the pulmonary artery (Fig. 1.19(a)). A similar maneuver of the transducer to that which moves from the four-chamber plane to left ventricular outflow, performed at the level of the arterial duct, allows the duct and arch to be seen in the same section, and therefore be compared in size and relative position (Fig. 1.19(b) and (c)). Thus, the transverse planes of the heart, which are the most basic, involve a sweep in a horizontal plane across the fetal trunk, from the abdomen to the inlet of the thorax, with small adjustments from the transverse to demonstrate the aortic outflow tract more clearly and the transverse arch and duct simultaneously. A combination of those transcriptions movements, which conserve the plane of imaging, will allow each plane to be viewed from a different aspect, and optimization of the image to define specific structures most clearly.

In an alternative approach to cardiac scanning, using some of the new 3D/4D ultrasound machines, a cardiac volume can be obtained. A machine-acquired cardiac volume is like obtaining an automated form of the manual sweep and should be started about the level of the aortic outflow, with the settings on the machine optimized for the fetal size, that is, a smaller angle of sweep for a smaller fetus and vice versa. Using tomographic imaging (TUI), a series of planes from the stomach to the aortic arch can then be displayed, on 2D and color (Fig. 1.20(a)–(h)). Narrowing the distance between each slice can allow closer examination of each part of the heart and varying the distance can select each ideal view of the five essential cuts. This

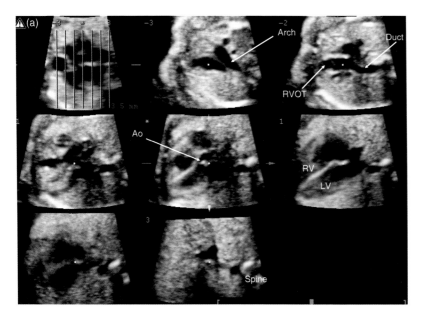

Fig. 1.20(a). The images are obtained from a volume set. The heart is sliced in seven sections at 3 mm distances, from the upper thorax (top row) to the abdomen (bottom row). Thus, there are only 21 mm between the abdomen and arch in this 20-week fetus. The reference image (top left) shows the relationship of the cuts to the fetus in a long-axis projection. The first slice (middle of the top row) shows the arch and duct, 3 mm below this (right panel of top row) is the pulmonary artery and its connection to the duct. The central image in the display shows the origin of the aorta from the left ventricle and the middle row right panel, the four-chamber view. The middle slice in the bottom row shows the abdominal situs. The display demonstrates that the aorta is only 3 mm above the four-chamber view, whereas the pulmonary artery is 9 mm above it. Similarly, the stomach and vessels in the abdomen are 6 mm below the four-chamber view. The fetus lies HF.

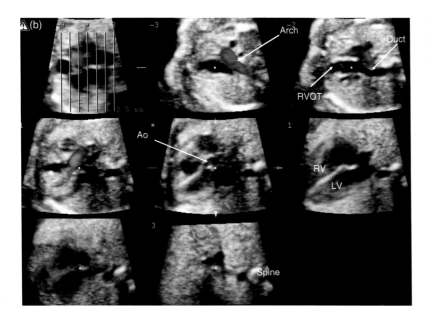

Fig. 1.20(b). The same image as in Fig. 1.20(a), with color added, shows a systolic frame. Forward flow is clearly seen in the ascending aorta and transverse aortic arch. No flow is seen in the pulmonary artery (despite this being a systolic frame) because the direction of flow within it is at right angles to the color flow beam.

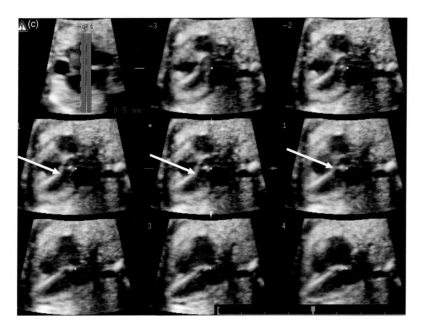

Fig. 1.20(c). In the same fetus, the slices are taken at 0.5 mm distances (compare the top left image with the top left in Fig. 1.20(a)), in order to focus on the crux of the heart and the origin of the aorta. This allows, for example, close examination of the perimembraneous part of the ventricular septum, which is seen here in the middle row of images (arrows).

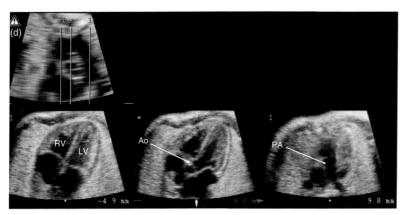

Fig. 1.20(d). In a larger fetus at 31 weeks, the four-chamber view (bottom left) is 4.9 mm below the aorta (middle) and 14.7 mm below the pulmonary artery (bottom right). The fetus lies HB.

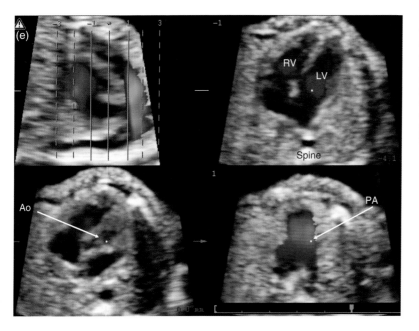

Fig. 1.20(e). The three most fundamental sections for fetal heart examination are obtained from a volume sweep and the relationship of each cut in the long-axis view is shown in the upper left panel. The first slice (upper right) demonstrates the four-chamber view, the next moving cranially, the aortic origin (bottom left) and the third, the pulmonary artery (bottom right). The fetus lies HB.

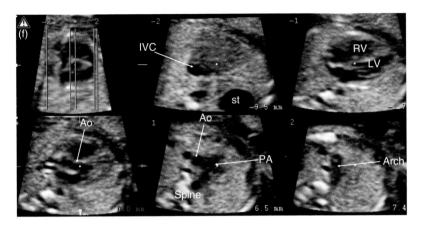

Fig. 1.20(f). The five views, essential for a basic fetal echocardiogram, are displayed as tomographic images from a volume sweep. The fetus lies HB. The position of each slice has been adjusted (image on top left) to display an ideal image of each cut. Note how close the sections are between the four-chamber view and the origin of the aorta and between the three-vessel view and the arch. The five views comprise: abdominal situs (middle top), four-chamber view (upper right), origin of the aorta (lower left), three vessel view (lower middle) and transverse aortic arch (lower right).

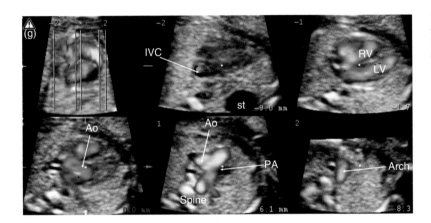

Fig. 1.20(g). The same set of tomographic images shown in Fig. 1.20(e), with the color information added, allows the identification of the 2D structures more clearly.

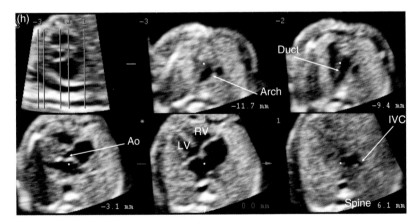

Fig. 1.20(h). The five essential views are displayed from tomographic images, where the fetus lies HF, from the transverse arch in the middle of the top row to the abdomen on the bottom right. The four-chamber view in the center of the bottom row seems to show a ventricular septal defect but this is artifact.

method of heart examination can improve the understanding of how each view is achieved and also how the heart is constructed.

In the majority of cases, the transverse views of the fetal heart are sufficient to identify all the normal features and to exclude cardiac malformation. However, long-axis views of the heart are sometimes useful adjuncts to analysis, especially in cardiac anomalies. The transducer is turned from a four-chamber view through 90° and then the beam is "swept", in a similar fashion to

17

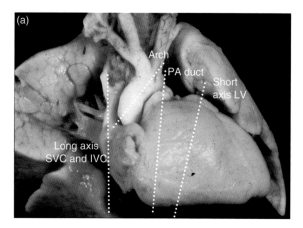

Fig. 1.21(a). The heart specimen is viewed from the front. The successive cuts across the specimen in order to achieve standard sagittal planes are shown. Note that there is some variation in the angle of the cut, and therefore transducer angulation, necessary in order to show the typical views. Thus, in a mechanically acquired volume sweep, depending on the starting angle, either the perfect arch is achieved or the perfect duct, but not both in the same longitudinal sweep. Note that the short-axis of left ventricle, pulmonary artery and duct, IVC and SVC views are almost coronal cuts, whereas the aortic arch is not.

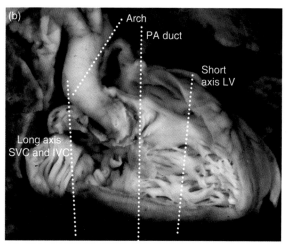

Fig. 1.21(b). The cuts necessary to produce the standard long-axis views are shown on an opened specimen.

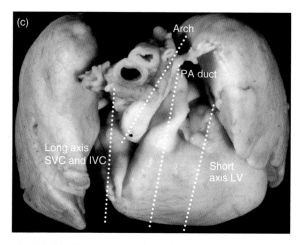

Fig. 1.21(c). The heart is seen from above allowing the sagittal cuts to be seen from a different perspective.

the horizontal sweep, across the fetus, to display successive sagittal planes from one side of the fetus to the other, making fine adjustments of the beam in order to show standard views (Fig. 1.21(a)–(c)). The standard views, from the left to right of the fetus successively are: the short-axis view of the left ventricle, the long-axis view of the duct, the long axis of the aortic arch, to the long-axis view of the superior and inferior vena cava (Figs. 1.22–1.25). A common view to find in a sagittal plane is the so-called tricuspid-aortic view, where the beam cuts in front of the right side of the ventricular septum (Fig. 1.26). Although not very useful for analysis, this view is commonly obtained and the operator should understand how to move the transducer from

this plane to a more informative view. The longitudinal views obtained in long-axis volume sweeps are seen in Fig. 1.27(a) and (b). They tend to be a little less satisfactory than the transverse sweeps, as the angle for a perfect arch is slightly different from that necessary for a perfect ductal arch. However, they are useful to help in understanding the relationship of the long-axis views to each other.

Once the mechanism to obtain the cardiac views is understood and practiced, cardiac evaluation can become very rapid and easy and achieved in every case, even when image quality is difficult. The details of the normal features to be identified in the views obtained, are described in the following chapters.

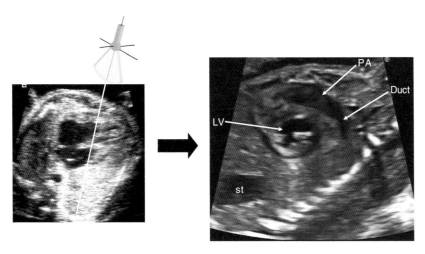

Fig. 1.22. On the left-hand panel, the position of the ultrasound beam relative to the four-chamber view is shown in order to produce the image on the right-hand panel. The right-hand panel shows the short axis view of the left ventricle which is obtained by turning the transducer through 90° on this line through the four-chamber view. Note the beam passes through the stomach (st) on the left side of the abdomen.

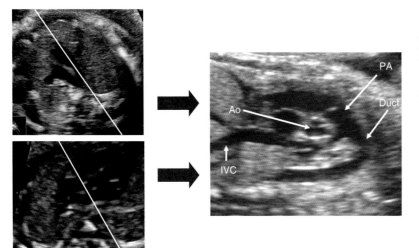

Fig. 1.23. On the left-hand panels, the position of the ultrasound beam relative to the view of the transverse arch or the view of the aortic origin is shown in order to produce the image on the right-hand panel. The right-hand panel shows the long axis view of the duct, obtained by turning the transducer through 90° on either line on the left panel. (This view is called the short-axis view of the great arteries in postnatal echocardiography, although it is only the aorta that is seen in short axis.)

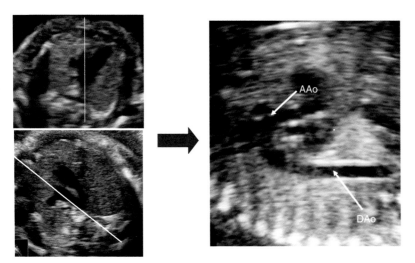

Fig. 1.24. The left-hand panels show that the angulation of the beam necessary to obtain the image seen on the right-hand panel will vary with the position of the fetus. The view on the right-hand panel is the long axis of the aortic arch, obtained by turning the transducer through 90° along the line of the transverse arch.

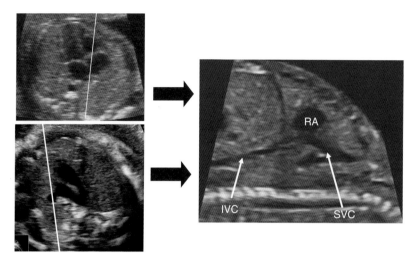

Fig. 1.25. In the upper left panel, the fetus lies with the head in front of the screen. The position of the beam relative to the four-chamber view is shown in order to produce the image on the right-hand panel. In the lower left panel, the position of the beam relative to the view of the transverse arch is shown in a fetus lying with the head behind the screen. Turning the transducer through 90° along either line will show the long axis view of the inferior and superior cava veins.

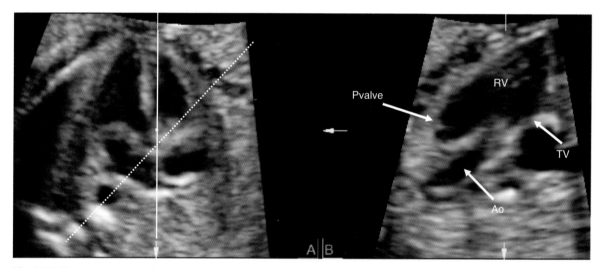

Fig. 1.26. These two views are obtained as part of a 4D volume set. The position of the solid line in the left-sided image is just anterior to the right side of the ventricular septum. The image obtained at right angles to this view is seen on the right. The aorta comes into the scan plane as it sweeps out of the left ventricle towards the right, before it turns leftwards again. Below (caudal to) the aorta, the beam cuts through the tricuspid valve. This "tricuspid-aortic" view is a commonly obtained, although not very informative view. To obtain more useful long-axis views, the ultrasonographer must move further to the right side of the fetal thorax and angle back towards the heart. The image obtained by the dotted line, for example, would show the long-axis view of the arterial duct.

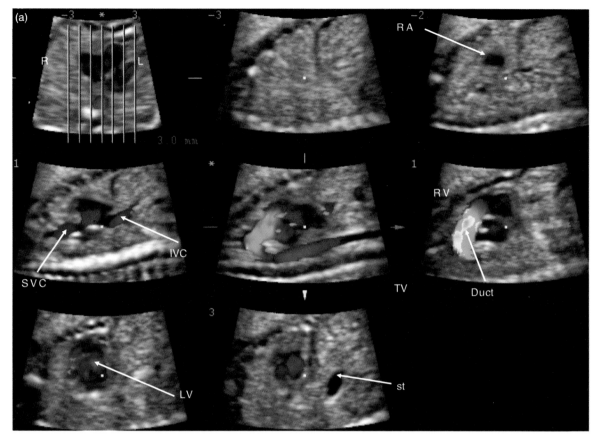

Fig. 1.27(a). In the volume illustrated, the beam sweeps from the right side of the chest to the left, starting with the middle image on the top row to the middle image in the bottom row. The first (most right-sided) cardiac structure seen in the top right image is the right atrium. The drainage of the superior and inferior vena cava to the right atrium is seen on the left image of the middle row. Part of the aortic arch is seen in the central frame, although it is not perfectly imaged at this orientation. In contrast, the ductal arch is seen well on the right-sided image in the middle row. The short-axis views of the left ventricle are seen in the two views on the lower row, with the stomach coming into view in the most leftward section.

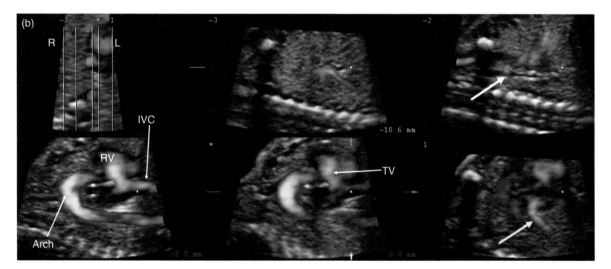

Fig. 1.27(b). In this volume sweep, the angle is perfect for a complete aortic arch (lower left image) but not quite right for a perfect ductal arch, the closest being the middle image in the lower row. These five slices are 14.8 mm apart, from the hilum of the right lung (middle image on the top row) to the left side of the left atrium, where the junction of a pulmonary vein (yellow arrow) is seen (bottom row, right). Note the azygous vein (white arrow) draining to the superior cava vein just to the right of the trachea, in the right-sided image in the upper row. Forward flow across the tricuspid valve is seen in the middle frame of the lower row.

Chapter 2

The four-chamber view: normal and abnormal

Introduction

It is customary to start fetal cardiac evaluation with the four-chamber view. This is not only the easiest view to obtain, but also the most crucial of the cardiac examination, as it displays many of the features of normality, or alternatively, of abnormality. The correct method of obtaining the four-chamber view has been described in the previous chapter. Now we shall describe the method of analysis of the view.

Normal appearance of the four-chamber view

There are four aspects of normality to evaluate in the four-chamber view: size, position, structure, and function.

Normal size

The heart occupies about one-third of the area of the chest or about one half of the circumference. Once the operator is experienced, in general, the heart size can simply be assessed by eye. However, if there is doubt, the circumference of the heart and thorax should be measured in the four-chamber section and the ratio

compared to the normal range, which is 0.55 ± 0.05 (Fig. 2.1(a)). Although this is rather a crude method of measuring heart size, and the reference range should not be interpreted too precisely, measurement can be useful in confirming or refuting an impression of cardiomegaly.

Normal position

The heart lies in the left chest with its axis, (the angle of the ventricular septum to the midline of the thorax) at approximately 45 degrees (Fig. 2.1(b)), although there is some variation in this value in the normal fetus, from about 30 degrees to 60 degrees. Note which structures within the heart lie to the right of the midline and which normally to the left.

Normal structure

(1) There are two atria and two ventricles of approximately equal cavity size and wall thickness (Fig. 2.2(a)–(i)). The size relationships can usually be estimated by eye, but numerical estimates of atrial width, ventricular length, and width, septal and wall thickness can be obtained by measuring the atria and ventricles and the thickness of the walls

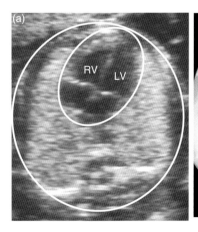
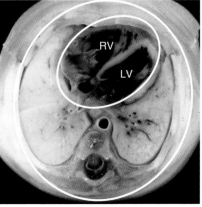

Fig. 2.1.(a). The heart is seen in the four-chamber view on echocardiography and in a correlating anatomical section. It occupies about one-third of the thorax. If there is doubt on visual inspection about the normality of the heart size, the circumference can be measured and compared to the thoracic circumference, as shown. The normal ratio is 0.55 ± 0.05.

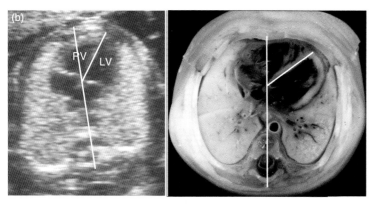

Fig. 2.1.(b). Contd. The normal angle between the interventricular septum and the midline of the thorax is about 45 degrees. Note that about half the right ventricle, the whole left ventricle, more than half of the left atrium and the descending aorta normally lie in the left chest. The right atrium normally lies entirely to the right of the midline.

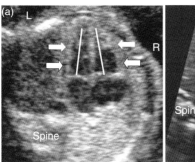
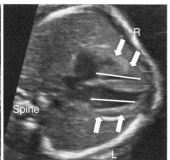

Fig. 2.2.(a). Two atria and two ventricles are seen in both an apical and a lateral projection of the normal four-chamber view. The atria and ventricles are of approximately equal cavity size in area, length and breadth. Because of the apical trabeculation in the right ventricle, however, it often appears slightly shorter than the left. Note the slightly different appearance of the four-chamber view in the apical (left-hand panel) and lateral (right-hand panel) projections. The ventricular walls (thick arrows) and septum always appear thicker in a lateral projection.

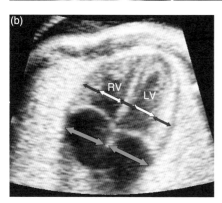

Fig. 2.2.(b). The ventricular walls and septum (red lines) are of approximately equal thickness, but can be measured at mid-cavity as shown. The yellow lines measure ventricular cavity width, and the green lines, atrial width.

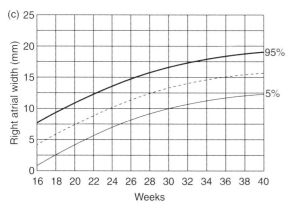
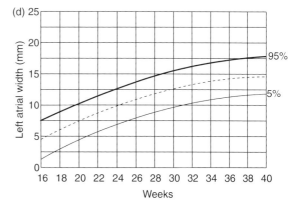

Fig. 2.2.(c). The right atrial width, measured as shown in Fig. 2.2(b), is plotted against gestational age. It tends to be slightly bigger than the left atrium at any time in gestation.

Fig. 2.2.(d). The left atrial width, measured as shown in Fig. 2.2(b), is plotted against gestational age.

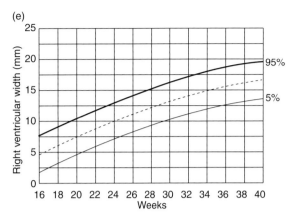

Fig. 2.2.(e). The right ventricular width, measured as shown in Fig. 2.2(b), is plotted against gestational age.

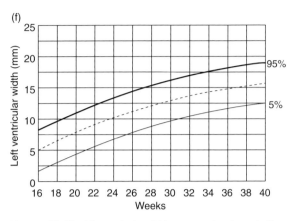

Fig. 2.2.(f). The left ventricular width, measured as shown in Fig. 2.2(b), is plotted against gestational age.

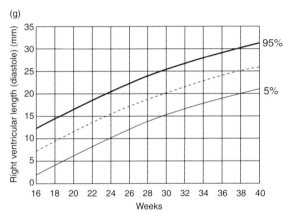

Fig. 2.2.(g). The right ventricular length, measured as shown in Fig. 2.2(a), is plotted against gestational age.

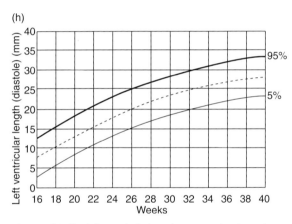

Fig. 2.2.(h). The left ventricular length, measured as shown in Fig. 2.2(a), is plotted against gestational age.

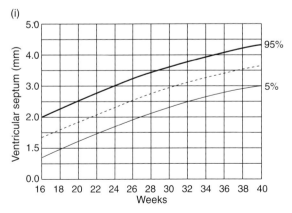

Fig. 2.2.(i). The interventricular septum, measured as shown in Fig. 2.2(b), is plotted against gestational age. This graph can also be used for ventricular wall thickness, as the measurements are similar throughout gestation.

and septum at mid-cavity (Fig. 2.2(b) and 2.2(i)). It should be appreciated that all the graphs shown are somewhat inaccurate, especially in late gestation, when the data points used for creating the graphs are few. However, they can serve as a rough guide.

(2) There are two atrioventricular valves, the tricuspid valve opening into the right ventricle and the mitral valve opening into the left ventricle. Both should open freely, which is best appreciated in the moving image, particularly if a cine loop is acquired in the four-chamber view and the speed of display slowed. The orifice size of the two valves is similar if they are measured at the valve rings, although the tricuspid valve tends to be larger than the mitral, especially in the last 10 weeks of gestation (Fig. 2.3(a)–(c)).

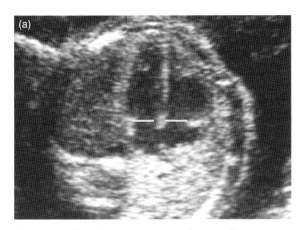

Fig. 2.3.(a). The atrioventricular valve orifices are of approximately equal size. Although measurement is not necessary as a routine, if a measurement is made, the valves should be measured at the level of the valve rings in diastole as shown.

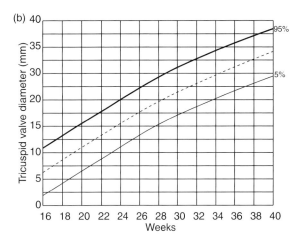

Fig. 2.3.(b). The tricuspid valve diameter, measured as shown in Fig. 2.3(a), is plotted against gestational age.

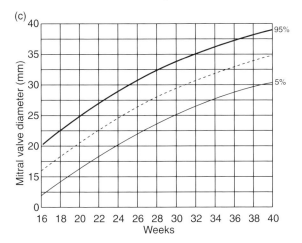

Fig. 2.3.(c). The mitral valve diameter, measured as shown in Fig. 2.3(a), is plotted against gestational age.

(3) The "crux" or center of the heart is the point at which the atrial septum meets the ventricular septum and at which the atrioventricular valves also insert. The septal leaflet of the tricuspid valve is attached to the septum slightly more apically than the mitral (so-called differential insertion) such that the cross at the center of the heart is not straight but shows "off-setting" (Fig. 2.4(a)–(b)). This appearance is more readily appreciated in the apical than in the lateral four-chamber view. This difference is a matter of millimeters in the early fetal heart, but it still is usually appreciable as early as 12 weeks of gestation.

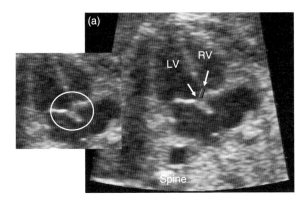

Fig. 2.4.(a). The crux of the heart is enlarged to emphasize the appearance of "off-setting" of the atrioventricular valves, which occurs because the septal leaflet of the tricuspid valve is inserted lower (more towards the apex) in the ventricular septum than the mitral. The difference in the level of the valves (denoted in red) is a matter of millimeters.

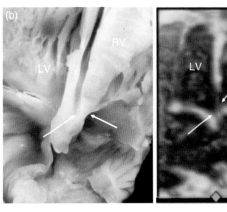

Fig. 2.4.(b). A magnified view of the off-setting in a normal 18-week gestation fetal heart, oriented as in Fig. 2.4(a), is shown in the left-hand panel. Note that the mitral valve within the left ventricle effectively hinges from the atrial septum (yellow arrows) whereas the tricuspid valve (white arrows) hinges more apically from the ventricular septum. On the right-hand panel, a rendered image of the crux shows the off-setting clearly. Note also the typical pattern of apical trabeculation seen in the right ventricle in the echocardiographic image.

25

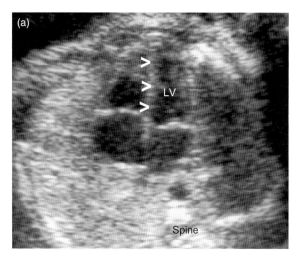

Fig. 2.5.(a). The heart is seen in an apical four-chamber view. In this view, the ventricular septum appears intact from apex to crux. However, the septum is seen with the ultrasound beam parallel to it, which is less ideal than a more lateral view, for excluding a ventricular septal defect.

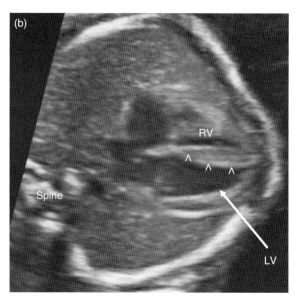

Fig. 2.5.(b). The heart is seen in a lateral four-chamber view. In this view, the ventricular septum is seen with the ultrasound beam perpendicular to it, which allows it to be more confidently confirmed as intact from apex to crux.

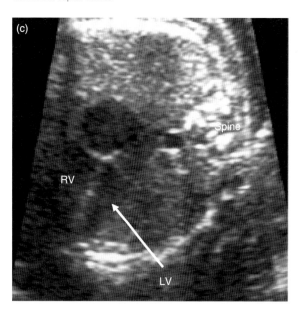

Fig. 2.5.(c). The heart is seen in a "back-up" apical four-chamber view, where the fetal position is less favorable for cardiac analysis. Nevertheless, despite this, most of the normal features of four-chamber view size, position, structure, and function can still be appreciated, albeit less clearly.

(4) The ventricular septum appears intact from the apex to the crux, in all projections of the four-chamber view (Fig. 2.5(a)–(c)).

(5) Three distinct parts of the atrial septum can be recognized in the four-chamber view (Fig. 2.6(a)–(c)). Furthest from the apex of the heart is a short section of atrial septum arising from the posterior wall of the atrium. Next is the foramen ovale itself, together with its covering flap, which billows into the left atrium. Third is that portion, often referred to as the primum septum, between the foramen ovale and the crux of the heart, where the atrioventricular valves take origin. The foramen ovale is an opening in the middle third of the atrial septum, which is "guarded" by a flap valve, a mobile piece of tissue, which lies usually in the body of the left atrium. The flap valve normally allows blood to pass freely from the right to left atrium although it closes against the atrial septum briefly during the cardiac cycle, at the end of atrial systole. The foramen ovale itself occupies about one-third of the atrial septum, although it appears smaller in size in the lateral than in the apical four-chamber view projection (Fig. 2.6(a) and (b)). If the foramen is accurately measurable, it is normally about equal in size to the aortic diameter at any gestation. Patency of the foramen ovale is an invariable feature of the normal fetal circulation.

(6) The apex of the right ventricle is more coarsely trabeculated than the left giving it the appearance of being more "filled-in" than the left. The moderator band is a particularly thick band of trabeculation, which is seen at the right ventricular apex (Fig. 2.7(a)). The tricuspid valve has septal and free wall chordal attachments to its supporting

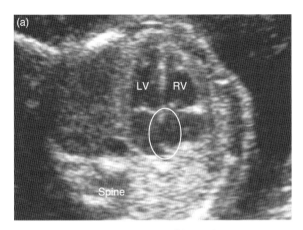

Fig. 2.6.(a). The three components of the atrial septum are seen in an apical four-chamber view, the posterior third of the atrial septum, the foramen ovale defect and the primum portion, which reaches the crux. The foramen ovale usually looks larger in this orientation than in the lateral view seen in Fig. 2.6(b).

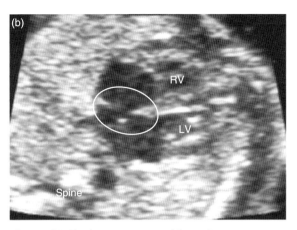

Fig. 2.6.(b). The three components of the atrial septum are seen as in Fig. 2.6(a) but, in this projection, the limits of the foramen ovale defect are usually more clearly seen. The flap valve, which "guards" the foramen defect, can be best seen in this lateral orientation. It "flickers" in the body of the left atrium throughout the cardiac cycle.

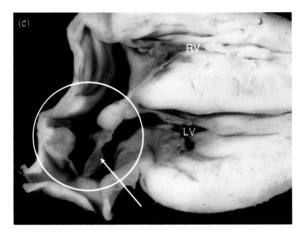

Fig. 2.6.(c). A close-up view of the opening in the atrial septum (oval foramen) is shown on the anatomical section, which has been oriented to match the echocardiogram seen in Fig. 2.6(b). The two rims of the defect can be clearly seen at the left and right sides of the circle, and the cut edge of the flap valve (arrow), which is thin and membranous, is seen below the defect, within the cavity of the left atrium.

papillary muscles, in contrast to the mitral valve, which only has free wall attachments. This aspect is not easy to see (Fig. 2.7(b)) but can sometimes be appreciated in the moving image. Normally, the right ventricle lies anterior and to the right and the left posterior and to the left, but the distinctive trabecular patterns of the left and right ventricles, and the different attachments of their intimately related mitral and tricuspid valves respectively, allow the ventricles to be distinguished from each other morphologically, even when the ventricles are not in their normal position within the thorax.

(7) Upper and lower pulmonary veins enter the left atrium from each side of the thorax. A pair of pulmonary veins (usually the lowermost pair) can be seen to connect to the back of the left atrium on either side of the descending aorta, both on two-

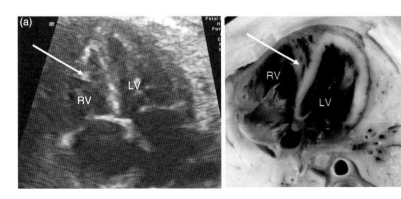

Fig. 2.7.(a). The moderator band, seen here in similar echocardiographic and anatomical sections (arrows), is a thick muscle bundle in the apex of the right ventricle, which can often be a useful marker to distinguish the morphological right from the morphological left ventricle. Note that the right ventricular apex appears more "filled-in" than the left, which appears "empty" by comparison.

27

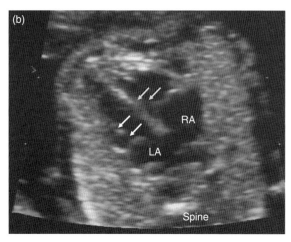

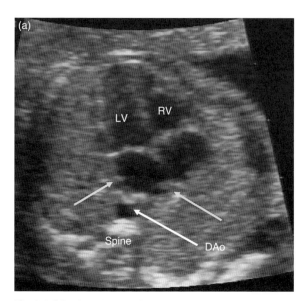

Fig. 2.7.(b). Contd. The tricuspid valve has chordal attachments to the papillary muscles, which lie on the septal surface (yellow arrows) as well as the apex and anterior wall of the right ventricle. In contrast, the papillary muscles of the mitral valve only lie on the free wall of the left ventricle (white arrows). Sometimes, in a complex malformation, these atrioventricular valve attachments can help to distinguish a morphological right from a morphological left ventricle, as the mitral valve is always associated with the left ventricle and the tricuspid with the right.

Fig. 2.8.(a). The right and left lower pulmonary veins are seen connecting to the back of the left atrium (yellow arrows) on either side of the descending aorta (DAo) on the 2D image.

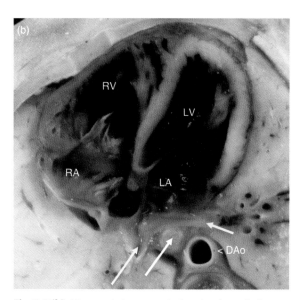

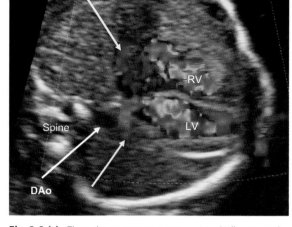

Fig. 2.8.(b). The correlating anatomical section shows the lower right and left pulmonary veins (yellow arrows) joining the left atrium. Note how they lie in relation to the esophagus (white arrow) and descending aorta.

Fig. 2.8.(c). The pulmonary venous connections (yellow arrows) to the left atrium must be confirmed on color flow mapping as seen here. The descending aorta lies between the left pulmonary vein and the spine.

dimensional imaging and color flow mapping of the four-chamber view (Fig. 2.8(a)–(c)).

(8) There is one vessel seen in short axis in the posterior mediastinum, the descending aorta. It lies slightly to the left of the spine, close to the back of the left atrium (Fig. 2.8(a)–(c)).

(9) There is normally a little fluid in the pericardial sac, seen as a black line particularly around the ventricular chambers. This fluid acts as a lubricant to allow the heart to contract freely and is seen as moving fluid on the color flow map. It tends to appear more pronounced in lateral

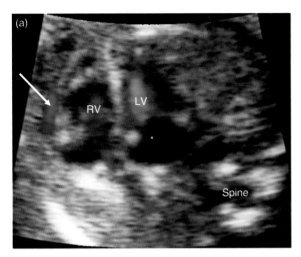

Fig. 2.9.(a). Movement of fluid within the pericardial cavity (arrow) can be detected by modern color Doppler equipment during the heart cycle. This is a normal amount of pericardial fluid and should not be mistaken for an effusion. There is equal inflow into the heart in diastole on color flow.

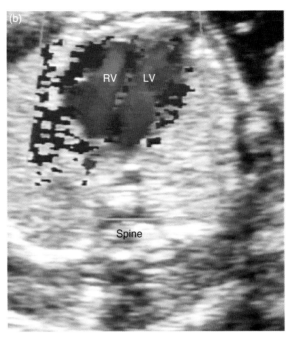

Fig. 2.9.(b). There is equal flow in diastole into both ventricles across the atrioventricular valves, seen on color flow mapping. No atrioventricular valve regurgitation should be seen on colour flow mapping during systole.

than in apical views. Its normal appearance without color is seen, for example, in Figs. 2.5(b) and 2.7(a), and with color flow mapping in Fig. 2.9(a).

Normal function

Both ventricles contract equally and vigorously, which can only be appreciated in the moving image. In diastole, there should be approximately equal flow across the atrioventricular valves on color flow mapping (Fig. 2.9(a) and (b)) and in systole there should be no regurgitation of blood (or color flow in the opposite direction) into the atria through either the mitral or tricuspid valve.

Possible deviations of four-chamber view from normal

Abnormalities of size

The cardiothoracic ratio may be abnormal, either increased or decreased (Fig. 2.10). An increased cardiothoracic ratio usually indicates an increased heart size (cardiomegaly) but may also arise when the absolute heart size is normal, but the chest is abnormally small. This is usually obvious as the underlying cause is either oligohydramnios, in the setting of renal

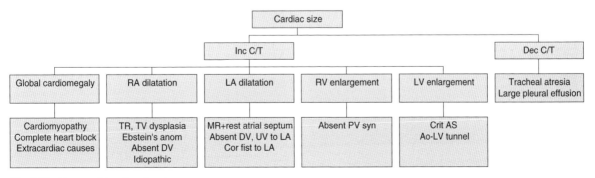

Fig. 2.10. Abnormalities of cardiac size.

disease (Fig. 2.11) growth retardation, or a thoracic dysplasia.

Heart smaller than normal

If the heart appears small, this is due to **cardiac compression** from extracardiac structures within the confines of the chest. This can occur in tracheal atresia, (Fig. 2.12), in diaphragmatic hernia or with a large pleural effusion. Tracheal atresia obstructs the normal

free flow of fluid between the lungs and the amniotic cavity, causing lung distension and enlargement.

Heart larger than normal

The heart may be globally enlarged, when all the chambers are enlarged to a similar extent, or the enlargement may affect only one cavity or side of the heart. Defining which cavity or side is enlarged, helps to establish the cause.

Heart globally enlarged

Global enlargement of the heart occurs either in the setting of increased stroke volume and/or cardiac output, or in reduced contractility of the myocardium. When the stroke volume is increased, the contraction of the heart will appear more vigorous than normal. This occurs in **high-output states** including **anemia, sacrococcygeal teratoma, arteriovenous malformation, chorioadenoma, and TRAP sequence** (Fig. 2.13(a),(b)). In **complete heart block**, increased stroke volume (and therefore increased heart size) serves to maintain adequate cardiac output with a very slow rate. This can occur with a structurally normal heart (isolated complete heart block) or in association with structural heart disease, most commonly left atrial isomerism (Fig. 2.13(c)).

Cardiomegaly resulting from **reduced contractility** of the myocardium occurs in **myocarditis, cardiomyopathy** (Fig. 2.13(d)–(f)) or **severe hypoxia**. A rare cause of cardiomyopathy is myocardial non-compaction where the apex or both apices are thick-walled,

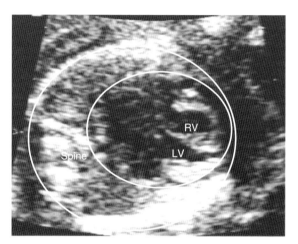

Fig. 2.11. The heart appears to be enlarged (compare with Fig. 2.1) but this is due to a small thorax and lungs in the setting of severe oligohydramnios as a result of renal disease. The cardiac anatomy is difficult to see because of the lack of fluid.

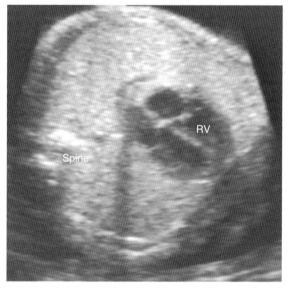

Fig. 2.12. The heart appears small within the thorax but this is due to enlarged lung fields compressing the heart. The lungs are more echogenic than normal. The underlying diagnosis is tracheal atresia.

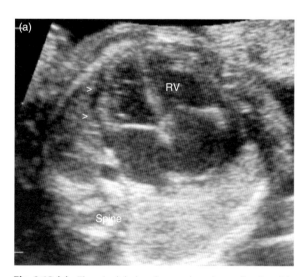

Fig. 2.13.(a). There is global cardiomegaly and a small pericardial effusion (arrowheads) in this fetus with anemia. The function on the moving image was hyperdynamic.

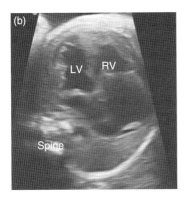

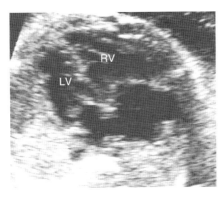

Fig. 2.13.(b). Contd. There is fairly marked cardiomegaly with right heart dominance in both examples, secondary to intracerebral arteriovenous malformations (also called vein of Galen aneurysms). The function on the moving image was hyperdynamic.

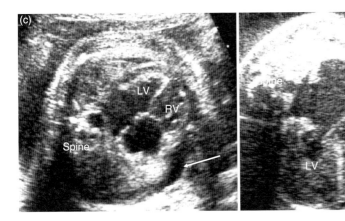

Fig. 2.13.(c). Both fetuses had complete heart block and global cardiomegaly. The fetus shown on the left-hand panel has a structurally normal heart and a small pleural effusion. The fetus shown on the right-hand panel has associated structural heart disease in the form of an atrioventricular septal defect and left atrial isomerism.

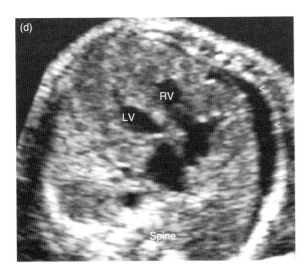

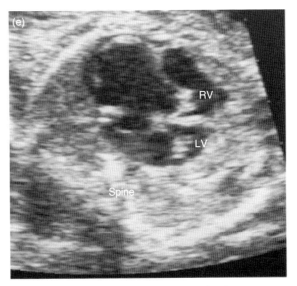

Fig. 2.13.(d). The heart is enlarged and there is a small pleural effusion (arrows). There is biventricular hypertrophy and, on the moving image, the contraction was poor. This was due to a cardiomyopathy of unknown origin, probably a storage disease.

Fig. 2.13.(e). There is global cardiomegaly and on the moving image, both ventricles contracted poorly. There was fetal hydrops secondary to cardiac failure, in turn occurring as a result of a cardiomyopathy. The predominance of atrial dilatation indicates a degree of restrictive cardiomyopathy.

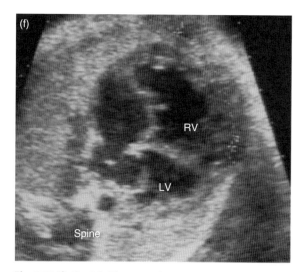

Fig. 2.13.(f). Contd. There is cardiomegaly, mainly due to right-sided dilatation in this 34-week fetus. On the moving image, the right ventricle was very poorly contracting although there was still forward flow into the pulmonary artery. After birth, right ventricular dysfunction recovered somewhat and the child survived in the short term, but with a global cardiomyopathy.

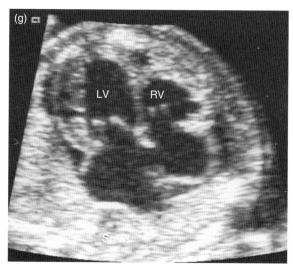

Fig. 2.13.(g). There is cardiomegaly and biventricular hypertrophy in this recipient fetus in twin–twin transfusion syndrome. There is also a small pericardial effusion. This appearance is fairly typical for this condition.

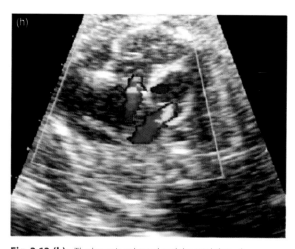

Fig. 2.13.(h). The heart is enlarged and there is bilateral atrioventricular valve regurgitation. There was increased echogenicity of the myocardium and, on the moving image, cardiac function was diminished in this case of cardiomyopathy.

there is diminished contraction and, on the color flow map, color is seen to penetrate in deep recesses in the ventricular wall. Some conditions, for example severe fetal anemia, may demonstrate a progression from an initial high output state with hyperdynamic circulation and vigorous contraction to a low output state with reduced contractility and further dilation of the heart, as hypoxia supervenes. Myocardial hypertrophy and cardiomegaly can occur in the recipient fetus in the **twin–twin transfusion syndrome**

(Fig. 2.13(g)). Tricuspid and mitral regurgitation frequently occur as a consequence of dilation of the heart from whatever cause (Fig. 2.13(h)). This should be distinguished from the situation where anatomical abnormality of the atrioventricular valves results in mitral or tricuspid regurgitation, or rarely both, and therefore are themselves the cause of cardiac dilatation. In the latter situation, dilatation of the related atrium will normally predominate.

If cardiomegaly is not global but due to a chamber or chambers enlarged, the first step is to define which chamber is affected.

Right atrial enlargement

If the right atrium is enlarged (Fig. 2.14(a)), this usually indicates **tricuspid regurgitation**. Tricuspid regurgitation can be secondary to a non-structural cardiac cause, such as a tachycardia, or an extracardiac cause such as an arteriovenous malformation, constriction of the arterial duct or twin–twin transfusion syndrome. A rare extracardiac cause of right atrial enlargement is **absence of the ductus venosus** where the umbilical vein connects directly to the right atrium (Fig. 2.14(b)). Alternatively, the cause may be intracardiac due to **dysplasia of the tricuspid valve leaflets** (Fig. 2.14(c),(d)) resulting in varying degrees of valve regurgitation. In pathological terms, dysplasia is associated with nodularity of the valve leaflets. **Ebstein's anomaly** is a relatively uncommon but well-recognized condition

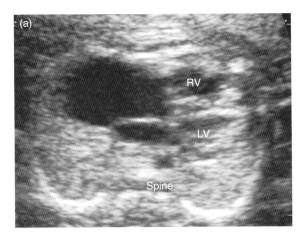

Fig. 2.14.(a). There is cardiomegaly but this is mainly due to right atrial dilatation, in this case because of tricuspid valve dysplasia and regurgitation.

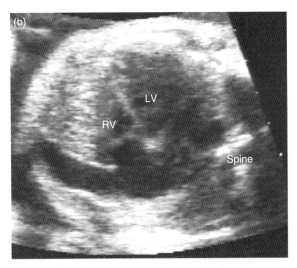

Fig. 2.14 .(b). The ductus venosus was absent and in this view the abnormal connection of the umbilical vein to the right atrium is seen. In other views, the right atrium could be seen to be enlarged producing cardiomegaly.

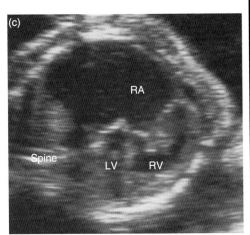
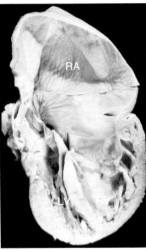

Fig. 2.14.(c). There is massive cardiomegaly as a result of right atrial dilatation, due in turn to tricuspid regurgitation. On both the echocardiographic and matching anatomical section, the tricuspid valve leaflets can be seen to be thickened and dysplastic but the degree of offsetting is normal. Note the abnormal cardiac axis, with the septum at right angles to the midline.

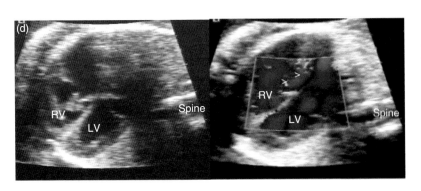

Fig. 2.14.(d). The tricuspid valve leaflets can be seen to be thickened and there is regurgitation (arrows) on color flow mapping, producing right atrial enlargement. This is mild tricuspid valve dysplasia.

33

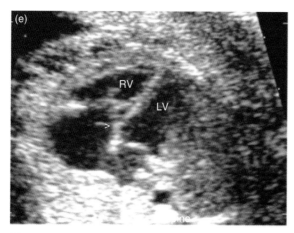

Fig. 2.14.(e). Contd. There is mild cardiomegaly here, due to mild right atrial dilatation. The tricuspid valve is mildly displaced into the right ventricle (Ebstein's anomaly). The septal leaflet of the tricuspid valve (arrowhead) could be seen to be tethered to the septum throughout the cardiac cycle on the moving image.

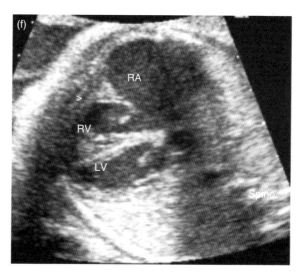

Fig. 2.14.(f). The right atrium, particularly the appendage, is massively enlarged but the tricuspid valve is normal with no dilatation of the valve ring or regurgitation. This is idiopathic dilatation of the right atrial appendage, a rare condition and a diagnosis of exclusion.

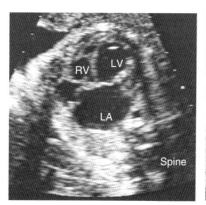 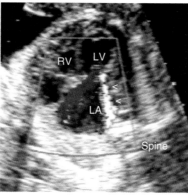

Fig. 2.15. There is left ventricular dilatation due to a critically obstructed aortic valve. In addition, there is left atrial dilatation due to the combination of mitral regurgitation (arrowheads), seen on color flow mapping on the right-hand panel, and a restrictive foramen ovale defect. Note that there is no obvious foramen ovale on the 2D image and no interatrial jet on the color flow map supporting the diagnosis of a restrictive atrial septum secondary to left heart disease.

in which the septal leaflet of the tricuspid valve is displaced or positioned further down the septum in the right ventricle than normal (Fig. 2.14(e)). The abnormal valve is often also dysplastic and regurgitant, thus enlarging the right atrium. It is illustrated further later in the chapter. There is a rare condition in which the right atrial appendage is grossly enlarged in the absence of an identifiable cause, the tricuspid valve is completely normal, with a normal sized valve ring and no regurgitation. This is called **idiopathic dilatation of the right atrial appendage** (Fig. 2.14(f)).

Left atrial enlargement
The left atrium can be enlarged in the setting of moderate to severe **mitral regurgitation**, but only if flow (or off-loading) across the foramen ovale defect is restricted. Mitral regurgitation can be due to intrinsic malformation of the mitral valve leaflets, which is rare, or secondary to a severely obstructed aortic valve (aortic stenosis or atresia), which is more common (Fig. 2.15). Rare extracardiac causes of left atrial enlargement include **absence of the ductus venosus**, where the umbilical vein connects directly to the left atrium, or a **coronary artery fistula** draining to the left atrium.

Right ventricular enlargement
The right ventricle can be enlarged producing cardiomegaly if there is severe pulmonary regurgitation, which usually occurs in the setting of the **absent pulmonary valve syndrome**, an uncommon variant of tetralogy of Fallot (Fig. 2.16). It may also be enlarged in conditions which produce volume overload to the right

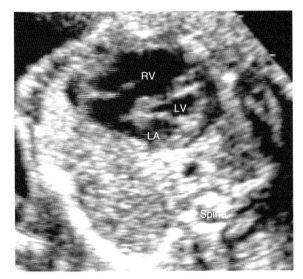

Fig. 2.16. The right ventricle is dilated due to severe pulmonary regurgitation in the absent pulmonary valve syndrome. Note the displacement of the cardiac axis towards the left. The typically associated outlet ventricular septal defect and aortic override is not seen in this section.

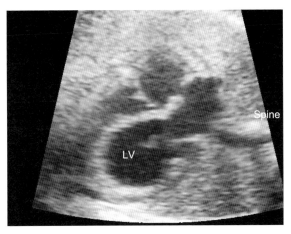

Fig. 2.17. The left ventricle is dilated and "globular" in shape. In the moving image, the contraction was poor. This appearance is typical of critical aortic stenosis.

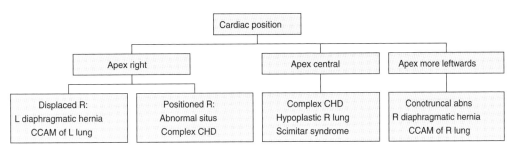

Fig. 2.18. Abnormalies of cardiac position.

side, such as coarctation or total anomalous pulmonary venous drainage which will be discussed under disproportion.

Left ventricular enlargement

The left ventricle can be enlarged producing cardiomegaly as a result of **critical aortic stenosis** (Fig. 2.17) or severe aortic regurgitation in the setting of an **aorto-left ventricular tunnel**, a rare condition (see Chapter 3).

Abnormalities of position

In describing the position of the heart, we need to consider not only if the heart lies mainly in the right or the left chest, but also the angle of the axis of the heart to the midline and the position of the apex. An abnormal position of the heart may arise as a result of an intrinsic problem with embryonic heart development, or as a consequence of displacement by other structures. The heart can lie in the left chest with an abnormal axis, predominantly in the right chest, or centrally in the thorax (Fig. 2.18).

Apex more leftwards than normal

The position of the heart can be displaced leftwards by an abnormal space-occupying lesion in the right chest, such as a **right-sided diaphragmatic hernia** (Fig. 2.19(a)) or **congenital cystic malformation of the right lung**. Alternatively, the axis can be displaced leftwards until the septum is almost at right angles to the midline. This can occur in right heart dilatation or in the setting of some great artery malformations, such as tetralogy of Fallot or common arterial trunk, although the mechanism of this is unclear (Fig. 2.19(b)). Note

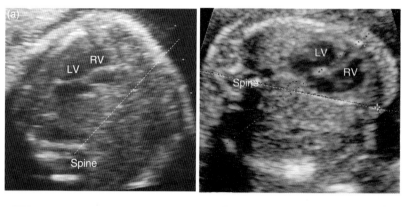

Fig. 2.19.(a). The heart lies entirely in the left chest in both examples. The dotted line represents the midline (compare with the normal in Fig. 2.2). This is due to cardiac displacement by the liver in the right thorax, as a result of a right-sided diaphragmatic hernia. This is an important diagnosis not to miss, as, although tracheal balloon placement can be successful, the natural history of this defect without treatment carries a very poor prognosis for postnatal survival.

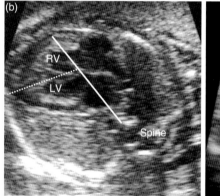
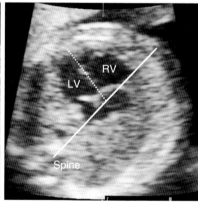

Fig. 2.19.(b). The apex of the heart lies more to the left than normal with the angle of the septum almost 90 degrees to the midline in both panels. The fetus on the left-hand panel had tetralogy of Fallot, the fetus on the right-hand panel had a structurally normal heart and was normal at birth.

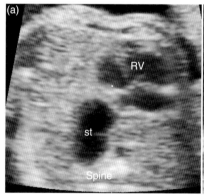
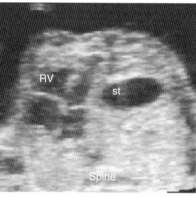

Fig. 2.20.(a). In both examples, the heart is displaced into the right chest by the abdominal organs herniated through a left-sided diaphragmatic defect. The stomach (st) is seen in the left chest, although in a different position in each example. Typically, the right ventricle is pushed against the right chest wall and the left ventricle is smaller than the right, as here. Study of Fig. 1.11 shows that, normally, a significant proportion of the right lung lies between the right ventricle and right chest wall, in contrast to the situations illustrated here.

that an unusually leftwards axis can occur in an otherwise normal fetus, where no explanation for the abnormal axis is found.

Apex in the right chest

The heart can lie in the right chest because of displacement by an abnormal space-occupying lesion in the left chest, such as a **left-sided diaphragmatic hernia** or **congenital cystic adenomatous malformation of the left lung**. In this case, the axis of the heart is often almost parallel to the midline (Fig. 2.20(a) and (b)).

Alternatively, the heart can be in the right chest in association with **abnormal laterality**, disorders which occur at a very early stage of embryonic development. These conditions are more fully described in Chapter 4. One example of abnormal laterality is complete **situs inversus**, or mirror image arrangement. In this condition, the morphological left atrium lies on the right and the morphological right atrium on the left. Most commonly, the ventricles and great arteries are connected appropriately to the atrial arrangement, so that the heart appears as a mirror image of the normal. It

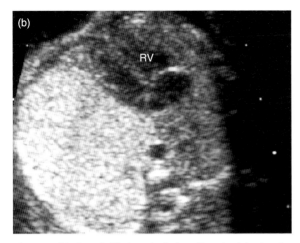

Fig. 2.20.(b). Contd. The heart is displaced into the right chest by a hyperechogenic left lung, due to congenital cystic adenomatous malformation of one lobe.

usually occurs in association with a similar mirror image arrangement of the lungs and bronchi and the abdominal organs, with the stomach bubble being visible on the right, but it may sometimes only affect the thoracic organs. **Right and left isomerism** fall within the same category of abnormalities of laterality, and are usually associated with complex intracardiac malformations. Abnormal heart position is not an essential feature of either condition, but is often present and may or may not be associated with an abnormal position of the stomach bubble (Fig. 2.20(c)). The heart may sometimes be predominantly right-sided in complex intracardiac defects where the atrial arrangement is normal.

Apex central

The heart can be positioned centrally in the chest, usually in the setting of **complex heart disease** (Fig. 2.21(a)), or in **hypoplasia of the right lung**, which is often associated with Scimitar syndrome (Fig. 2.21(b)). Scimitar syndrome is a condition in which there is

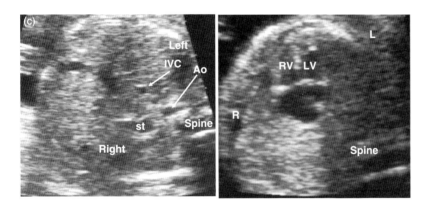

Fig. 2.20.(c). Both the left and right panels are obtained in the same patient during a sweep. In the abdomen, the stomach lies on the right and the aorta and inferior vena cava on the same side, to the left of the midline. In the thorax, the apex is to the left. Note the associated atrioventricular septal defect in this case of right atrial isomerism.

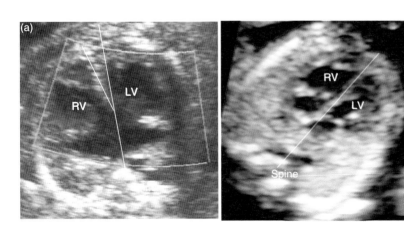

Fig. 2.21.(a). In the left-hand panel, the heart lies centrally in the chest with the line of the septum almost parallel with the midline. There is cardiomegaly due to complete heart block. There is also a complete atrioventricular septal defect in this case of left atrial isomerism. The right-hand panel illustrates a central heart of unknown etiology, where the septum lay completely under the midline. There was no lung lesion in the left chest pushing the heart rightwards, although there were findings suspicious for coarctation. This was found in the donor fetus of a monochorionic twin pair, with severe growth retardation after laser treatment. Primary right lung hypoplasia was perhaps the explanation.

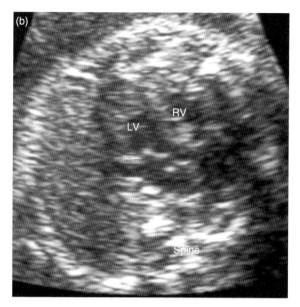

Fig. 2.21.(b). Contd. The heart is displaced into the right chest because of hypoplasia of the right lung. This is commonly associated with hypoplasia of the right pulmonary artery, collateral arterial supply to the right lung from the aorta, and anomalous pulmonary venous drainage of part of the right lung. This condition is known as the scimitar syndrome, because of a characteristic radiological sign of scimitar shape found after birth.

partial anomalous pulmonary venous drainage of the right lower lobe of the lung, usually to below the diaphragm, with either a small or absent right pulmonary artery. Some, or all, of the right lung derives blood supply directly from the aorta. The etiology of an abnormal heart position is not always explicable. Primary lung hypoplasia is a diagnosis of exclusion (Fig. 2.18).

Miscellaneous other abnormalities of position

Some additional unusual forms of abnormal heart position include **criss-cross or upstairs/downstairs AV connections, pentalogy of Cantrell, ectopia cordis, and absence of the pericardium**. In criss-cross atrioventricular valves or upstairs/downstairs connections, the four-chamber view cannot be imaged in the usual transverse orientation. Two atrioventricular valves can be found but they tend to lie in inferior/superior arrangement instead of side-by-side (Fig. 2.22(a) and (b)). Both conditions have a ventricular septal defect, usually large. In criss-cross connections, the blood flow may be from left atrium to right ventricle and right atrium to left ventricle, through the ventricular septal defect. Alternatively, the atrioventricular connections

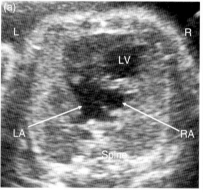
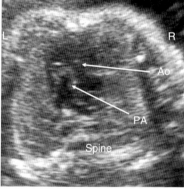

Fig. 2.22.(a). In the left-hand panel, the four-chamber view is clearly abnormal. The fetus lies HF, so the apex points to the right. The atrial situs is normal with the right atrium to the right of the left atrium. Only a left ventricle, lying to the right, is seen in this plane. On the right-hand panel, both great arteries were found arising above the left-sided right ventricle, which in turn lay above the level of the left ventricle.

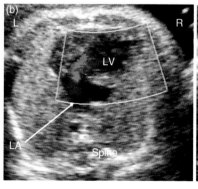
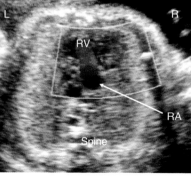

Fig. 2.22.(b). In the same fetus as illustrated in Fig. 2.22(a), on the left-hand panel, color flow mapping showed that blood in the left atrium flowed through the mitral valve into the right-sided and lower morphological left ventricle. In a different plane of section, more superior to that shown on the left-hand panel, the right atrium could be seen to connect via a tricuspid valve to the anterior and superior morphological right ventricle. There was a large ventricular septal defect in addition.

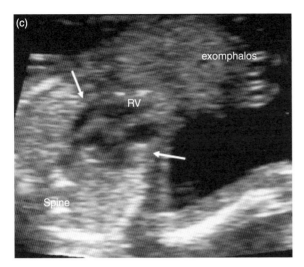

Fig. 2.22.(c). Contd. This fetus was first seen at 16 weeks and had an exomphalos, with protrusion of the cardiac apex through an anterior sternal wall defect.

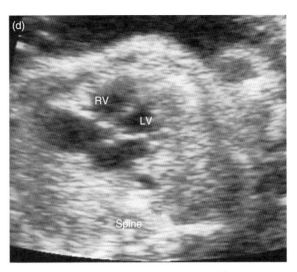

Fig. 2.22.(d). The four-chamber view, in the same fetus as is illustrated in Fig. 2.22(c), is seen at 25 weeks. Note that the heart is now completely within the thorax. At birth, the complete picture of pentalogy of Cantrell was confirmed, with exomphalos, an anterior sternal wall defect, an anterior defect in the diapragm and pericardium in addition to congenital heart disease, in this case a ventricular septal defect.

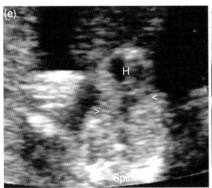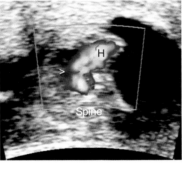

Fig. 2.22.(e). In this 14- week fetus, in the four-chamber cut, the whole heart (H) could be seen completely outside the thoracic cavity and swinging freely on its "stalk," made up of the great vessels (right-hand panel) in the amniotic cavity. The arrows mark the extent of the anterior thoracic defect.

may be concordant but lying in infero-superior relations to each other. Both conditions tend to have a double outlet connection of the great arteries, but each case must be described by identifying the connection at each level of the heart in this complex abnormality. Most cases are not suitable for a biventricular repair.

The pentalogy of Cantrell is a severe midline defect, which results in an omphalocoele, a defect in the diaphragm and lower sternum, protrusion of some or all the cardiac apex outside the thoracic cavity (Fig. 2.22(c)) and, often, although not always, congenital heart disease. The degree of protrusion of the heart is varied and can appear more severe in early pregnancy than later in gestation (Fig. 2.22(d)). The associated congenital heart disease is usually a ventricular or atrial septal defect or tetralogy of Fallot, but there may be other lesions, or the heart may be structurally normal. Ectopia cordis is when the whole heart lies outside the chest cavity (Fig. 2.22(e)). The heart swings freely within the amniotic cavity on the "stalk of the great arteries" and the pericardium is absent (Fig. 2.22(f)). There may be associated intracardiac malformation.

When the pericardium is absent as an isolated anomaly, the heart can lie in an unusual position within the thorax, either more leftwards or more centrally. This diagnosis can only be made definitively at cardiac surgery for associated intracardiac lesions, which can occur but are not invariable.

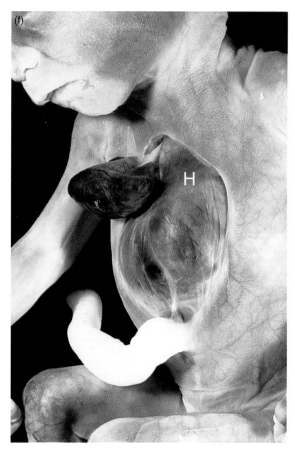

Fig. 2.22.(f).Contd. The pathological specimen shows a large anterior thoracic and abdominal wall defect, similar to the example in Fig. 2.22(e), with the heart lying freely outside the chest, and not protected by a pericardial sac. In contrast, the abdominal contents and liver are enclosed in a membrane.

Abnormalities of structure

Unequal atrial chambers

One or other atrium can be enlarged but this usually produces cardiomegaly and the causes are detailed above.

Right atrium small

In our experience, the right atrium is rarely smaller than normal although it can appear a little small in **tricuspid atresia** (Fig. 2.23(a)). This is because there is normally a large foramen ovale allowing all the systemic venous return to "off-load" freely across it to the left atrium.

Left atrium small

If the left atrium is smaller than normal, this may indicate **total anomalous pulmonary venous drainage**

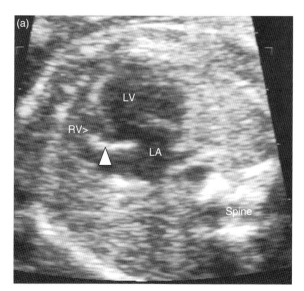

Fig. 2.23.(a). The right atrium appears smaller than the left. The right ventricle is much smaller than the left and smaller than normal for the gestation. There is muscular tissue reaching the crux of the heart (arrowhead) in the position of the tricuspid valve. There is no opening tricuspid valve seen. There is a small inlet ventricular septal defect. These findings are characteristic of tricuspid atresia.

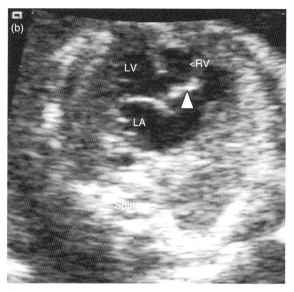

Fig. 2.23.(b). In this example of tricuspid atresia, the right ventricle is a little bigger than in Fig. 2.23(a), as the ventricular septal defect is larger. The arrowhead indicates the atretic tricuspid valve.

(see Fig. 2.48(b)). A small left atrium is also usually seen in the **hypoplastic left heart syndrome**, in association with other abnormal features, and in conjunction with **disproportion of the ventricles** as described below.

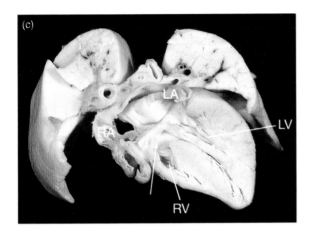

Fig. 2.23.(c). Contd. An anatomical specimen of tricuspid atresia is seen in a four-chamber view. The left atrium and left ventricle are connected via the mitral valve but the pathway between the right atrium and a diminutive right ventricle is blocked by thickened fibrous tissue (arrow). A moderate-sized ventricular septal defect allows communication between the two ventricles.

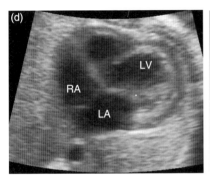 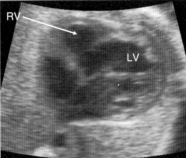

Fig. 2.23.(d). The four-chamber view is seen in systole on the left and diastole on the right. In diastole, the mitral valve opens but there is no opening valve on the right side of the crux of the heart. The small right ventricular cavity and ventricular septal defect, which are always associated with a diagnosis of tricuspid atresia, are clearly seen.

Unequal ventricular chambers

One or other ventricle can be enlarged but this usually produces cardiomegaly and the differential diagnoses in cardiomegaly have been discussed above.

A normal volume of flow is a stimulus for growth, so a structure which is smaller than normal, is usually receiving diminished blood flow.

Small right ventricle

A small right ventricle occurs in **tricuspid atresia** or **pulmonary atresia with intact ventricular septum**. In tricuspid atresia, the tricuspid valve does not open. Anatomically usually, the leaflets are absent and muscular tissue extends to the crux of the heart (Fig. 2.23(a)–(e)), although membranous tricuspid atresia can also rarely occur. On the color flow map, there is no flow between the right atrium and the right ventricle and there is always a ventricular septal defect, although it may be sometimes be small and difficult to see (Fig. 2.23(e)). Pulmonary atresia with intact septum can be difficult to distinguish from tricuspid atresia in some cases, but, by definition, there

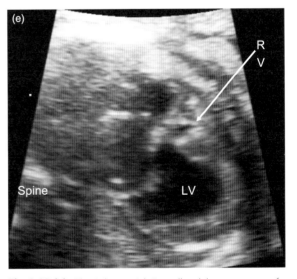

Fig. 2.23.(e). The right ventricle is small and the appearance of the four-chamber view is very similar to that seen in the example of pulmonary atresia with intact septum seen in Fig. 2.24(a). However, this is tricuspid atresia but the ventricular septal defect was small and found in a more cranial plane of section than this view.

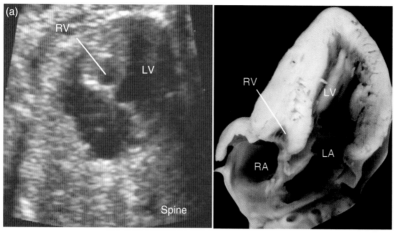

Fig. 2.24.(a). On the left panel, there is a small right ventricular cavity on the echocardiogram with thickened walls. Note the difference in appearance between this, which is pulmonary atresia with intact ventricular septum, and the typical examples of tricuspid atresia, seen in Figs. 2.23(a)–(e). On the right, the anatomical specimen shows a similar example of pulmonary atresia, with a minute right ventricle, which was only 1–2 mm in length.

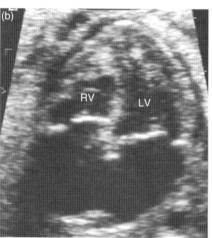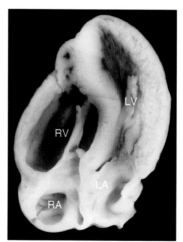

Fig. 2.24.(b). In the left-hand panel, the right ventricular cavity is only slightly smaller than normal in this example of pulmonary atresia, but the walls of the right ventricle appear thickened. Because of the obstructed pulmonary valve, there is high pressure in the right ventricle and the septum bulges into the left ventricular cavity, a characteristic appearance with this diagnosis. The septum is straight in the normal fetus (compare with Figs. 2.1–2.8). The panel on the right is from a similar fetus seen to have pulmonary stenosis initially and a thick-walled rounded right ventricle, which bulged into the left ventricle. By the time of autopsy, the pulmonary valve had become atretic.

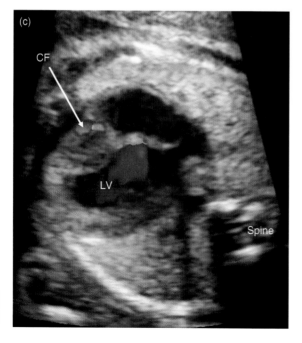

Fig. 2.24.(c). The right ventricle is small and thick walled in this case of pulmonary atresia with intact ventricular septum. On color flow mapping, a coronary fistula (CF) could be seen connecting the right ventricular cavity with the right coronary artery, with bidirectional flow within it during the cardiac cycle. Areas of high velocity representing stenoses are sometimes seen in these vessels (see Fig. 5.13(b)).

is no ventricular septal defect, the tricuspid valve is patent (although it is usually small and very restricted in its opening) and the right ventricular cavity is thick walled. The differentiation is important as the two conditions have rather different implications for management and prognosis. In pulmonary atresia, the right ventricle sometimes shows increased echogenicity and it contracts poorly (Fig. 2.24(a) and (b)). In some cases, careful examination of the right ventricle with color flow mapping can demonstrate fistulous connections between the right ventricle and the coronary arteries (Fig. 2.24(c)). Such cases form a subset of this malformation which carries a poorer prognosis for successful

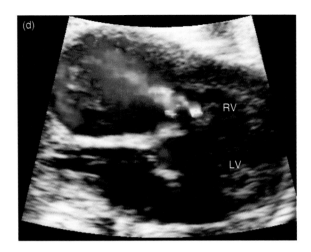

Fig. 2.24.(d). Contd. In this fetus at 35 weeks' gestation, the right ventricle was small and thick walled and there was no forward flow across an atretic pulmonary valve. In the four-chamber view, there was tricuspid regurgitation at high velocity, filling the right atrium and causing dilatation of the right atrium.

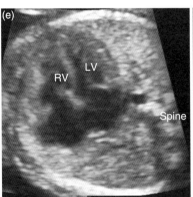 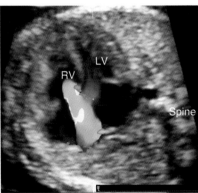

Fig. 2.24.(e). In the still 2D image of the four-chamber view on the left-hand panel, the heart is fairly unremarkable. However, on the moving image, the right ventricle contracted poorly and there was also limited excursion of the tricuspid valve. On the color flow map, shown in the right-hand panel, there was moderate tricuspid regurgitation and this was at high velocity on pulsed Doppler, indicating a high pressure within the right ventricular cavity. Knowing this, the right ventricular walls now appear a little thickened on the 2D image.

postnatal management. There is often tricuspid regurgitation, which helps to distinguish pulmonary atresia with intact ventricular septum from tricuspid atresia (Fig. 2.24(d)), in cases where the differential diagnosis is difficult.

Pulmonary atresia can occur as a consequence of the twin–twin transfusion syndrome (Fig. 2.24(e)). The mechanism is thought to be related to systemic hypertension in the recipient twin, resulting in diminished function of the right ventricle and tricuspid regurgitation. The poorly functioning right ventricle fails to open the pulmonary valve completely or at all, resulting, in turn, in pulmonary stenosis or even atresia. By the end of pregnancy, the pulmonary valve may become anatomically obstructed, either partially or completely. Thus, a functional hemodynamic disorder can be observed to produce an anatomical abnormality during the course of gestation.

Note the contrast in the findings between pulmonary atresia with intact ventricular septum described

here and pulmonary atresia with ventricular septal defect, described in Chapter 3, in which the right ventricle is of normal size and contracts normally.

A small right ventricle can occur in the setting of a **common atrioventricular junction** when the common valve drains mainly to the left ventricle, a so-called unbalanced atrioventricular septal defect (Fig. 2.25(a)). **Tricuspid stenosis** is an additional rare cause of a small right ventricle, although the diminution in size may be subtle. It is a difficult diagnosis to make prenatally, as blood reaching the right atrium will preferentially pass across the atrial septum to the left atrium. This increase in right to left shunt is not possible to distinguish from the right to left shunt which occurs normally at the foramen ovale. The tricuspid valve leaflets may appear thickened and restricted in excursion. Blood reaching the right atrium "off-loads" across the atrial septal defect, resulting in diminished flow into the right ventricle and thus relative hypoplasia (Fig. 2.25(b)).

43

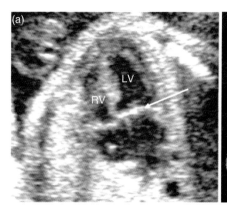
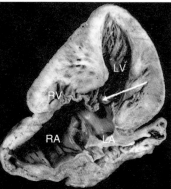

Fig. 2.25.(a). On the echocardiogram on the left-hand panel, the right ventricle is smaller than the left and at first glance this might be an example of tricuspid atresia. However, closer examination shows that there is a common atrioventricular valve (arrow) with an unbalanced connection to the ventricles, in this case mainly draining to the left ventricle. The defect in the atrioventricular septum could be more readily seen when the common valve was open. A similar specimen, is shown in the right-hand panel, positioned to match the echocardiogram. The right ventricle is extremely small and the anatomy could be confused with tricuspid atresia, but the off-setting at the crux of the heart is absent. There is a atrioventricular septal defect with a common atrioventricular valve extending at the same level from right to left across the crest of the ventricular septum, but draining mainly into the left ventricle.

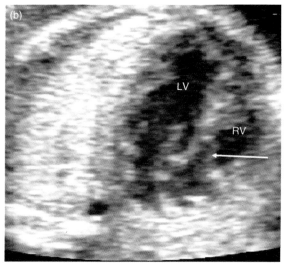

Fig. 2.25.(b). The right ventricle is smaller than the left and did not reach the apex. The mitral valve is widely open in this diastolic frame whereas the tricuspid valve is not (arrow). This is a case of tricuspid stenosis.

Small left ventricle

A small left ventricle indicates **mitral stenosis** or **atresia**. In atresia, there is no flow across the mitral valve, in stenosis, it is reduced. Both mitral atresia and stenosis are commonly associated with aortic atresia, in the setting of the **hypoplastic left heart syndrome**, a relatively common form of congenital heart disease (Fig. 2.26(a) and (b)). Alternatively, less commonly, mitral atresia can occur with a concordant patent aorta and a ventricular septal defect (Fig. 2.26(c)) or with a double outlet connection. A rare cause of a small left ventricle is **isolated mitral stenosis**, which is a difficult diagnosis to make prenatally. Blood entering the left atrium is off-loaded across the foramen ovale, resulting in diminished flow into the left ventricle and thus decreased

left heart growth. There would be bidirectional flow at the atrial septum, more than normal (see Chapter 5), but this may be difficult to detect (Fig. 2.26(d)). The mitral valve leaflets may be restricted in motion and thickened and the mitral valve attachments may be abnormal. The most common abnormality of mitral valve attachment is a parachute mitral valve where the papillary muscles are positioned more closely together than normal (see Fig. 4.21(a)), limiting the normal opening of the mitral valve.

Small posterior ventricle, anterior morphological left ventricle

This uncommon but well-recognized condition is a form of **tricuspid atresia**, but there is in addition a **discordant atrioventricular connection**, such that the anterior morphological right atrium connects to an anterior morphological left ventricle (Fig. 2.27(a)–(c)). The characteristics which denote the left ventricle are a relatively "empty" apex without the thick trabeculations normally found in the apex of the right ventricle, only septal attachments of the mitral valve, and the great artery which arises from this ventricle is "wedged" into the center of the heart, close to the crux. The wedging of the great artery arising from the left ventricle can be seen in Fig. 2.27(b), where flow in the left ventricular outflow tract is seen on color flow mapping in the four-chamber view. The left-sided connection (the tricuspid valve) is absent and the great arteries are almost invariably transposed. The aorta, which arises from the

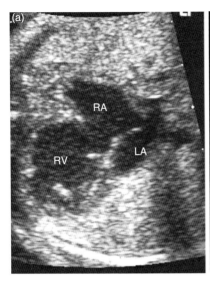
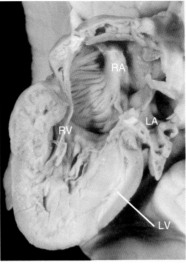

Fig. 2.26.(a). In the hypoplastic left heart syndrome, the left ventricle varies in size depending on the degree of patency of the mitral valve. In the echocardiographic example, there is complete mitral atresia and the left ventricular cavity cannot be seen. The left atrium is smaller than the right. In the anatomical specimen in the right panel, it is just possible to see the vestigial left ventricle, as a small slit.

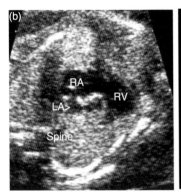
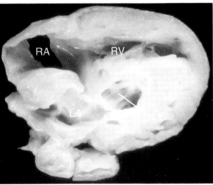

Fig. 2.26.(b). In the echocardiogram, there is a small left atrium and left ventricular cavity, although no flow could be demonstrated across the mitral valve. Note that the flap valve of the foramen ovale lies in the right atrium because of the obligate left-to-right shunt. The specimen in the right panel is in the same orientation and shows a small, thick-walled left ventricle with the right ventricle curving around it to form the apex. The atrial septum in the anatomical specimen was thick and intact and bulging to the right.

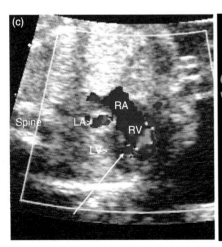
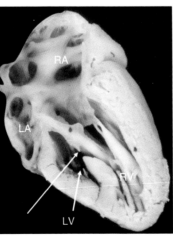

Fig. 2.26.(c). The left side of the heart is smaller than the right although it reaches the apex in the echocardigraphic image on the left. During diastole, blood flow crosses the tricuspid valve but not the mitral. The left ventricle and normally connected aorta were supplied with blood through quite a large mid-muscular ventricular septal defect. Flow in the ventricular septal defect (yellow arrow) is seen passing from the right to left ventricle on color flow mapping. In the right-hand panel, a similar specimen shows thick muscular tissue between the left atrium and left ventricle (mitral atresia). The left ventricle does not quite reach the apex, because the ventricular septal defect (yellow arrow, right-hand panel) is relatively small allowing little blood to flow from right to left ventricle.

45

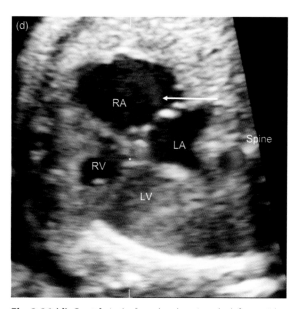

Fig. 2.26.(d). Contd. In the four-chamber view, the left ventricle is smaller than the right. In the arch views, the findings were suspicious for coarctation. Close examination of the mitral valve suggested that the papillary muscles were closer together than normal and that the valve was opening poorly. On the color flow map, most of the shunt through a small foramen ovale was left to right (arrow). This suggests a significant morphological abnormality of the mitral valve (mitral stenosis) in association with the arch anomaly.

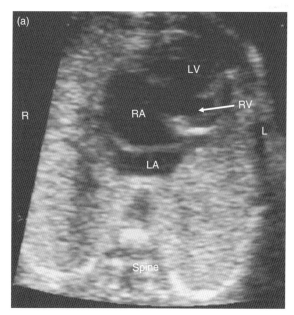

Fig. 2.27.(a). The atria lie in a normal relationship to each other, with the right atrium anterior to the left atrium. The posteriorly positioned left-sided atrioventricular valve is atretic. There is one main ventricle lying anteriorly, connected to the right atrium, but it had the morphological characteristics of a left ventricle. The small, posterior, morphological right ventricle receives blood from the main chamber via a ventricular septal defect. This is atrioventricular discordance with tricuspid atresia (or absent left connection).

hypoplastic right ventricle, receives blood through a ventricular septal defect from the main left ventricle. The aortic valve lies anterior and to the left of the pulmonary valve, which is typical of atrioventricular and ventriculo-arterial discordance (see Chapter 3).

Disproportion of the ventricles

There may be what is termed "disproportion" of the ventricles, where the sides of the heart are unequal, but the atrioventricular valves are functionally normal. This term should be confined to those cases where the cause of unequal ventricles is not immediately obvious, therefore excluding conditions such as mitral or tricuspid atresia or tricuspid regurgitation. Disproportion is a purely descriptive term with several different causes. Usually, the whole left side of the heart, both atrium and ventricle, is smaller than normal and the right heart is larger than normal. Both ventricles are usually within the normal range for size but their ratio, whether the LV/RV cavity size or mitral/tricuspid orifice size is used for measurement, is abnormal (Figs. 2.2 and 2.3). This can occur in a number of different situations. It can be within normal limits for the ventricles to appear

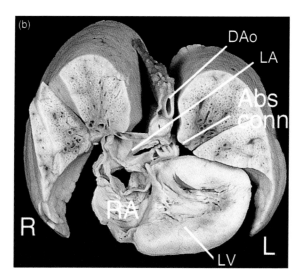

Fig. 2.27.(b). The heart is shown in a four-chamber cut. There is no connection between the left-sided, morphological left atrium and a left-sided ventricle. The main ventricle is connected to the right atrium but is morphologically a left ventricle, identified from the trabecular pattern, the mitral valve attachments and the wedging of the arising great artery.

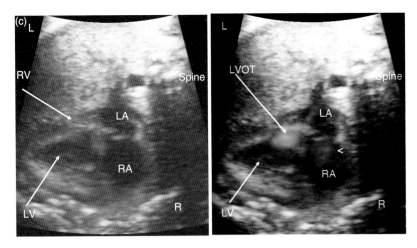

Fig. 2.27.(c). Contd. In the four-chamber view, the atria were normally positioned with the left atrium on the left and the right atrium to the right. The left-sided ventricle was barely visible and all the flow at the atrial septum (arrowhead in the right-hand panel) was from left to right indicating atresia of the left-sided atrioventricular valve. Close examination of the main ventricle indicated it was a left ventricle, connected to the right atrium. Typically in this condition, the left ventricular outflow tract (LVOT) gave rise to the pulmonary artery. This therefore was a discordant atrioventricular and ventriculo-arterial connection with left sided atrioventricular valve atresia.

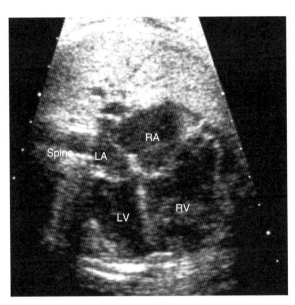

Fig. 2.28. The right side of the heart is larger than the left and there appears to be a pericardial effusion. However, this appearance is within normal limits for 36 weeks, which was the gestational age at the time of this scan. The heart was normal after birth.

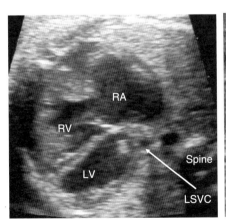
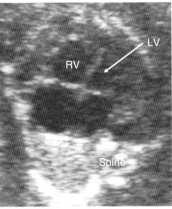

Fig. 2.29. In the fetus illustrated in the left-hand panel, the right atrium and ventricle were dilated relative to the left heart structures from an early gestational age. There was a small pericardial effusion but the chromosomes were normal. There was early growth retardation but nothing specific otherwise. There was no tricuspid regurgitation to account for the right atrial dilatation. The left atrium was particularly small, yet the pulmonary veins drained normally and the aortic arch was a good size. There was a persistent left superior caval vein draining to the coronary sinus. The heart was otherwise normal after birth, although the child has an undiagnosed syndrome postnatally, resulting in severe developmental delay at 5 years of age. In the example illustrated in the right-hand panel, there was cardiomegaly and mild disproportion in this fetus, secondary to severe intrauterine growth retardation due to placental insufficiency.

47

unequal after about 30 weeks' gestation, with right ventricular dominance (Fig. 2.28). Alternatively, disproportion can be associated with extracardiac causes such as growth retardation, diaphragmatic hernia (Fig. 2.20(a)), absent ductus venosus (Fig. 2.14(b)), or unusual syndromes (Fig. 2.29).

The most common cardiac cause of disproportion is **coarctation of the aorta**, where the narrowed area of aorta in the aortic arch leads to an increased afterload in the left ventricle, resulting in turn in a diminished right to left shunt at the atrial septal defect, reducing left heart flow and thus size (Fig. 2.30(a)–(e)). The degree of disproportion in size can be quite variable in coarctation, depending on the severity of arch obstruction.

Further features of coarctation on examination of the great arteries and transverse arch are described in Chapters 3 and 4, respectively. Ventricular disproportion can also be a feature of **totally anomalous pulmonary venous drainage**, where the pulmonary veins drain to the right side of the heart instead of the left atrium, resulting in diminished blood flow to the left ventricle and increased flow to the right (Fig. 2.31). Even when identified prior to 30 weeks of gestation, a fetus with ventricular disproportion will sometimes have a normal outcome. However, the finding indicates the necessity to positively exclude an underlying cause, such as coarctation of the aorta, by serial assessment of the child after birth.

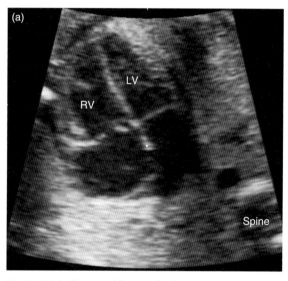

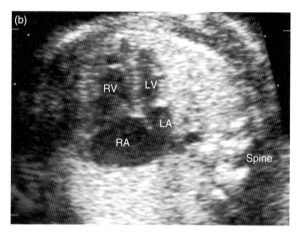

Fig. 2.30.(b) and (c). The difference in ventricular sizes is more impressive in these further echocardiographic examples of coarctation than that shown in Fig. 2.30(a), with the left side of the heart much smaller than the right.

Fig. 2.30.(a). There is mild ventricular disproportion in this fetus at 20 weeks' gestation. This is suggestive of a coarctation lesion, which proved to be present after birth.

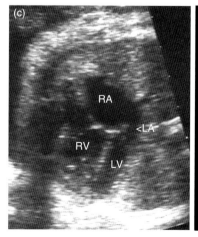

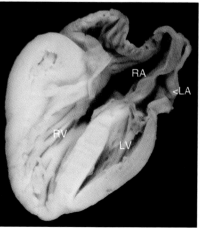

Fig. 2.30.(c). The anatomical section of a fetus with confirmed coarctation of the aorta, is positioned to match the similar echocardigraphic cut. There is marked disproportion, with the left atrium, mitral valve, and left ventricle all smaller than the corresponding right heart structures. The left ventricle is a little short of the apex of the heart.

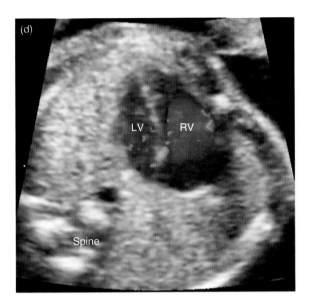

Fig. 2.30.(d). Contd. The color flow map accentuates the difference in ventricular sizes, in this example of disproportion of the ventricles due to coarctation of the aorta.

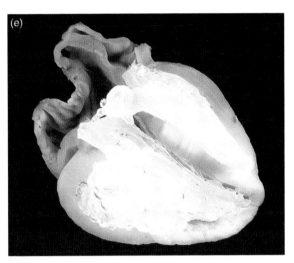

Fig. 2.30.(e). The cast made from the anatomical specimen emphasizes the difference in cavity sizes, in this example of coarctation of the aorta in the mid-trimester fetus.

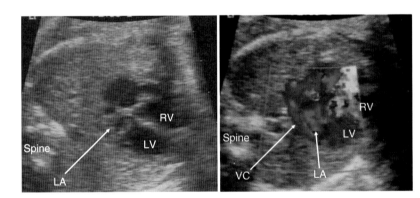

Fig. 2.31. On the left-hand panel, the heart is seen in a four-chamber view. It could easily pass as normal but there was mild disproportion of the ventricles, with the right slightly bigger than the left and the left atrium in particular appears a little small. On the right-hand panel, in the same plane, the color flow map shows a vessel behind the heart with flow going from the left of the thorax to the right across the midline. This was a venous confluence (VC) in total anomalous pulmonary venous drainage. Note there is an increased distance between the descending aorta and the left atrium as a clue to this difficult diagnosis. However, all the 2D findings here are subtle and easily overlooked. Color flow mapping is essential to make the diagnosis.

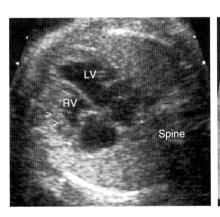

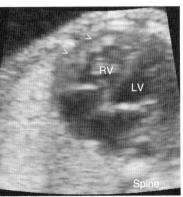

Fig. 2.32. The right ventricular wall (arrowheads) appears thickened in comparison with the left in each panel, with the right ventricular cavity reduced in size. Both fetuses illustrated had significant pulmonary stenosis.

49

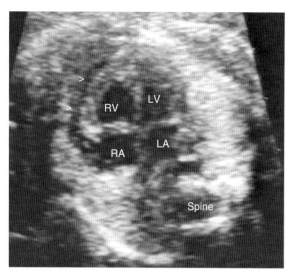

Fig. 2.33. The right ventricular walls appear thickened in the presence of a small pericardial effusion (arrows). However, this is an artifact, the heart was normal.

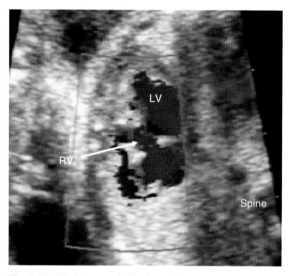

Fig. 2.35. The left ventricle fills during diastole to the apex, whereas there is much less flow across the tricuspid valve in this case of tricuspid stenosis.

Unequal ventricular thickness

The thickness of the ventricular walls should be approximately equal to each other and to the thickness of the ventricular septum. Increased pressure within the ventricle can result in increase in the wall thickness of a ventricle but this can be difficult to appreciate if it is mild. Obstruction to outflow in either ventricle can produce increased pressure, causing **left ventricular hypertrophy** in aortic stenosis and

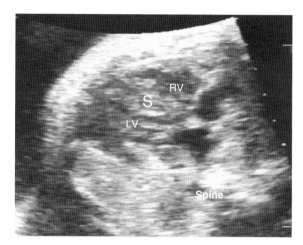

Fig. 2.34. There was biventricular hypertrophy with thickening most marked in the septum (S). The cavity of both ventricles was almost obscured during systole. This fetus had Noonan's syndrome after birth.

right ventricular hypertrophy in pulmonary stenosis (Fig. 2.32). Sometimes the ventricular walls can appear falsely thickened in the presence of a pericardial effusion (Fig. 2.33). **A thickened septum** is a fairly common finding in late gestation with **maternal diabetes** and it usually is of no consequence. It is unusual to see isolated septal hypertrophy as an in-utero manifestation of **hypertrophic obstructive cardiomyopathy**, as this condition, although well recognized in children and adults, is very rare prenatally and also in infancy. However, some cases of fetal biventricular hypertrophy, usually seen in later gestation, have proved to have **Noonan's syndrome** (Fig. 2.34). A few cases of apparent ventricular and septal hypertrophy have been seen in fetal life, which have not been evident postnatally, so counseling when these are found must be cautious.

Unequal AV valve opening

The two atrioventricular valves may not open freely and equally, either due to an abnormality of the valve itself or due to an abnormality further "downstream." In **tricuspid or mitral atresia**, the appropriate valve will not open at all and there will be no color flow across the valve. In **tricuspid or mitral stenosis**, the valve may appear thickened and restricted in motion, with less flow across the valve on color flow mapping than on the other side (Fig. 2.35). These valve abnormalities will result in a smaller than normal related ventricle, and have been described above. If there is a higher than normal pressure in a ventricle, as would occur in **aortic** or **pulmonary stenosis or atresia**, the related atrioventricular valve will not open freely.

Abnormalities at the crux

The crux or center of the heart is essential to image precisely so that it can be evaluated correctly. The coronary sinus lies just below the mitral valve at the atrioventricular junction and this normal structure can give a false appearance of an atrioventricular septal defect if the crux is not imaged exactly (Fig. 2.36(a) and (b)). Note how close these sections are in the mid-trimester fetus.

Loss of off-setting

Loss of off-setting at the crux, where the atrioventricular valves appear to lie "straight" across the crux, usually implies the presence of a common atrioventricular valve in an **atrioventricular septal defect**. This is where, instead of two discrete atrioventricular valve rings with separate leaflets, there is one shared ring with leaflets in common, or shared, between the sides of the heart across the crest of the ventricular septum. This type of atrioventricular valve is associated with a deficiency in the central septal structures of the heart. This deficiency (nearly) always results in an abnormal communication ("hole") between the atria, adjacent to the crux of the heart and distinct from the normal foramen ovale. If there is only an atrial defect, this is sometimes called a partial atrioventricular septal defect or an ostium primum atrial defect (Fig. 2.37(a) and (b)). In this situation, the common valve is attached to the crest of the ventricular septum, so that there is no

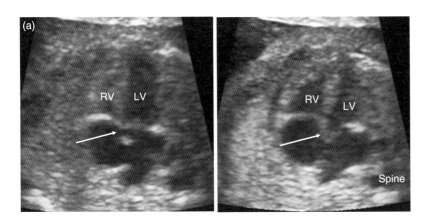

Fig. 2.36.(a). On the left-hand panel, the heart is imaged just below a true four-chamber view section. There is an apparent defect in the atrial septum on the atrial side of the atrioventricular valves (arrow). This is the mouth of the normal coronary sinus, which drains into the right atrium. The atrioventricular valves could be interpreted in this cut to be in a straight line across the septum without differential insertion. However, in the right-hand panel, in the same fetus, the crux is imaged correctly in a section just above the left-hand image, clearly demonstrating differential insertion or off-setting (arrow) of the atrioventricular valves. Compare the left-hand panel of this figure with the left-hand panel of Fig. 2.37(a).

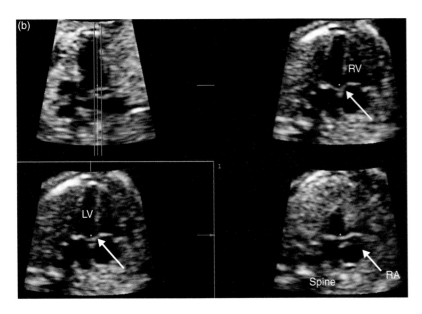

Fig. 2.36.(b). This 20-week heart is cut in tomographic slices 0.8 mm apart, from a true four-chamber view (top right), cutting caudally to the opening of the coronary sinus (white arrow, bottom left), and then to the course of the sinus below the left atrium (bottom right). The slice on the bottom right could be misinterpreted to show lack of differential insertion, although the crux in the true four-chamber view clearly shows off-setting (yellow arrow).

51

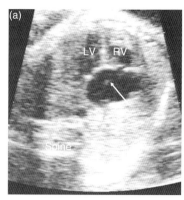 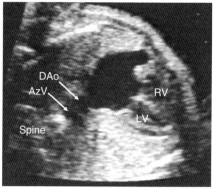

Fig. 2.37.(a). Both panels illustrate a partial atrioventricular septal defect. On the left-hand panel, the portion of the atrial septum, which is normally attached to the crux, is seen (arrow), whereas in the right panel no atrial septum at all can be seen (which can be termed a common atrium). In the example shown in the right-hand panel, there is also a dilated azygous vein (AzV) seen behind the heart, indicative of interruption of the inferior vena cava in left atrial isomerism.

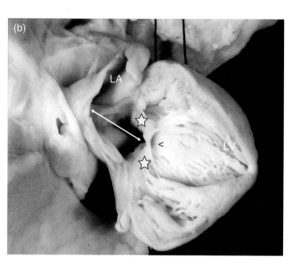

Fig. 2.37.(b). This heart has not been sectioned in a four-chamber plane but is opened from the left side to show the features of this defect. There is a large "partial" atrioventricular septal defect otherwise know as an ostium primum "ASD." It is easy to mistake the valve for a normal mitral valve. In fact, it cannot be, as it is fused to the crest of the ventricular septum (arrowhead) and the atrioventricular component of the atrial septum is missing, creating a large defect on the atrial side of the common valve (double-headed arrow). The appearance is formed by fusion of the superior and inferior bridging leaflets (starred).

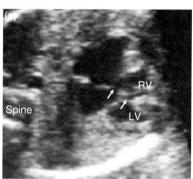 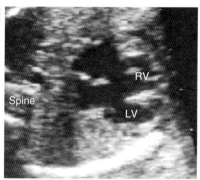

Fig. 2.38.(a). The heart is seen in a lateral four-chamber view. In systole, seen on the left-hand panel, when the common valve is closed, a small atrial and ventricular defect is seen above and below the valve (arrow heads). There is loss of differential insertion such that the valve lies straight through the center of the heart. In the diastolic frame on the right side, the valve is open, revealing the large size of the defect, involving both atrial and ventricular septums.

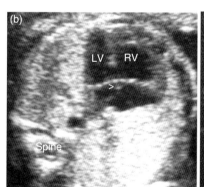 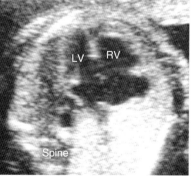

Fig. 2.38.(b). The heart is seen in an apical four-chamber projection in systolic and diastolic frames, on the left and right, respectively. Note the difference in the appearance of an atrioventricular septal defect in this view as compared to that in Fig. 2.37. In this example there is s relatively small atrial defect but quite a large ventricular defect. Note again the straight, not offset, appearance of the atrioventricular valve at the crux, particularly when the valve is closed.

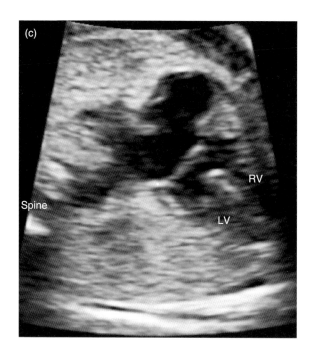

Fig. 2.38.(c). Contd. The heart is seen in a lateral four-chamber view. There is a large primum atrial septal defect and a moderate sized inlet ventricular septal defect, with a common valve positioned straight across the crux of the heart. This is an atrioventricular septal defect.

associated ventricular septal defect. However, if, as is most common, there is also a communication between the ventricles at their inlets, adjacent to the crux and contiguous with the atrial septal deficiency, it is termed a complete atrioventricular septal defect (Fig. 2.38(a)–(c)). This is an important defect to recognize, partly because it is a common condition and partly because it has important associations and implications (see Chapter 8), although the diagnosis may sometimes be very difficult (Fig. 2.38(d) and (e)). An atrioventricular septal defect is a frequent component of more complex heart disease, such as left heart disease (Fig. 2.38(f)) and isomerism syndromes (Fig. 2.38(g) and (h)). When the heart is unevenly divided in the

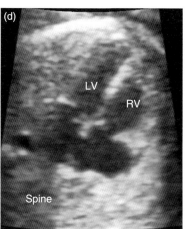
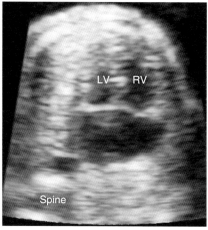

Fig. 2.38.(d). It is crucial to image the four-chamber view correctly in order to be sure of excluding an atrioventricular septal defect. In the left-hand panel, the crux appears normal but the view is slightly oblique. In the same patient, in the correct orientation seen on the right-hand panel, there is a common atrioventricular valve, positioned straight across a small atrioventricular septal defect.

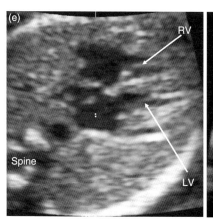
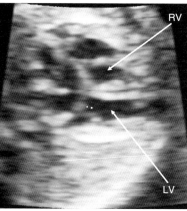

Fig. 2.38.(e). A normal lateral four-chamber view is seen on the left-hand panel. Note the normal appearance of the crux in this projection. On the right-hand panel, a lateral four-chamber view is seen in an example of a small atrioventricular septal defect. Note the differences in appearance at the crux.

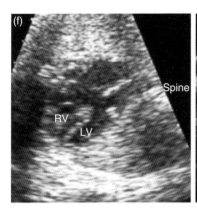
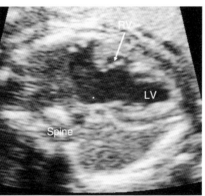

Fig. 2.38.(f). Contd. In both panels, the atrioventricular septal defect is seen in the typical central position in the heart with the common valve open in diastole. However, in addition, on the left-hand panel, the left heart is smaller than the right, due to associated coarctation of the aorta. On the right-hand panel, the right ventricle is small, as the common valve drains mainly to the left ventricle. In the context of an atrioventricular septal defect, these are termed unbalanced ventricles.

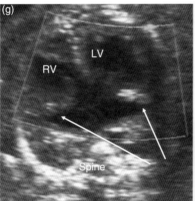
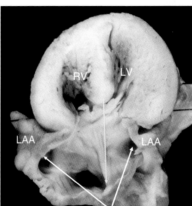

Fig. 2.38.(g). In the normal heart, the atrial appendages have a different morphology, with the right-sided appendage being broad and blunt, and the left-sided appendage, narrow and pointed. On the echocardiogram on the left hand panel, the heart is enlarged and in an abnormal position in the thorax and there is an atrioventricular septal defect. Both atrial appendages are narrow and pointed (white arrows), therefore of left morphology, indicating left atrial isomerism. The specimen shown in the right-hand panel correlates well with the echocardiogram. Both of the atrial appendages are narrowed and pointed and anatomically of left type (left isomerism). There is a large atrioventricular septal defect (yellow arrow) and some hypertrophy of the ventricular walls due to complete heart block, a not uncommon association with left atrial isomerism.

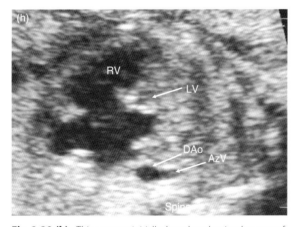

Fig. 2.38.(h). This case was initially thought to be simply a case of a typical hypoplastic left heart. However, closer inspection reveals a common valve connected to a dominant right ventricle. In addition, there is a dilated azygous vein behind the heart indicating left atrial isomerism. This detail would influence counseling and prognosis for the treatment of the hypoplastic left heart syndrome.

context of a common valve, the ventricles are termed "unbalanced." Alternatively, the heart is said to be left or right ventricular dominant.

The typical off-setting at the crux is also lost in **double inlet ventricle**. This is a fairly unusual condition where both atrioventricular valves open into one main ventricular chamber (Fig. 2.39(a)–(c)). This gives the appearance of "absence" of the ventricular septum in the four-chamber view, or no ventricular septum reaching the crux of the heart. There is in fact a ventricular septum in this condition but it does not divide the heart equally and also lies above the four-chamber view, therefore is not visible in this section. In the majority of cases of double inlet ventricle, the main chamber is a morphological left ventricle, which can be distinguished by the lack of dense apical trabeculation. However, a double inlet connection to a morphological right ventricle, though rare, can occur (Fig. 2.39(d)).

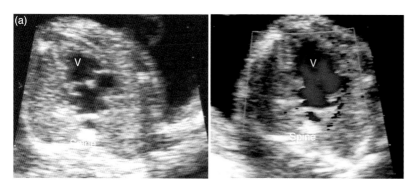

Fig. 2.39.(a). Two atria and two atrioventricular valves are seen, but they open into a single ventricular chamber (V). Note the loss of off-setting at the crux. The ventricular septum is not seen reaching the crux in the normal way (compare with Fig. 2.8, for example). The apex does not appear to be heavily trabeculated (compare with Fig. 2.39(d)), suggesting the main chamber is a morphological left ventricle.

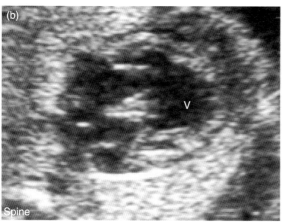

Fig. 2.39.(b). Similarly in a lateral four-chamber projection, both atrioventricular valves are seen, but not the ventricular septum, which is readily seen in this projection (compare with Fig. 2.5(b) or 2.6(b)). In this case, both valves drain to a single morphological left ventricle.

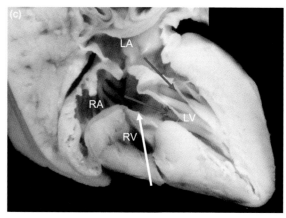

Fig. 2.39.(c). In the anatomical specimen, there are two patent atrioventricular valves (red arrows) but both are connected to the posterior anatomically left ventricle. The ventricular septum is malaligned anteriorly and as a result the right ventricle is hypoplastic. In this view, the ventricular septal defect (white arrow), which is part of the malformation, can also be seen.

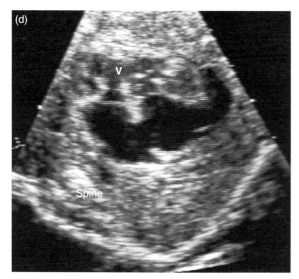

Fig. 2.39.(d). Both atrioventricular valves open into a single heavily trabeculated ventricle. This is double inlet right ventricle. Compare the appearance of this apex with that of the single left ventricle shown in Fig. 2.37(a) and (b).

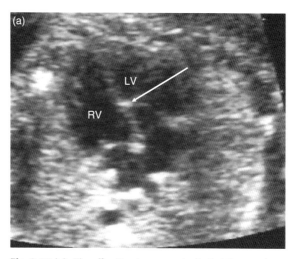

Fig. 2.40.(a). The off-setting is exaggerated in that the septal insertion of the tricuspid valve is further down into the right ventricle than normal (arrow). This is mild Ebstein's anomaly. Note the unusual size and shape of the right atrium in this condition.

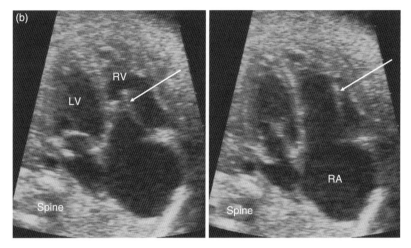

Fig. 2.40.(b). Contd. These panels illustrate a more severe degree of Ebstein's malformation than in Fig. 2.40(a). A systolic frame is shown in the left-hand panel, a diastolic in the right-hand panel. The long anterior leaflet (arrow) typical in Ebstein's malformation is seen. The septal leaflet is tethered (or stuck down) to the ventricular septum. The right atrium is larger than normal, partly because of displacement of the valve and partly because of tricuspid regurgitation.

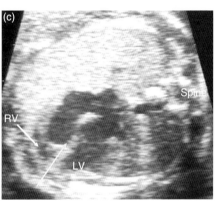 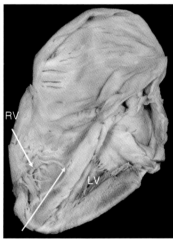

Fig. 2.40.(c). In this example, the tricuspid valve on the echocardiogram is so displaced (yellow arrow) that there is very little right ventricle visible beyond it. Note the deviation of the ventricular septum, flattening the left ventricle. This is severe Ebstein's anomaly. The specimen shown on the right-hand panel is very similar. The right side of the heart is dilated and compresses the left atrium and left ventricle. The mural and septal leaflets of the tricuspid valve are attached firmly to the right ventricular wall rather than being freely mobile. Thus in a four-chamber section, the septal leaflet is positioned more apically than normal (yellow arrow) and the degree of offsetting of the tricuspid valve as compared to the mitral valve is much more pronounced than usual.

Exaggerated off-setting

Another abnormality with a key feature seen at the crux is Ebstein's malformation. In this anomaly, the insertion of the septal leaflet of the tricuspid valve is lower in the ventricular septum than normal, displaced towards the apex. The off-setting therefore is exaggerated compared with the normal (Fig. 2.40(a)–(c)). The degree of displacement is highly variable and this corresponds loosely with the severity of the condition. The coaptation point of the valve is displaced into the body of the right ventricle and there is commonly a variable degree of regurgitation, which starts further into the body of the right ventricle than it would do in a normal tricuspid valve (Fig. 2.41). If the regurgitation is severe, the right atrium will be dilated, sometimes grossly, producing cardiomegaly (see above).

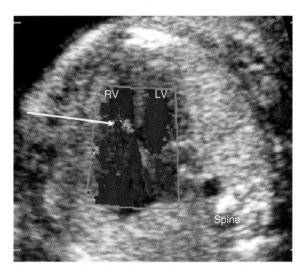

Fig. 2.41. Usually in Ebstein's anomaly, there is some degree of tricuspid regurgitation. As seen here, regurgitation starts (arrow) further into the right ventricle than in a normally positioned valve, at the displaced coaptation site of the tricuspid valve cusps.

Reversed off-setting

The offset at the crux can appear reversed, with the atrioventricular valve in the left-sided ventricle arising nearer to the apex than that of the right-sided ventricle. As it is always the tricuspid valve that arises nearest the apex, this finding implies that the tricuspid valve, and its intimately associated morphological right ventricle, is on the left side and the morphological left ventricle on the right. As a result, the ventricle with the more coarsely trabeculated apex and moderator band (denoting it the right ventricle) will lie on the left side of the heart or in the more posterior ventricle. If the arrangement of the atria is normal, there will be a discordant connection of the atria to the ventricles, **atrioventricular discordance** (Fig. 2.42(a)–(c)). This rare anomaly usually occurs in association with discordance of the ventriculo-arterial connection as well, in the condition known as "congenitally corrected" transposition of the great arteries, where the morphological left atrium is connected to the morphological right ventricle. The right ventricle in turn is connected to the aorta, thus the flow of blood from the pulmonary veins reaches the aorta as in the normal, but does so through the right ventricular chamber. Conversely, the morphological left ventricle is connected to the right atrium and pumps to the pulmonary artery. This defect has important long-term consequences in terms of cardiac function. In addition, there are often associated intracardiac lesions, such as Ebstein's

anomaly (Fig. 2.42(b)), a ventricular septal defect or pulmonary stenosis.

Defects in the ventricular septum

The ventricular septum is an uneven quadrilateral in shape. Only part of the base of the quadrilateral, made up of part of the **muscular** ventricular septum and the

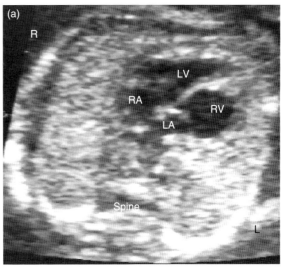

Fig. 2.42.(a). The lower atrioventricular valve (which is always the tricuspid valve) lies in the more posterior, left-sided ventricle. Note that this is the more trabeculated ventricle also, further denoting it as the right ventricle. The atria, however, are in their normal positions. This is atrioventricular discordance but its characteristics are quite subtle in this four-chamber view.

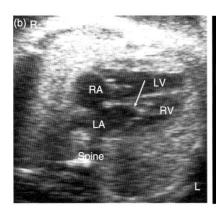
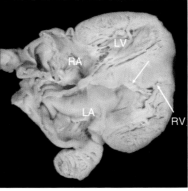

Fig. 2.42.(b). In this example of atrioventricular discordance, reversed differential insertion is more pronounced due to mild Ebstein's malformation of the tricuspid valve. The anatomical specimen is very similar to the ultrasound image. The right atrium connects to the anatomic left ventricle and left atrium to the anatomic right ventricle, so there are discordant atrioventricular connections. The atrioventricular valves follow the pattern of the ventricles so the mitral valve is anterior and the tricuspid valve posterior resulting in reversal of off-setting at the crux of the heart. The displaced hinge point of the "Ebsteinoid" tricuspid valve (yellow arrows) emphasizes the reversed off-setting.

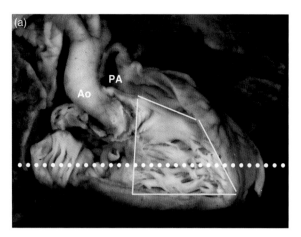

Fig. 2.43.(a). The heart is opened from the front, so that the anterior surface of the right side of the ventricular septum is seen. The shape of the ventricular septum is a quadrilateral shown in yellow. The dotted line represents the four-chamber view section. It can be seen that a ventricular septal defect could be in any position above or below this line, and not be seen on the four-chamber projection. However, when the beam is swept from the abdomen to the arch in a continuous fashion, the whole septum can be examined.

inlet septum, is seen in a true four-chamber view. The whole septum from the base of the heart as it sits on the diaphragm up to the pulmonary valve should be "swept" by the ultrasound beam in order to exclude a defect (Fig. 2.43(a)). In the apical four-chamber view, as the septum thins towards the crux, dropout can give the impression of a defect, which is artifactual (Fig. 2.43(b)). If there is doubt about the integrity of the septum in the apical view, the transducer must be moved so that the ultrasound beam is perpendicular to the septum. A true defect often has bright margins, the so-called T-sign (Fig. 2.43(c)). In Fig. 2.43(d), the four-chamber view is normal but the muscular defect lies just below (or caudal to) the level of the correct four-chamber view. In fetal life, there is normally bidirectional flow across a ventricular septal defect on color flow mapping (Fig. 2.43(e)). Apparently unidirectional flow is either overlap from another structure, usually the pulmonary artery or atrioventricular valve

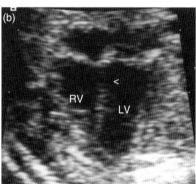
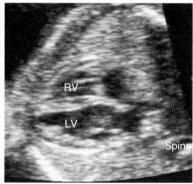

Fig. 2.43.(b). On the left-hand panel, the heart is imaged in an apical projection. The ultrasound beam is parallel to the ventricular septum and fails to resolve the septum as it thins towards the crux, giving an appearance suggestive of a ventricular septal defect at this point (arrowhead). The right-hand panel is the same fetus with the same part of the ventricular septum imaged but with the ultrasound beam perpendicular to the septum. The septum is clearly seen to be intact.

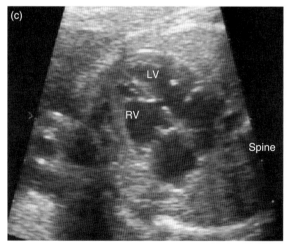

Fig. 2.43.(c). The heart is seen in a four-chamber projection. There is a moderate-sized mid-muscular ventricular septal defect. There are bright margins at the edges of the defect, the so-called "T sign."

inflow, or can occur if there is associated obstruction to outflow from one or other ventricle. However, the findings must make sense, for example, if flow across a convincing ventricular septal defect appears all left-to-right, this would indicate left ventricular outflow tract obstruction or coarctation, for which there would be other evidence. Conversely, if flow across a ventricular septal defect appears to be all right-to-left, this would imply right ventricular outflow obstruction, which would be evident from other features. A ventricular septal defect can be varied in size but, in general, those which are readily seen prenatally, particularly if they come to attention from routine screening obstetric ultrasound, tend to be in the moderate to large range.

A rare complicating finding in a ventricular septal defect is a **straddling atrioventricular valve**. This usually only occurs in large ventricular septal defects in

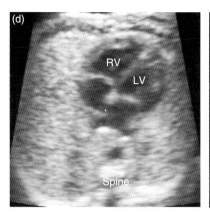 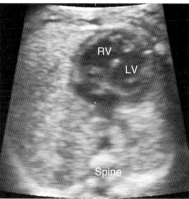

Fig. 2.43.(d). Contd. In the correct four-chamber view, seen on the left-hand panel, the ventricular septum appears intact. However, a moderate sized apical muscular ventricular septal defect is seen as the ultrasound beam is swept down from the four-chamber view to the base of the heart as it sits on the diaphragm.

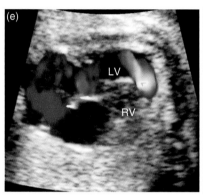 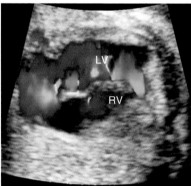

Fig. 2.43.(e). There is left-to-right flow in the left-hand panel and right-to-left flow in the right panel in this moderate sized apical muscular ventricular septal defect.

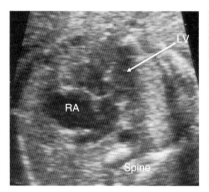 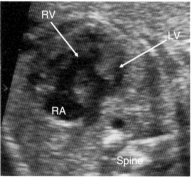

Fig. 2.44. In the left-hand panel, in the systolic frame, the closed atrioventricular valves are seen. There is an inlet ventricular septal defect and the left ventricle is smaller than the right. In the diastolic frame on the right panel, the anterior leaflet of the mitral valve opens into the right ventricle, as it was attached to papillary muscles on the right side of the septum. In this fetus with transposition of the great arteries, this complication prevented the possibility of a biventricular repair.

association with complex malformations such as double outlet right ventricle. In a straddling atrioventricular valve, the attachments of the valve, either mitral or tricuspid, cross through the ventricular septal defect to attach to papillary muscles in the opposite ventricle (Fig. 2.44). Closure of such a ventricular septal defect surgically may be difficult or impossible to achieve without compromising the function of the straddling atrioventricular valve.

Abnormalities of the atrial septum

A defect in the distal part of the atrial septum at the entry point of the superior vena cava is termed a **sinus venosus defect**. It is a relatively rare form of atrial septal defect in postnatal life and, to our knowledge, there are no cases reported in the literature diagnosed prenatally, although a case seen by us is illustrated in Fig. 2.45. A secundum atrial septal defect is a very common cardiac lesion after birth and is due to the failure

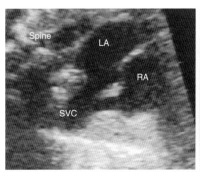
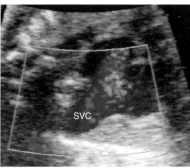

Fig. 2.45. In the 2D image, the superior vena cava "overrides" an atrial septal defect. On the right-hand panel, on color flow mapping, the flow from the superior vena cava is seen to drain mostly to the left atrium with a smaller stream draining to the right atrium. This is a sinus venosus atrial septal defect.

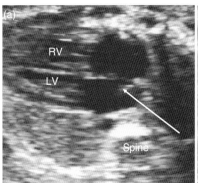
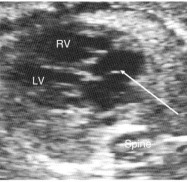

Fig. 2.46.(a). The four-chamber view appears normal in this case of transposition of the great arteries. However, the movement of the foramen ovale flap was unusual. Note that it lies in the left atrium in a fairly normal position in the left-hand panel and in the right atrium on the right panel (arrows).

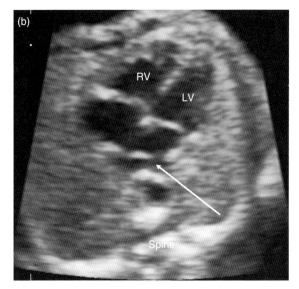

Fig. 2.46.(b). The flap valve in this normal fetus had a wide excursion, coming in contact with the atrial wall at some points in the cardiac cycle. Although this appearance has been linked to the detection of ectopic beats, it is probably coincidental, as both are common in late pregnancy.

of the flap valve to adequately seal over the foramen ovale, a process which occurs progressively during the first year of life. Thus, this type of heart disease cannot be diagnosed prenatally or even in early infancy, unless the defect is very large. Sometimes the foramen ovale appears wider than normal in the fetus, especially in an apical four-chamber view (Fig. 2.6(a)) but this does not indicate the future presence of a secundum atrial septal defect. The type of defect sometimes referred to as an **ostium primum atrial septal defect**, where the atrial septum does not reach to the crux of the heart, is an integral **part of a common atrioventricular valve** and is described above under defects at the crux (Figs. 2.37, 2.38).

Normally the flap valve of the foramen ovale lies open, wholly in the body of the left atrium, only closing briefly at the end of atrial systole. Some **abnormalities of the motion of the flap valve** can be observed. In great artery abnormalities, particularly transposition of the great arteries, the foramen flap may prolapse back and forward through the atrial defect during the cardiac

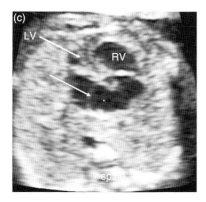

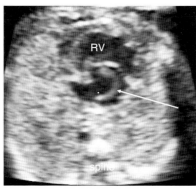

Fig. 2.46.(c). Contd. In the four-chamber view, the left ventricle is hypoplastic in this case of mitral atresia. The flap valve (yellow arrows) lies in the left atrium in the left-hand panel and almost reaches the tricuspid valve in the right-hand panel, as it herniates to the right in the diastolic frame.

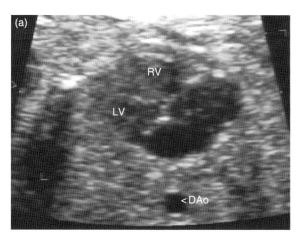

Fig. 2.47.(a). The back of the left atrium is not the normal shape but is more rounded. This is because it is not receiving pulmonary veins, as they drained anomalously to the innominate vein. Note the increased distance between the descending aorta and the left atrium (compare with the normal in Fig. 2.8(a).

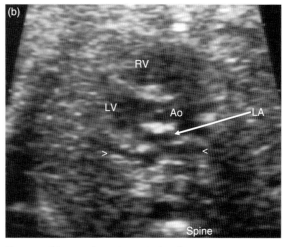

Fig. 2.47.(b). Just above the level of the four-chamber view, the venous confluence lies behind the left atrium but not connecting to it. The left atrium itself is small. A pulmonary vein is seen joining the confluence from each side (arrow heads).

cycle (Fig. 2.46(a)). Why this should be so is not clear, but it is not uncommonly noted. Alternatively, the flap valve can be continuously opposed to the atrial wall, or show more limited excursion, in conditions of increased left atrial pressure. This will occur in the setting of left heart obstruction, such as mitral or aortic stenosis. The flap valve can appear "**aneurysmal**" in that it bulges towards the left atrial wall and sometimes almost into the mitral valve. This is a fairly common appearance, especially in late pregnancy and appears to have no pathological significance (Fig. 2.46(b)). Alternatively, the flap valve can appear aneurysmal in mitral atresia when the flap valve will herniate almost into the tricuspid valve (Fig. 2.46(c)).

A defect, which we have never identified but which is widely quoted, although rarely reported in the

literature, is **primary restriction of the foramen ovale**. The foramen is said to appear small with a high velocity jet across it. This is said to lead to right heart dilatation and even fetal hydrops. This is in distinction to secondary restriction or closure of the atrial septum, which is not uncommonly seen in left heart disease (see Fig. 2.15).

Abnormalities of pulmonary venous drainage

There are usually four pulmonary veins in total, an upper and lower vein on each side. Usually it is the left and right lower veins that are seen on the four-chamber view. In **total anomalous pulmonary venous drainage**, the pulmonary veins cannot be seen connecting to the left atrium. The back of the atrium (Fig. 2.47(a)) looks rounded and smooth in contrast to the usual appearance (compare with Fig. 2.8). A confluence of veins usually forms behind the left atrium but does not actually connect with it (Fig. 2.47(b)). Instead, either an ascending channel drains the confluence to the superior vena cava or innominate vein, or, a descending channel passes through the diaphragm to connect to the portal system (see Fig. 4.15), or third, the confluence is connected to the coronary sinus. Much less commonly, the pulmonary veins all connect directly to the right atrium (Fig. 2.48(a) and (b)). The fact that a significant volume of blood, which normally goes directly to the left ventricle, drains to the right heart, can lead to ventricular disproportion with right ventricular dominance. However, this is not an invariable sign of total anomalous pulmonary venous drainage, perhaps because of the presence of a widely patent foramen ovale in many cases. In right atrial isomerism, by definition, there is total anomalous pulmonary venous drainage as there is no morphological left atrium (see more on isomerism syndromes in Chapter 4), but in about 50% of cases, the veins connect directly to the atrial mass, so do not cause a hemodynamic problem. However, the connection is often rather different from normal, in that the veins form a confluence, which then drains into one or other side of the atrial mass (Fig. 2.49).

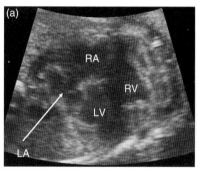
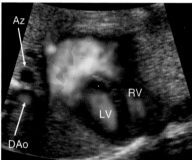

Fig. 2.48.(a). On the left-hand panel, the four-chamber view appeared somewhat abnormal with ventricular and particularly atrial disproportion but this was in late gestation and the fetus had left atrial isomerism so the findings were attributed to this, especially as the pulmonary veins (right-hand panel) were identified and appeared to be related to the left-sided atrium. Note the two vessels behind the heart, the descending aorta on the left and the dilated azygous vein on the right, as a result of interruption of the inferior caval vein, suggestive of left atrial isomerism.

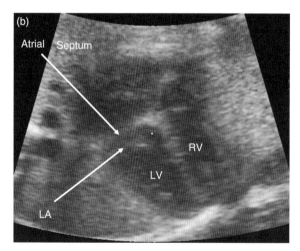

Fig. 2.48.(b). This is the same frame as in the right-hand panel of Fig. 2.48(a) with the color information removed. The atrial septum can be seen to be deviated to the left. The left atrium is very small in this frame and lies below the plane of section in which the pulmonary veins are seen. The pulmonary veins therefore all drained directly to the right-sided atrium, an unusual form of anomalous drainage, and an unusual malformation in association with left atrial isomerism.

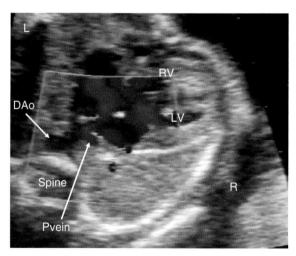

Fig. 2.49. The heart is seen in the four-chamber view, but the fetus lies HF instead of HB as expected. The apex, therefore, points to the right in this case of right atrial isomerism. The descending aorta lies to the left of the spine in a normal position. The pulmonary veins formed a confluence, which drained closer to the atrial septum than the separate pulmonary veins normally drain (compare with Fig. 2.8).

Abnormalities in the posterior mediastinum

The descending aorta behind the left atrium may lie more rightwards than normal (Fig. 2.50). This may occur when there is a **right-sided aortic arch**, as, in this setting, the aorta usually descends on the right in the thorax, crossing the midline to continue on the left at about the level of the diaphragm. However, sometimes in a right arch, the aorta crosses higher in the thorax and the position of the descending aorta in the four-chamber view is normal.

The aorta may lie more posteriorly, further away from the left atrium than normal. This can occur in **total anomalous pulmonary venous drainage** as the venous confluence behind the left atrium, which is not always directly visible in the four-chamber view, displaces the aorta posteriorly (Fig. 2.47). However, this is not an invariable feature of total anomalous pulmonary venous drainage.

In the normal fetus, only one large vessel is seen behind the heart in a four-chamber view (see Fig. 2.1). However, in Fig. 2.51(a) two vessels can be seen lying behind the left atrium, one being the aorta and one a **dilated azygous vein**. This occurs in the setting of an interrupted inferior vena cava, where venous flow from the lower body is forced to take an alternative route to the heart. This additional blood flow dilates the normally small and almost invisible azygous vein. An interrupted inferior caval vein can occur in an otherwise normal fetus but more often it is associated with

left atrial isomerism, with or without additional intracardiac malformation (see Chapter 4). A rare cause of azygous vein dilation is absent ductus venosus with direct drainage of the umbilical vein to the azygous vein. In this setting the inferior vena cava would also be found. In Fig. 2.51(b), there appear to be three vessels lying behind the heart. The color flow map demonstrates that only two of the three vessels are vascular. The central vessel was a **dilated esophagus** and the right-sided vessel part of a **pulmonary venous confluence** (Fig. 2.51(c)) in this complex case of right atrial isomerism.

Additional structural abnormalities seen in the four-chamber view

There can be a small "cyst-like" structure seen indenting the left lateral wall of the left atrium (Fig. 2.52). This is a **persistent left superior caval vein**. It can also be seen in longitudinal views (See Chapter 4). This is a vein which is present in embryological life, but which normally involutes. However, it persists in about 1 in 300 normal people, although it does have an increased

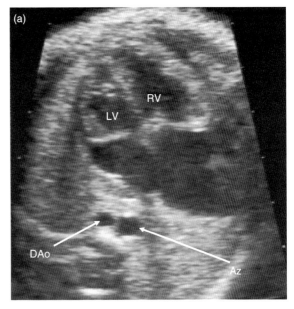

Fig. 2.51.(a). There are two large vessels seen in cross-section behind the left atrium in the four-chamber projection. One is the descending aorta (DAo) and the larger one is a dilated azygous vein (Az), as result of interruption of the inferior vena cava. This is indicative of left atrial isomerism. The right heart, particularly the right atrium, was dilated. The appearance of the foramen ovale, although wide, is within normal limits, but after birth there was a secundum atrial septal defect. This was anticipated prenatally, as the fetus had other features of the Holt–Oram syndrome. There was also severe pulmonary hypertension in the newborn, which has persisted.

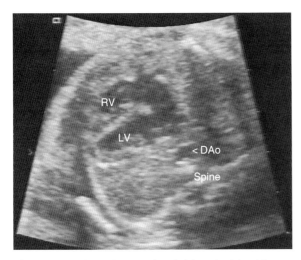

Fig. 2.50. The descending aorta lies slightly to the right of the spine at the level of the four-chamber view (compare with, for example, Figs. 2.6 and 2.8), because of a right-sided aortic arch. Note in addition, the abnormal axis of the heart in this fetus with tetralogy of Fallot.

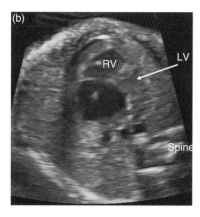

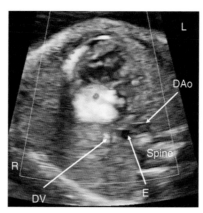

Fig. 2.51.(b). Contd. On the left-hand panel, the four-chamber view can be seen to be abnormal. There is an unbalanced atrioventricular septal defect, as a common valve drained predominantly to the right ventricle. There appear to be three "vessels" behind the heart in the posterior mediastinum but on the color flow map on the right hand panel, only two of the three structures were shown to be vascular. The central structure was the esophagus (E), dilated due to malrotation of the gut. The most right-sided vessel proved to be the descending vein (DV) from a pulmonary venous confluence.

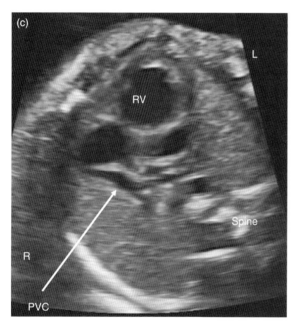

Fig. 2.51.(c). In a slightly more cranial view than that seen in Fig. 2.51(b), the vessel to the right in the posterior mediastinum connected to a pulmonary venous confluence (PVC), which lay behind the atria and drained via the descending vein below the diaphragm. This fetus had right atrial isomerism.

association with congenital heart disease. The left superior caval vein drains to the coronary sinus, which is the venous drainage of the myocardium. The coronary sinus is seen just below the four-chamber view lying in the atrioventricular groove (Fig. 2.36(a) and (b)). When the coronary sinus is dilated, it can distort the appearance of the four-chamber view in such a way that the atrioventricular junction appears "straight", giving a false appearance of an atrioventricular septal defect (Fig. 2.53). However, if the transducer beam is directed cranially, the true crux is seen above the level of the coronary sinus and can be correctly evaluated. A persistent left superior vena cava and atrioventricular septal defect can however, co-exist (Fig. 2.52, right hand panel). A dilated coronary sinus has been implicated in partially obstructing flow into the mitral valve leading to benign left ventricular "smallness," although there is no convincing evidence that this is a real pathological entity.

A rare abnormality is the detection of redundant dysplastic valve tissue in the body of the right atrium (Fig. 2.54). This is usually attached to the Eustachian valve, a ridge of tissue on the floor of the right atrium,

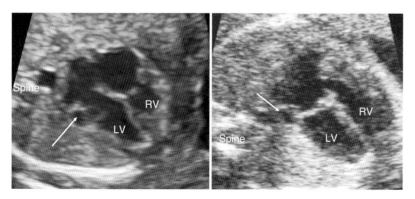

Fig. 2.52. In both left- and right-hand examples, there is a cyst-like structure seen adjacent to the left lateral wall of the left atrium, close to the atrioventricular junction. This is a persistent left-sided superior vena cava. It usually drains to the coronary sinus, which will be dilated as a result. Note that in the right-hand example, there is also a partial atrioventricular septal defect (or primum atrial septal defect).

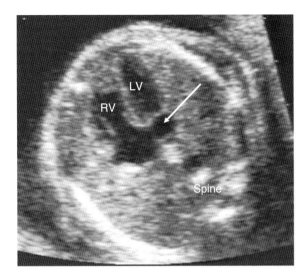

Fig. 2.53. The coronary sinus is dilated due to a persistent left superior vena cava draining into it. This image can be misinterpreted as showing an atrioventricular septal defect, as the atrioventricular junction appears "straight," and the normal mouth of the coronary sinus draining to the right atrium can give the impression of an atrial septal defect. However, this view lies below (caudal to) the level of a true four-chamber plane.

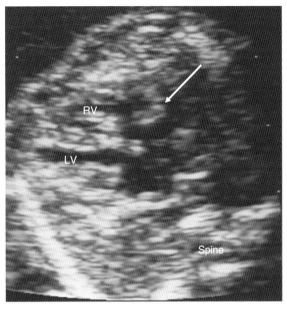

Fig. 2.54. Redundant tissue was seen in the right atrium (arrow), which prolapsed through the tricuspid valve during the cardiac cycle. This was much more readily appreciable on the moving image. This is a Chiari malformation.

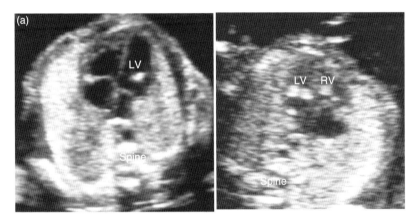

Fig. 2.55.(a). On the left-hand panel, there is an echogenic focus in the typical position in the body of the left ventricle. Histologically, it lies in the papillary muscles of the mitral valve. On the right-hand panel, there are multiple echogenic foci in both ventricular cavities in a case of trisomy 13.

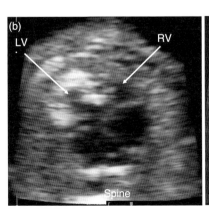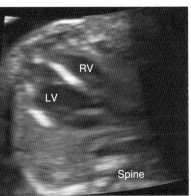

Fig. 2.55.(b). Both images were obtained from the same fetus at 21 weeks of gestation. There was extensive excess calcium deposition in the wall of the left ventricle, apex, and septum. However, cardiac function was completely normal and remained so throughout gestation. There were no other abnormal findings in the rest of the fetus. These findings are consistent with a normal outcome for the child.

65

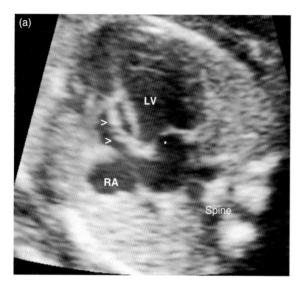

(a)

(b)

Fig. 2.56.(a). This is an example of pulmonary atresia with intact ventricular septum, with the right ventricle not reaching the apex. In the moving image, the right ventricle was thick walled and poorly contracting. The chordal apparatus and papillary muscles of the tricuspid valve were hyperechogenic due to calcification in this rather peculiar pattern along their length.

Fig. 2.56.(b). This is an example of critical aortic stenosis, which shows a similar pattern of chordal and papillary muscle calcification as is seen in Fig. 2.56(a) but on the other side of the heart. Note the globular shape of the left ventricle, which was poorly contracting in the moving image. There is bright echogenicity in a linear fashion along the length of the mitral valve attachments (arrowheads). Compare this appearance with a typical echogenic focus shown in the left-hand panel of Fig. 2.55(a).

which directs blood from the inferior vena cava across the foramen ovale. The excessive tissue is called a **Chiari malformation**. It is highly mobile within the right atrium and sometimes prolapses through the tricuspid valve. It is rarely obstructive but sometimes associated with tricuspid valve abnormalities.

A very commonly identified abnormality in the four-chamber view is an **echogenic focus** (Fig. 2.55(a)). It occurs in up to 20% of normal fetuses if carefully looked for. It is an area of increased calcification histologically, usually in one of the papillary muscles of the mitral valve, but an echogenic focus may be seen in the right ventricle or in the septum as well. There may also be multiple echogenic foci (Fig. 2.55(a)), which can be a marker for trisomy 13, as it was in the fetus illustrated in the right hand panel. Even when echogenic foci are very prominent, they have no pathological significance as far as the heart is concerned, although their level of association with chromosomal anomalies is still uncertain. Patchy echogenicity occurring in a heart which functions normally, appears to be non-pathological (Fig. 2.55(b)), but particularly if an echogenic focus has a more extensive or unusual form, a detailed anomaly scan is indicated to exclude extracardiac malformations. An echogenic focus is usually readily distinguishable from the echogenicity in the

papillary muscles or ventricular walls, which occurs in critical aortic stenosis, or less commonly, in pulmonary atresia with intact septum (Fig. 2.56(a) and (b)). Increased echogenicity of the atrial or ventricular walls, which may be uniform or patchy, can occur in complete heart block.

An echogenic focus can occasionally be confused with a tumor mass, although close examination usually easily distinguishes them. Cardiac **tumors** can be seen in the four-chamber view. They are most frequently rhabdomyomas histologically, although fibroma, and much more rarely hemangioma, lipoma and myxoma have also been reported prenatally. A rhabdomyoma can lie anywhere in the atrial or ventricular mass, are homogenous masses, slightly more echogenic than myocardium (and less echogenic than foci), and may be multiple. They usually bulge into the cardiac cavity (Fig. 2.57(a) and (b)) and may obstruct valve function. Some intracardiac masses have an unexpected or unpredictable course when they are not typical in appearance for rhabdomyomas or teratomas (Fig. 2.57(c) and (d)). Fibromas tend to be in the septum and are single masses (Fig. 2.57(d)). Teratomas tend to lie on the surface of the heart protruding into the pericardial sac and attached to the arterial roots. They tend to contain cysts of varying size (Fig. 2.58). There is frequently an associated pericardial effusion, which may be large.

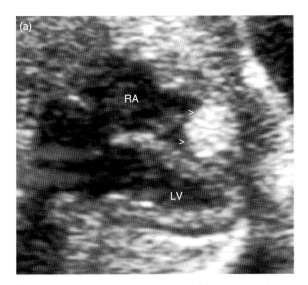

Fig. 2.57.(a). A single mass is seen in the left lateral ventricular wall indenting the left ventricular cavity. It is slightly more echogenic than myocardium in nature. Its appearance is highly suggestive of a rhabdomyoma.

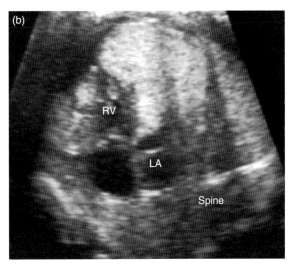

Fig. 2.57.(b). There are multiple masses in the right ventricle and a large single mass in the left so that the left ventricular cavity is almost obliterated. The multiplicity of the tumors is indicative of rhabdomyomas.

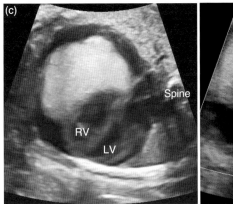
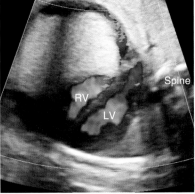

Fig. 2.57.(c). A tumor of unknown histology is seen. It appeared embedded in the right ventricular myocardium like a rhabdomyoma but it was single and extended superiorly to the arch vessels, unlike a rhabdomyoma. The speed of its growth was suggestive of perhaps a rhabdomyosarcoma.

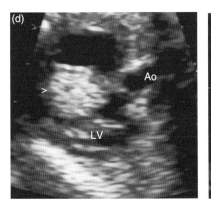
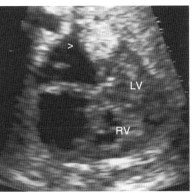

Fig. 2.57.(d). On the left-hand panel, there was a single mass in the septum (arrow head). This could have been a rhabdomyoma or a fibroma. It never caused obstruction to the left ventricular outflow tract. Postnatally, there was no evidence of tuberous sclerosis on investigation and the mass has become proportionately smaller as the child has grown. The child is now 3 years old and asymptomatic. On the right-hand panel, in a different patient, there was an echogenic mass in the left atrium (arrow head), which disappeared completely in the newborn, who remains asymptomatic.

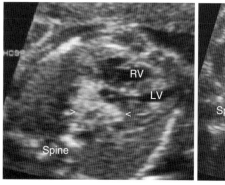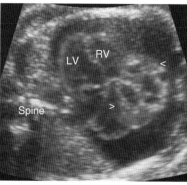

Fig. 2.58. On the left panel, there is an echogenic cystic mass in the mediastinum. Pathologically, it was a teratoma attached the base of the heart. Although this grew during pregnancy, fetal compromise did not develop and the mass was successfully removed in the neonate. On the right-hand panel, a similar multicystic mass is seen lying in a similar position, but in this case a marked pericardial effusion and ascites developed before 30 weeks of gestation.

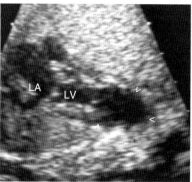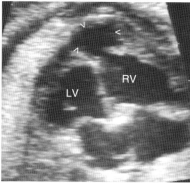

Fig. 2.59. In the left-hand panel, a large protrusion (arrow heads) is seen with a broad connection from the left ventricular cavity. In the right-hand panel, an abnormal contour is related to the right ventricular apex. These are two examples of ventricular aneurysms.

An **aneurysm or diverticulum** may be seen in the four-chamber view as a "bulge" in the wall of either ventricle (Fig. 2.59). A diverticulum is typically narrow-necked with muscular walls, whereas an aneurysm is thinner-walled, with a broad junction and shows either no, or asynchronous, contraction with the ventricle. In practice, the features in the fetus are often mixed between these two diagnoses.

Occasionally, "strands" of tissue can be seen crossing the left ventricular cavity (Fig. 2.60). These are called **left ventricular bands** and may be the source of innocent murmurs in childhood. They have no pathological significance.

Myocardial non-compaction can occur in isolation or in the setting of left atrial isomerism. The ventricles are thick-walled, dilated and poorly contracting (Fig. 2.13(c)) with the characteristic finding of color flow showing deep inlets into the thickened ventricular walls. **A pericardial effusion** can occur in many settings in the fetus and usually can be best evaluated in the four-chamber view (Fig. 2.61). It is important to be familiar with the normal amount of pericardial fluid

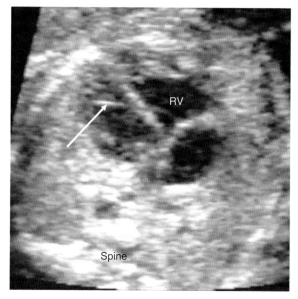

Fig. 2.60. There is a fibrous band crossing the apex of the left ventricular cavity. It is possible that this could give rise to a vibratory murmur in postnatal life. It is of no clinical significance.

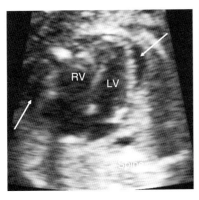 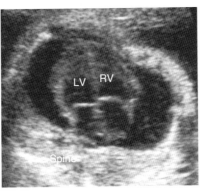

Fig. 2.61. On the left-hand panel, there is a small collection of pericardial fluid at the right atrioventricular junction and at the left apex (arrows). This was an isolated finding in a fetus with trisomy 21. In the right-hand panel, there is a large pericardial effusion in the setting of an advanced case of twin–twin transfusion syndrome and calcification of the great arteries.

(see figures which illustrate a normal four-chamber view and Fig. 2.9(a)). A pericardial effusion can occur as part of the complete picture of fetal hydrops from whatever cause, but particularly occurs in fetal anemia. A small pericardial effusion not uncommonly occurs with a congenital heart malformation, although it is not usually a manifestation of cardiac failure in this setting. A small pericardial effusion can be a sign of trisomy 21 and other markers for this condition should be carefully sought. It also occurs when there is some form of "irritant" in the pericardial sac, such as a cardiac tumor. A small effusion is seen in the left-hand panel of Fig. 2.61.

Cardiac failure is not synonymous with fetal hydrops, which has many causes. The only primarily cardiac causes of cardiac failure in utero are an abnormal rate (bradycardia or tachycardia) or abnormal function (cardiomyopathy). Some of the other causes of hydrops are associated with heart failure due to excess demand on a normal heart, although the primary cause is extracardiac, for example, anemia or an arteriovenous malformation, including twin-to-twin transfusion syndrome or vein of Galen aneurysm.

Summary of structural anomalies seen in the four-chamber view

No pulmonary venous drainage to left atrium

Abnormal mitral valve: stenosis, atresia, dysplasia

Abnormal tricuspid valve: stenosis, atresia, dysplasia, Ebstein's malformation

Common atrioventricular junction: with atrial component, ventricular component or both

Discordant AV junction
   with two patent AV valves
   with tricuspid atresia

Double inlet AV junction

Ventricular septal defect

Additional lesions: Persistent left superior vena cava, dilated azygous vein, sinus venosus atrial septal defect, Chiari mechanism, tumor, echogenic focus, ectopia, ventricular aneurysm, criss-cross or upstairs/downstairs connections, straddling AV valve, pericardial effusion.

Abnormalities of function

The **direction of blood flow at the atrial septum** will be **reversed** (left-to-right instead of the normal right to left) on color flow mapping or pulsed Doppler, if there is obstruction within the left heart at the level of the mitral or aortic valves (Fig. 2.62). In addition, in some severe cases of coarctation, it may be possible to appreciate some degree of left-to-right shunt at the foramen.

The **degree of excursion of the mitral or tricuspid valve** may be decreased either in intrinsic mitral or tricuspid valve disease or in aortic or pulmonary stenosis or atresia respectively. Isolated atrioventricular valve stenosis is uncommon but frequently there is an element of mitral stenosis with aortic stenosis and tricuspid stenosis with pulmonary stenosis. The limited opening of the respective atrioventricular valve is because of the high intraventricular pressure in arterial valve stenosis or atresia. There is usually also a small cavity size. Unequal excursion of the atrioventricular valves is manifested by unequal flow into the ventricles on **color flow mapping** (Fig. 2.63).

Contraction should be equal in both ventricles and the scanner needs to become familiar with the appearance of normal contraction. If the **ventricles contract unequally**, it suggests an obstruction to outflow of the respective ventricle, aortic or pulmonary stenosis. If both ventricles contract poorly, this indicates a **cardiomyopathy** and the heart will be dilated. Left ventricular

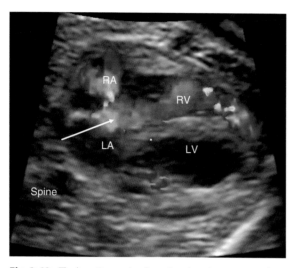

Fig. 2.62. The heart is seen in a four-chamber view in a case of critical aortic stenosis. The shunt across the foramen ovale is almost exclusively left-to-right (arrow). Note how little blood is reaching the left ventricular cavity, in contrast to the filling of the right ventricular cavity in this diastolic frame.

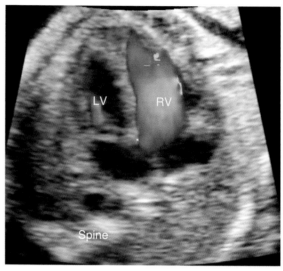

Fig. 2.63. The color flow map clearly shows unequal filling of the ventricles, with less flow into the left ventricle. This indicates either mitral valve stenosis (an uncommon diagnosis in isolation) or, more likely aortic valve stenosis or, not infrequently, a combination of the two. In this fetus, the high pressure in the left ventricle, due to a stenosed aortic valve, limits the amount of blood entering the left ventricle through the mitral valve. The left ventricle is a fairly good size despite the diminished flow, although it falls just short of the apex. Compare this with the normal inflows in Fig. 2.9.

dysfunction, usually with dilatation, is typical of critical aortic stenosis. A small poorly contracting left ventricle occurs in aortic atresia. Right ventricular dysfunction and dilatation secondary to critical pulmonary stenosis can occur but is uncommon. A small poorly contracting right ventricle occurs in pulmonary atresia. Abnormalities in valve excursion or of ventricular contraction are really only appreciated in the moving image.

Mitral regurgitation is an uncommon finding in utero and is seen on color flow mapping or pulsed Doppler. It is sometimes possible to see trivial mitral and tricuspid valve regurgitation using modern sensitive ultrasound machines (Fig. 2.64). Mild mitral regurgitation may be seen as benign finding, which resolves spontaneously, but the aortic valve and arch in this setting must be even more carefully checked than usual. More significant mitral regurgitation may occur in extracardiac disease such as renal disease or twin–twin transfusion syndrome, or in the setting of aortic stenosis (see Fig. 2.15).

Tricuspid regurgitation is a less common finding in fetal life than it is postnatally but can be seen on color flow mapping (Fig. 2.65(a)) and pulsed Doppler. It has special significance in the fetus before 14 weeks

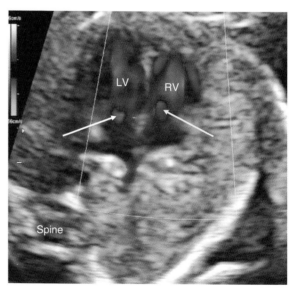

Fig. 2.64. There is trivial mitral (white arrow) and tricuspid (yellow arrow) regurgitation seen on color flow mapping in the diastolic frame in the four-chamber view. This is quite commonly found with modern sensitive equipment, but an even more careful check of the appearance of the aortic and pulmonary valves, arch and duct should follow, as well as ascertaining the arterial velocities.

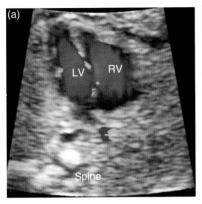
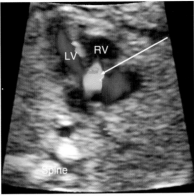

Fig. 2.65.(a). On the left-hand panel, the diastolic frame shows equal flow across the two atrioventricular valves on color flow mapping. On the right-hand panel, in systole, there is regurgitation back through the tricuspid valve (arrow). The blue flow in the left ventricle is blood being ejected during systole out the left ventricular outflow tract.

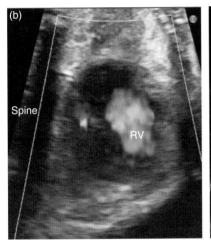
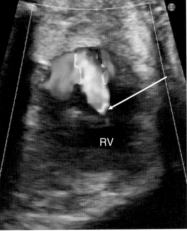

Fig. 2.65.(b). On the left-hand panel, in a diastolic frame, blood flows only across the right side, through the tricuspid valve. The small jet of blood seen in the left atrium is passing across the foramen ovale, as it cannot cross the mitral valve in this case of mitral and aortic atresia (the hypoplastic left heart syndrome). On the systolic frame seen in the right-hand panel, there is moderately severe tricuspid regurgitation, which is producing right atrial dilatation. As a result of tricuspid regurgitation, this fetus will be a poor candidate for surgical repair by the Norwood procedure.

gestation (see Chapter 6). It can occur in tricuspid dysplasia, Ebstein's malformation, pulmonary atresia with intact ventricular septum or as a result of constriction of the arterial duct. However, when the morphology of the tricuspid valve and the rest of the heart are otherwise normal, it tends to be a benign, transient finding. When tricuspid regurgitation occurs in the setting of the hypoplastic left heart syndrome (Fig. 2.65(b)), it is a poor prognostic feature for surgical treatment by the first stage Norwood procedure. In this form of surgery, the right ventricle will become the systemic ventricle and incompetence of the tricuspid valve is difficult to treat or repair surgically and will severely compromise the functional outcome.

Bilateral atrioventricular valve regurgitation may occur in tachycardias or in cardiomyopathy (Fig. 2.13(h)) or may be due to extracardiac disease such as anemia or arteriovenous malformation.

Summary

The four-chamber view is the most useful and informative of all the cardiac views. It is therefore essential to be able to obtain it quickly and correctly and to be thoroughly familiar with the features which denote normality during systematic evaluation. If any abnormal findings are then accurately defined, the correct diagnosis can be readily achieved.

Chapter 3

Great arteries and arches: normal and abnormal

Introduction

The great arteries and their connections are best seen in a series of transverse planes, imaged in a continuous sweep moving cranially from the four-chamber plane as described in Chapter 1. The aorta arises just above the level of the four-chamber plane, in the so-called "wedge" position, because of its close proximity to the two atrioventricular valve rings. To image the left ventricular outflow tract perfectly, it is often necessary to rotate the transducer slightly in order to "open out" the origin of the aorta as shown more fully in Chapters 1 and 4. Scanning more cranially than the aortic origin brings the right ventricular outflow tract into view in the three-vessel plane. Above the level of the three-vessel plane, the transverse arch is seen. Angling the transducer slightly on this plane can allow the duct and arch to be seen in the same section and therefore compared (Chapters 1 and 4). When an abnormality of the great arteries is suspected, it may be useful to turn into long-axis or sagittal planes of the fetus (See Chapter 4), in order to improve understanding of the malformation. A combination of views sweeping above the level of the aortic arch in a transverse plane, together with longitudinal planes may demonstrate the pattern of branching of the head and neck vessels from the aortic arch.

Normal appearance of the great artery views

Imaging the left ventricular outflow tract, the anterior wall of the aorta is continuous with the ventricular septum and the posterior wall is continuous with the anterior leaflet of the mitral valve (Fig. 3.1(a) and (b)). The three-vessel view lies immediately cranial to the left ventricular outflow and demonstrates the right ventricular outflow tract and duct, with the aorta and superior vena cava cut in short axis and lying to the right of the pulmonary artery (Fig. 3.2(a)–(e)). The initial direction of the aorta, at its origin from the heart, is cranial and rightwards towards the right

shoulder, then it turns posteriorly and leftwards to form the aortic arch. In contrast to the aorta, the pulmonary valve is separated from the tricuspid valve by a complete muscular ring of tissue, the infundibulum, and its course is straight, just to the left of the midline, directed posteriorly towards the spine. As a result, the pulmonary artery "crosses over" the aortic origin, giving a spiral arrangement to the two arteries (Fig. 3.2(f)). Above the level of the three-vessel plane, the most superior "arch" is the true aortic arch (Fig. 3.3(a)). The ductal arch lies below and to the left of the aortic arch (Fig. 3.3(b) and (c)). The arteries should be assessed in terms of size, position, structure and function in a similar fashion to four-chamber view evaluation.

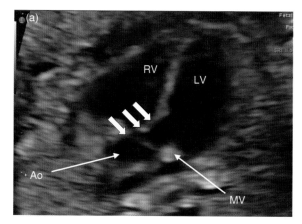

Fig. 3.1.(a). The aorta is seen arising from the left ventricle in a transverse section just above (cranial to) the four-chamber view. The ventricular septum is continuous with the anterior wall of the aorta (broad arrows). Note that the septum is straight between the ventricles but the line of continuity between the septum and the aorta is slightly curved, because of the initially anterior, sweeping course of the aorta. Note that the posterior wall of the aorta is continuous with the anterior leaflet of the mitral valve (HB).

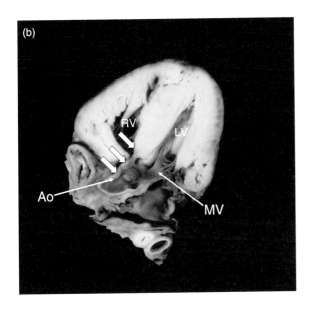

Fig. 3.1.(b). Contd. The anatomic correlate shows the same features. The anatomical specimen is oriented to match the position of the echocardiogram and show the same features. The aorta is seen arising wholly from the left ventricle, with the interventricular septum continuous with the anterior wall of the aorta and the posterior wall of the aorta continuous with the anterior leaflet of the mitral valve. Note that the septum between the right ventricle and left outflow tract is particularly thin at its junction with the aortic wall in this view (middle broad arrow). This is the normal atrioventricular component of the membranous septum.

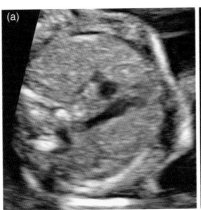
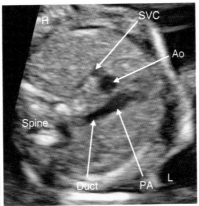

Fig. 3.2.(a). The left panel shows an unlabeled, and the right a labeled, example of a classic three-vessel view, with the pulmonary artery and duct seen lying to the left of the aorta, which lies to the left of the superior vena cava. The largest and most anterior vessel is the pulmonary artery, the smallest and most posterior of the three vessels is the superior caval vein. Note that, because of the arrangement of the great arteries, the pulmonary artery is seen in its long axis and the ascending aorta and superior vena cava are cut in their short axis.

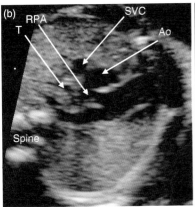
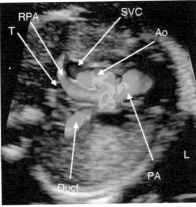

Fig. 3.2.(b). The three-vessel cut is made in a slightly lower plane than that of Fig. 3.2(a) so that the origin of the right pulmonary artery is seen, passing behind the ascending aorta and superior vena cava. The color flow map on the right demonstrates the right pulmonary artery more clearly.

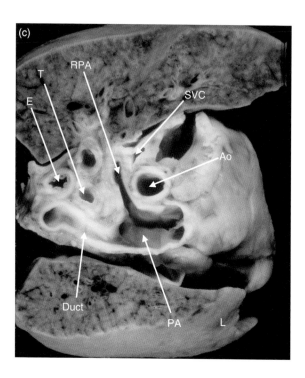

Fig. 3.2.(c). Contd. The anatomical specimen is oriented to match the echocardiogram shown in Fig. 3.2(b). The position of the trachea (T) and esophagus (E) relative to the other structures is more clearly seen.

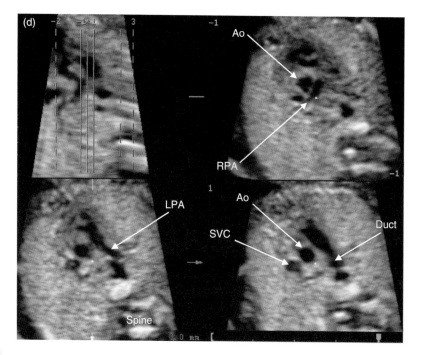

Fig. 3.2.(d). Three successive cuts of the pulmonary artery from an acquired volume set are shown. The most caudal plane is at the upper right and shows the origin of the right pulmonary artery, passing behind the aorta and superior vena cava. Slightly more cranially, on the left lower image, the origin of the left pulmonary artery is seen. Immediately above this cut, on the right lower image, the classic three-vessel view, showing the arterial duct is seen. This set demonstrates that, if the plane is angled down to the right, the right pulmonary artery and duct can be imaged in the same section. Alternatively, if the plane is angled down and to the left, the left pulmonary artery and the duct are seen, but it is not usually possible to image all three structures at once.

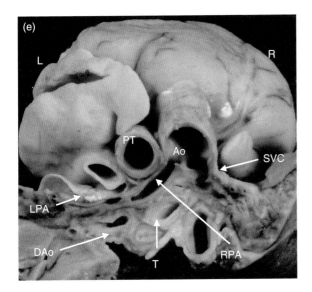

Fig. 3.2.(e). Contd. The heart is viewed from above in this 23-week gestation specimen. It has been sectioned just below the level of the duct and shows the origin of the right and left pulmonary arteries from the pulmonary trunk (PT). The trachea (T) lies between the right pulmonary artery (RPA) and the descending aorta (DAo).

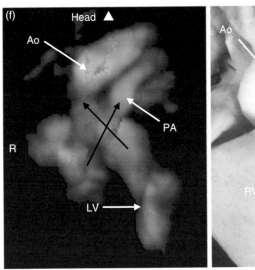
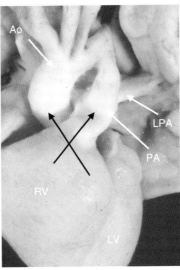

Fig. 3.2.(f). The left-hand panel shows a glass body reconstruction of the great arteries, demonstrating their spiral arrangement. The aorta arises from the left ventricle directed superiorly and rightwards, whereas the pulmonary artery arises more anteriorly and crosses over the aortic origin. The aorta then turns leftwards and forms the arch. The two great arteries are therefore at right angles at their origin and then run parallel until their junction just in front of the spine. A matching anatomical specimen is shown on the right-hand panel. The black arrows illustrate the direction of the great arteries at their origins.

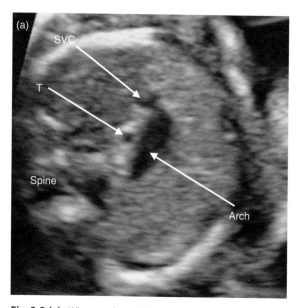

Fig. 3.3.(a). Whatever the position or orientation of the fetus, maintaining a horizontal projection, scanning cranial to the three-vessel view, the transverse aortic arch is seen, crossing the midline in front of the trachea (T) from right to left. The aortic arch is the most superior (or cranial) arterial vessel.

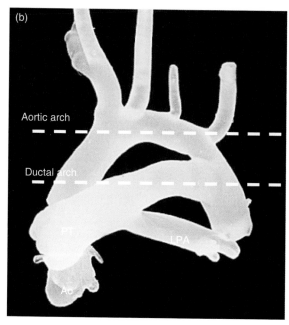

Fig. 3.3.(b). A cast of a 19-week gestation heart shows how the aortic arch and ductal arches lie at different levels. In the normal fetus, the aortic arch is always more cranial. Moving transversely in a cranial direction, the duct is seen before the arch. If the transducer is tilted slightly on either the duct or the aortic arch, both structures can be viewed simultaneously as they lie immediately on top of each other. Note there is a small fourth branch from the aortic arch arising in between the left common carotid and left subclavian arteries in this example. This is a normal variant.

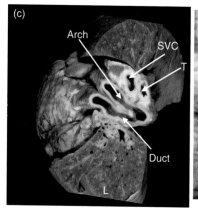 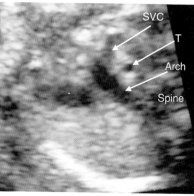

Fig. 3.3.(c). The anatomical specimen and echocardiogram are oriented to match. The transverse arch crosses the midline in front of the trachea (T). The cut must be slightly oblique in order to show the junction of the vessels. The echocardiographic section is slightly more transverse than the anatomical one.

Size

It is important to be aware of the normal size relationship of the two great arteries. This can usually be assessed visually but measuring the great arteries at the level of the valve in diastole should confirm the visual impression. At 12 weeks' gestation the great arteries are of equal size, but by about 16 weeks the pulmonary artery is slightly bigger than the aorta and this size relationship persists until postnatal life. For example, at 20 weeks, the mean aortic size is about 3 mm and the pulmonary artery about 3.5 mm. The transverse arch and arterial duct are similar in size and ideally are imaged simultaneously for direct comparison. The method of measuring the size of the great arteries, arch, and duct with normal growth charts is illustrated in Chapter 5.

Position

Sweeping up from the four-chamber plane towards the fetal head, the first great artery to be seen is the aorta (Fig. 3.4(a) and (b)) followed by the pulmonary valve lying above, or cranial to, the aortic valve. The aorta arises wholly from the left ventricle and the pulmonary artery from the right ventricle. The pulmonary trunk crosses over the aortic origin, such that the pulmonary valve lies to the left of the aortic valve. The duct lies to

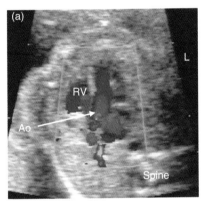
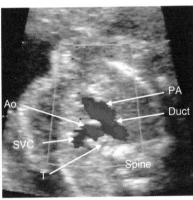

Fig. 3.4.(a). The two panels show sequential views from the same fetus lying HB. On the left-hand panel, the aorta is the first great artery seen cranial to the level of the four-chamber view. Flow in the ascending aorta is seen on color flow mapping to be arising wholly from the left ventricle. Flow in the main pulmonary artery is seen crossing over the aortic origin on the right-hand panel.

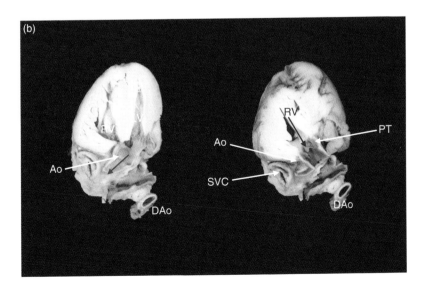

Fig. 3.4.(b). Analogous sections of a mid-trimester fetal heart are shown in the same orientation. In the left-hand image the aorta can be seen arising from the left ventricle, directed towards the right (red arrow). In the right-hand image, the pulmonary trunk (PT) arises from the right ventricle and heads towards the descending aorta (blue arrow). The two outflow tracts are at right angles.

the left of the transverse aortic arch and the aortic arch forms the most superior of the two arches (ductal arch and aortic arch) (Figs. 3.1–3.8).

Structure

There are two (equally) thin, mobile arterial valves. The great arteries are distinguished by their branching pattern. The first branches of the aorta are the coronary arteries, but these are usually too small to be seen in the fetus. The first visible branches of the aorta in the fetus, the arm, head, and neck vessels, arise some distance from the aortic valve and are initially directed superiorly from the aortic arch and therefore are not readily seen on the transverse views. In contrast, the pulmonary artery branches soon after its origin and its branches course laterally into each of the two lungs, therefore they are seen in transverse views. The arterial duct appears as a straight continuation of the pulmonary trunk (Figs. 3.7, 3.4, 3.2). Usually, the right pulmonary artery and duct are most readily seen on transverse views, as the left pulmonary artery is directed rather cranially, but it also can be seen, especially with color flow mapping. The pulmonary artery and duct and the transverse aortic arch both join the descending aorta in front of the spine. A slight tilt to the transducer allows the duct and transverse arch to be seen together (Chapter 4), forming a "V-shape" in the posterior thorax with the long arm being the pulmonary trunk and duct and the short arm being the transverse arch (Fig. 3.8). The transverse arch crosses the midline in front of the trachea and hooks over the left bronchus, forming a left arch (Figs. 3.3(a), 3.5).

Function

The arterial valves open freely – the valve cusps seem to "disappear" during systole as the valve cusps flatten against the arterial walls (Fig. 3.9). There is unaliased color flow across both valves (Fig. 3.4). The velocity of blood flow increases throughout gestation from about 30 cm/s at 12 weeks to about 1 m/s at term. In the same fetus, the velocity of flow tends to be slightly higher in the aortic than pulmonary artery but this is not consistent, as arterial velocities increase with fetal activity. In the normal heart, there is no regurgitation of flow seen on color flow mapping or on pulsed Doppler of

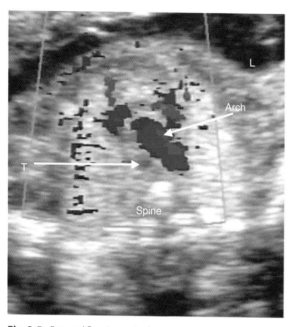

Fig. 3.5. Forward flow is seen in the transverse aortic arch as it crosses from right to left in front of the trachea (T). Note its uniform caliber.

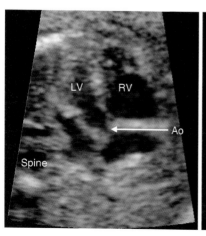
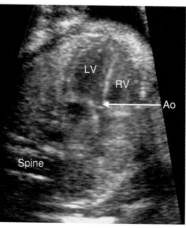

Fig. 3.6. Moving cranially from the four-chamber view, the first great artery to be found should be the aorta, wedged into the middle of the heart just above and in continuity with the atrioventricular valves. However, this vessel has to be proved the aorta by seeing no early branching, and in addition by showing early branching of the crossing great artery. The transducer beam needs to be tilted slightly in order to open out a length of aorta, as shown in the right-hand panel, to check that it has no early branches (HB).

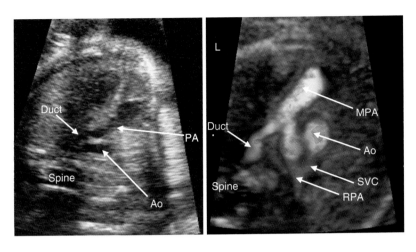

Fig. 3.7. The section cranial to Fig. 3.6 shows the main pulmonary artery crossing over the aortic origin. Depending on the precise orientation and the level of the section, the continuation of the main pulmonary artery is seen either into duct alone (left-hand panel), duct and right pulmonary artery (right-hand panel) or duct and left pulmonary artery (see Fig. 3.2(d)).

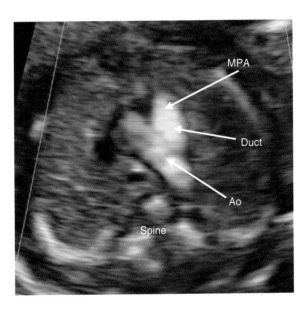

Fig. 3.8. Flow in the duct and arch should be in the same direction. This usually means, of course, that, in the normal, they will be the same color on flow mapping but it will depend on the orientation of the fetus to the ultrasound beam (see Fig. 5.11).

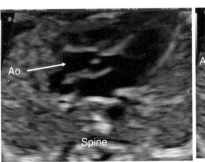 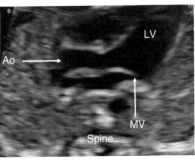

Fig. 3.9. In the diastolic frame on the left side, the mitral valve is open and the aortic valve cusps, seen as a line in the middle of the aorta, are closed. On the right-hand panel, the heart is seen in systole, when the mitral valve is closed and the aortic valve "disappears" as the valve cusps flatten against the arterial walls.

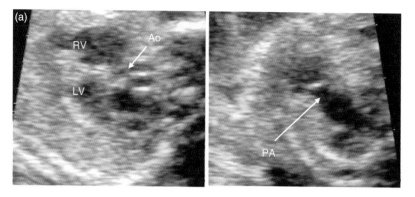

Fig. 3.10.(a). On the left-hand panel, the ascending aorta is very small and difficult to see, as it is atretic. On the right-hand panel, which is the same patient at the same magnification, note how easy it is to see the pulmonary artery, which is much bigger than the aorta. The pulmonary artery is usually somewhat easier to see, but an experienced sonographer will be suspicious if this is more marked than usual.

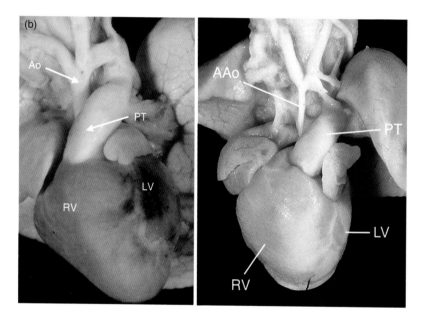

Fig. 3.10.(b). In both these hearts, the aorta is hypoplastic to a varying degree, consistent with the diagnosis of aortic atresia in the hypoplastic left heart syndrome. In contrast, the pulmonary trunk is enlarged.

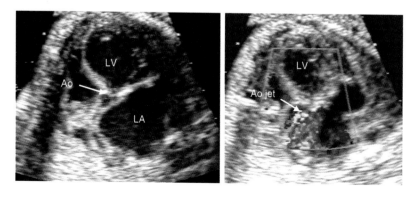

Fig. 3.11. The aortic root is smaller than normal. The aortic valve appears thicker than normal in the left-hand panel and it did not "disappear" during systole, when the valve normally opens freely. In the right-hand panel, due to the obstruction to flow at the valve level, there was aliasing of the color flow map in the ascending aorta and an increased velocity on pulsed Doppler.

the arterial valves. Flow in the duct and transverse arch is in the same direction (towards the spine) on color flow mapping (Fig. 3.8).

Possible deviations of great artery views from normal

Abnormalities of size

Aorta smaller than normal

The aorta can be smaller than normal. This is usually most evident from comparison with the size of the pulmonary artery and generally indicates that the aorta is receiving less blood flow than normal. This can occur in **aortic atresia, aortic stenosis, coarctation or interruption of the aorta**. Aortic atresia conventionally refers to complete obstruction at the level of the aortic valve

and aortic stenosis to a narrowing at or close to the level of the valve. In aortic atresia, there is no forward flow into the aorta from the left ventricle and the aorta is invariably small, often to the extent of being very hypoplastic and threadlike (Fig. 3.10(a) and (b)). In valvar aortic stenosis, the vessel is usually smaller than normal but the valve is also thicker than normal and does not "disappear" in systole (Fig. 3.11), in contrast to the normal valve, which seems to disappear during systole, as the valve opens and the cusps are flattened against the arterial walls. The color flow map shows aliasing and turbulence (Fig. 3.11) and the Doppler flow velocity is increased. Narrowing in the aortic arch, typically its distal portion is conventionally referred to as coarctation, and complete obstruction, typically with a loss of continuity of the arterial wall as well as the lumen, is known as interruption. In coarctation of the aorta,

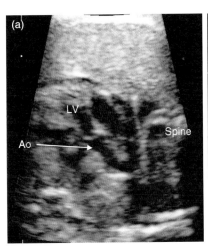
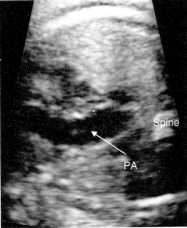

Fig. 3.12.(a). Comparing the vessels on sequential transverse views, measuring them and charting their ratio is a useful guide to distinguishing a normal from a pathological size relationship. The discrepancy of arterial sizes seen here is highly suspicious for an arch anomaly (HB).

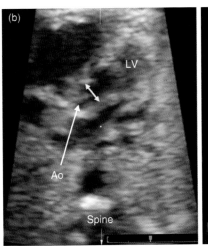
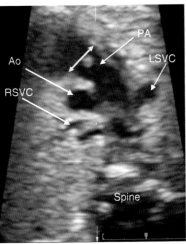

Fig. 3.12.(b). The great arteries are assessed in sequential transverse views. In this case of coarctation, there was in addition a left superior caval vein, not an uncommon association, but one which may confuse the diagnosis of coarctation a little. There is a discrepancy in the size of the aorta and pulmonary artery on measurement (yellow double-headed arrows). Note that the left superior vena cava (LSVC) is quite large and the right quite small (RSVC).

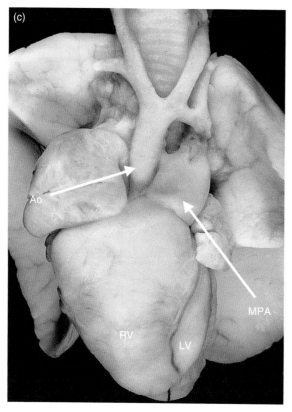

Fig. 3.12.(c). Contd. In the anatomical specimen there is a similar discrepancy in great artery sizes (compare with the normal size relationships in Fig. 3.2(f)), suggestive of coarctation. Note the additional sign of coarctation here, the discrepancy in ventricular sizes, with the left smaller than the right.

the aortic valve usually appears normal in the fetus, although a bicuspid aortic valve is a common association found postnatally. The aorta/pulmonary artery ratio is below the normal range (Fig. 3.12(a), (b) and (c)). This can usually be detected simply by observing the vessels sequentially, but measuring the great arteries at their origins and comparing the measurements with normal for the gestation, can confirm the visual impression. Measurement methods and charts are shown in Chapter 5. In interruption of the aorta, the aorta is usually more strikingly small, though patent (Fig. 3.13). **Subaortic stenosis**, where the obstruction, either muscular or membranous, lies in the left ventricular outflow tract below the level of the valve itself, is very rare in the fetus. When is does occur, the aorta is smaller than normal.

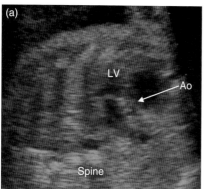

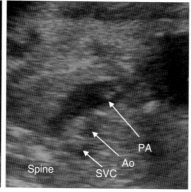

Fig. 3.13.(a). In this fetus, it was very difficult to find the aorta as it was markedly smaller than the pulmonary artery, which is shown on the right-hand panel at the same magnification. However, the aorta was patent with forward flow through it, in this case of interruption of the aorta. Note that on the three-vessel view, the aorta is very small relative to both the pulmonary artery and the superior vena cava (compare with Fig. 3.2)

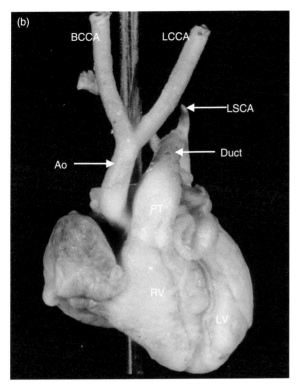

Fig. 3.13.(b). Contd. The ascending aorta is small in comparison to the pulmonary trunk. There is complete interruption of the aorta between the left common carotid and left subclavian arteries and as a result the brachiocephalic (BCCA) and left common carotid arteries (LCCA) form a characteristic "V" shape in front of the trachea (marked by a probe). The left subclavian artery (LSCA) arises from the descending portion of the aorta and is supplied by the arterial duct.

Pulmonary artery smaller than normal

The pulmonary artery can be smaller than normal, appearing to be the same size or even smaller than the aorta. This suggests that the pulmonary artery is receiving less blood flow than normal, and can indicate **pulmonary atresia or valvar stenosis** or alternatively less blood flow because of obstruction further "downstream," in **tricuspid valve obstruction**. The size of the pulmonary artery is quite variable in pulmonary atresia from near normal to threadlike (Fig. 3.14(a) and (b)), but no forward flow can be seen across the pulmonary valve on color or pulsed Doppler. In pulmonary stenosis, the valve cusps are thickened and restricted in opening. There is aliasing of the color flow map across the valve (Fig. 3.15), indicating turbulent flow, and an increase of the Doppler velocity. Pulmonary stenosis or atresia can be a common component of complex heart disease, such as double outlet right ventricle. **Subpulmonary (infundibular) stenosis** (Fig. 3.16), or narrowing below the valve ring itself, is characteristic of tetralogy of Fallot in postnatal life but this is not always readily apparent echocardiographically in the fetus.

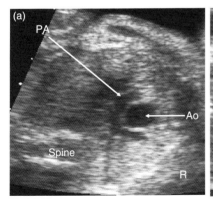

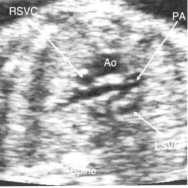

Fig. 3.14.(a). The pulmonary arteries shown on both panels vary from slightly smaller than normal to tiny but in neither of them was there forward flow across the pulmonary valve on pulsed Doppler or color flow mappng, indicating pulmonary atresia. In the fetus illustrated in the right-hand panel, there was, in addition, a persistent left superior vena cava (LSVC), seen as a fourth vessel in the three-vessel view.

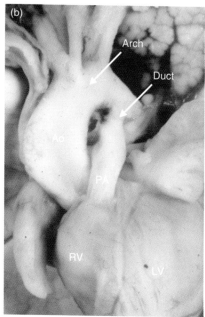
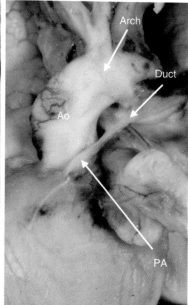

Fig. 3.14.(b). Contd. There is pulmonary atresia with intact septum in both specimens. There can be variation in the size of the pulmonary trunk in this setting. Note also that the right ventricle appears smaller than the left, as would be expected with this diagnosis. On the left-hand panel, the pulmonary trunk is smaller than normal but of reasonable size. In keeping with this, the duct is of good size and joins the aorta normally. On the right-hand panel, the pulmonary trunk is thread-like and is supplied by a severely hypoplastic arterial duct, which joins the underside of the aortic arch.

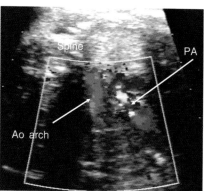
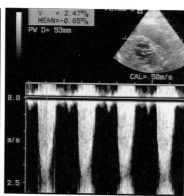

Fig. 3.15. There is aliasing of the color flow map across a stenosed and thickened pulmonary valve. On the right-hand panel, pulsed Doppler across the valve showed a velocity of nearly 2.5 m/s.

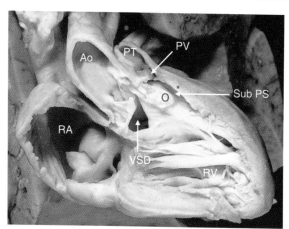

Fig. 3.16. The heart is opened from the front, to show the right side of the ventricular septum. The aorta is seen arising above a ventricular septal defect. There is marked subpulmonary muscular stenosis in this heart with tetralogy of Fallot. The stenosis is a result of blood being squeezed between the outlet septum (O), which is deviated anteriorly, and the free wall of the right ventricle (*). In this fetus, the pulmonary valve is also dysplastic and stenotic (PV) and there is marked hypoplasia of the pulmonary trunk, all common features of this diagnosis.

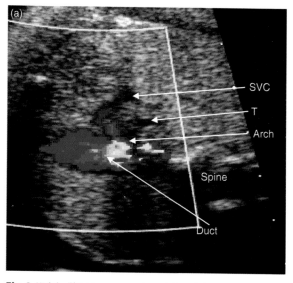

Fig. 3.17.(a). The transverse arch could barely be seen in its usual position on the 2D image as it was so hypoplastic. However, color flow mapping allows the vessel to be delineated by the reverse flow within it.

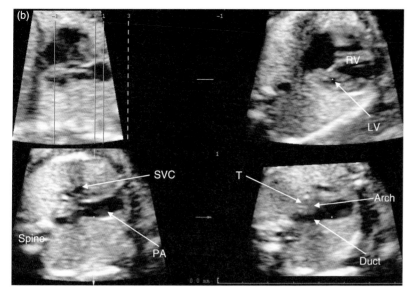

Fig. 3.17.(b). Contd. Three tomographic images were obtained in a case of the hypoplastic left heart syndrome. In the four-chamber view (upper right image), only a slit-like left ventricle could be found. The ascending aorta was so small, it could not be distinguished as the beam moved cranially from the four-chamber to the three-vessel view. In the three-vessel view (lower left panel) a good size pulmonary artery was seen but there was no visible vessel lying between the pulmonary artery and the superior vena cava in the normal position for the ascending aorta. As the beam progressed cranially above the duct (lower right panel), reverse flow could be seen in a tiny transverse arch.

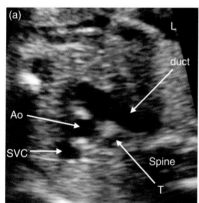
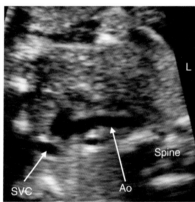

Fig. 3.18.(a). When the transverse arch and duct are directly compared in size in sequential views, it is clear that the aortic arch is significantly smaller than the duct.

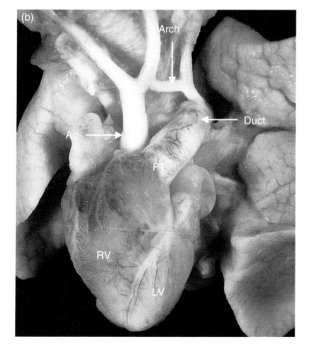

Fig. 3.18.(b). The anatomical specimen illustrates the same sort of findings as the echocardiogram shows in Fig. 3.18(a). The ascending aorta is about half the size of the pulmonary trunk. The transverse arch is even smaller and is also longer than normal (tubular hypoplasia). It joins the side of an enlarged arterial duct, a classical sign of coarctation of the aorta. Note also the discrepancy in ventricular sizes.

Aortic arch smaller than normal

The aortic arch is very hypoplastic in aortic atresia, and often cannot be seen on 2D imaging. However, it can be discovered by seeing reverse flow in the transverse arch, coming from the arterial duct (Fig. 3.17). It is smaller than normal and smaller than the duct in **coarctation** (Fig. 3.18(a) and (b)), although the direction of flow in the arch in coarctation is usually normal. The arch and duct are readily compared in transverse views. There is considerable overlap in the relative size of the aortic arch between normals and those demonstrated to have coarctation after birth.

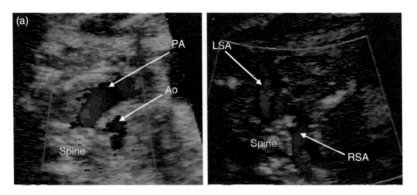

Fig. 3.19.(a). In the left-hand panel, the aorta is seen to be much smaller than the pulmonary artery on the three-vessel view. Scanning cranial to this level no vessel on 2D or color flow mapping could be found forming the transverse portion of the arch, due to aortic interruption. In the right hand panel, the left subclavian artery could be seen arising more posteriorly from the region of the ductal junction with the descending aorta, whereas the right subclavian arose from the ascending aorta. This is characteristic of aortic interruption type B.

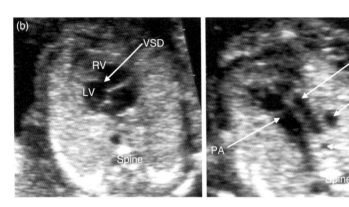

Fig. 3.19.(b). In the four-chamber view on the left-hand panel, the left ventricle is smaller than the right and there is a large ventricular septal defect. Immediately above this level, both great arteries were seen to be arising from the right ventricle as two parallel tubes, thus indicating double outlet right ventricle. The transverse arch was small and could not be completed but stopped short of the trachea, as it was interrupted.

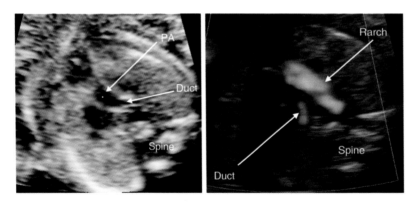

Fig. 3.20. In pulmonary atresia, the duct is usually smaller than normal as in the left-hand panel. In the example shown in the right-hand panel, the small duct is left sided, the arch right sided. The flow in the duct is in the opposite direction to normal and opposite to the aorta, so that the branch pulmonary arteries are being fed retrogradely.

Therefore a diagnosis of coarctation prenatally is generally a provisional diagnosis, to be confirmed or refuted postnatally. The **transverse arch is not found** at all echocardiographically in **interruption** of the aorta type B (Fig. 3.19(a) and (b), see also Fig. 3.13(b)). There is always a ventricular septal defect in an interrupted aortic arch, often large, but an interrupted arch can also occur with more complex intracardiac malformations (Fig. 3.19(b)).

Duct smaller than normal

The arterial duct is smaller than normal and blood flow in it is reversed in **pulmonary atresia** (Fig. 3.20). In pulmonary stenosis, the duct tends to be smaller than normal but the flow direction will depend on the severity of obstruction.

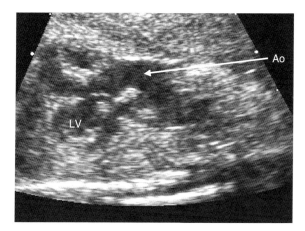

Fig. 3.21. The aorta is seen to arise astride the crest of the ventricular septum. It is measurably larger than normal and larger than the pulmonary artery. Use of the aorta/pulmonary artery ratio chart can demonstrate this more clearly.

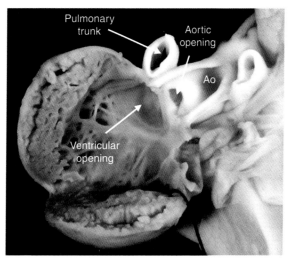

Fig. 3.22. An echocardiographic example of this defect has not been seen by us for over 10 years but a pathological specimen from our earlier series is shown here, viewed from the left ventricular outflow tract. The left ventricle was dilated and thick-walled and led into the aortic trunk via the aortic valve, which has been opened. On the septal side of the valve, there is an additional pathway, the tunnel, which has ventricular and aortic openings. This allowed blood to bypass the aortic valve and regurgitate into the ventricle.

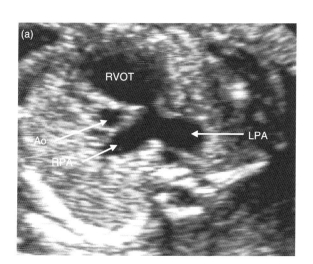

Fig. 3.23.(a). The right ventricular outflow tract (RVOT), main and branch pulmonary arteries are dilated due to regurgitation of blood flow through a dysplastic pulmonary valve. Note the absence of the arterial duct, a typical although not invariable feature of the absent pulmonary valve syndrome.

Aorta larger than normal

The aorta is often slightly larger than normal in **tetralogy of Fallot** and in the rare condition of an **aorto-left ventricular tunnel**. In tetralogy of Fallot, the increase in size is because the aorta receives more blood than the obstructed pulmonary artery (Fig. 3.21). An aorto-left ventricular tunnel is where there is an abnormal tunnel-like connection between the aorta above the level of the sinuses, and the left ventricular outflow tract. This produces marked aortic incompetence, readily seen on color flow mapping and leading to left ventricular dilatation (Fig. 3.22). Where there is a single great artery arising from the heart in the setting of a common arterial trunk, this artery is larger than a normal aorta or pulmonary artery would be for the gestational age, as it carries all the blood flow from the heart.

Pulmonary artery larger than normal

The pulmonary artery is larger than normal in the so-called **absent pulmonary valve syndrome**. This would be better named the dysplastic pulmonary valve syndrome, as there is valve tissue present, but it is abnormally formed and allows the valve to leak. This leads to dilatation of the right ventricle, pulmonary outflow tract and most particularly the branch pulmonary arteries (Fig. 3.23 (a) and (b)).

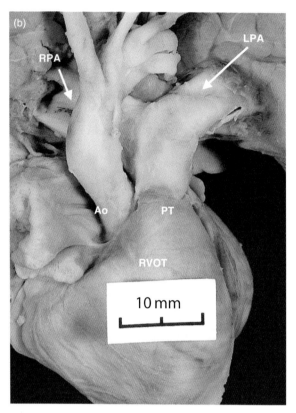

Fig. 3.23.(b). Contd. Note the gross enlargement of the branch pulmonary arteries in particular in this case of the absent pulmonary valve syndrome. Compare with the normal branch pulmonary artery size in Fig. 3.2(f). Normally they are less than half the size of the main pulmonary trunk (PT). There is no evidence of an arterial duct in this specimen either.

Both great arteries larger than normal

This occurs when there is excessive blood flow in the great arteries as would occur in an **arteriovenous malformation** in any site, but particularly in a vein of Galen malformation in the brain (Fig. 3.24).

Abnormalities of great artery position and structure

As the transducer beam is swept up from the four-chamber view, the ventricular septum should appear intact with the aorta arising completely from the left ventricle. Perimembranous ventricular septal defects can be seen in this view as a hole just below the aortic valve (Fig. 3.25).

The position of the great arteries, their relationship to each other and the way in which the ventricles connect to them are closely associated with each other. In the normal heart, the pulmonary artery origin is the more anterior, the great arteries "cross over" each other (this is termed "normally related"), and they connect with the ventricles in a concordant manner (aorta from left ventricle and pulmonary artery from right ventricle). In some types of abnormal connection, the normal relation of the great arteries is maintained and the pulmonary artery origin remains the more anterior. However, in others, the normal "crossing over" relationship of the great arteries is

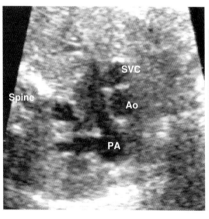

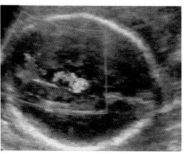

Fig. 3.24. In a three-vessel view, all the vessels appeared dilated. This was due to an arteriovenous malformation in the head, a vein of Galen aneurysm, resulting in excessive blood flow to and from the head. On the right-hand panel, the unusual intracranial vascularity, characteristic of this lesion, is seen.

lost and instead they are parallel to each other at their origins. A parallel arrangement of the great arteries nearly always indicates that the aorta is the more anteriorly arising vessel and that it arises from the right ventricle rather than the left ventricle.

Arterial override

As the transducer beam is swept up from the four-chamber view, the first great artery arising from the heart can be seen to sit astride the crest of the ventricular septum (Fig. 3.26(a)). In arterial override, there is always a ventricular septal defect. The great artery must be identified as an aorta or a pulmonary artery by its branching pattern. If it is an aorta, the most likely diagnosis is **tetralogy of Fallot**, in which case the pulmonary artery will be normally positioned and crossing over the aorta but significantly smaller than it (Fig. 3.26(a)–(g)). In the most extreme form of

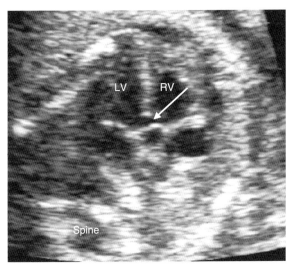

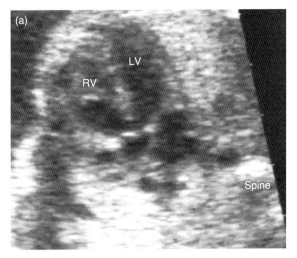

Fig. 3.25. Just above the four-chamber view, imaging the origin of the aorta, there appears to be a small ventricular septal defect, with bright echogenic edges, in the perimembranous region of the septum. This would need to be confirmed by imaging with the beam more perpendicular to the septum and by seeing color flow breaching the defect. Note that there is still a continuous, although curved, line between the ventricular septum and the anterior wall of the aorta as in the normal heart (compare with Fig. 3.1)

Fig. 3.26.(a). As the beam moves above the level of the atrioventricular valves, a valve is seen sitting astride the crest of the ventricular septum. There is no, even potential, continuity between the interventricular septum and the anterior wall of this vessel, in contrast to the example seen in Fig. 3.25. Only by scanning more superiorly, can this vessel be identified. It is an aorta if it forms the transverse aortic arch, or a pulmonary artery if it branches soon after its origin. Alternatively, if it does both, it is a common arterial trunk. If it proves to be an aorta, the diagnosis is a form of tetralogy of Fallot, if it is a pulmonary artery, the diagnosis will be transposition of the great arteries or double outlet right ventricle.

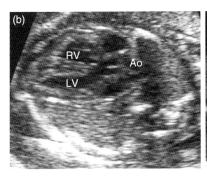
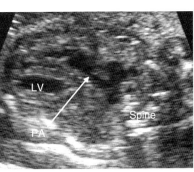

Fig. 3.26.(b). A great artery arises astride the crest of the ventricular septum. On the left-hand panel, there are no early branches to the vessel, indicating it is the aorta. There is no continuity between the ventricular septum and the anterior wall of the aorta. Above this level in the right-hand panel, the pulmonary artery can be seen to be crossing over the aorta in a normal fashion but it is smaller than normal, and smaller than the aorta. This combination of findings is typical of tetralogy of Fallot.

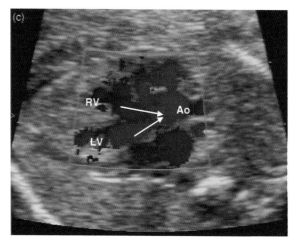

Fig. 3.26.(c). Contd. The overriding aorta receives blood flow (arrows) from both the right and the left ventricles.

tetralogy of Fallot, the pulmonary valve is completely obstructed (atretic) with no flow across it on pulsed Doppler or color flow mapping, and reverse flow in the arterial duct (Fig. 3.27(a)–(c)). Occasionally, **a subaortic ventricular septal defect with aortic override** can be associated with a normal size pulmonary artery. This combination has a high association with trisomy 18.

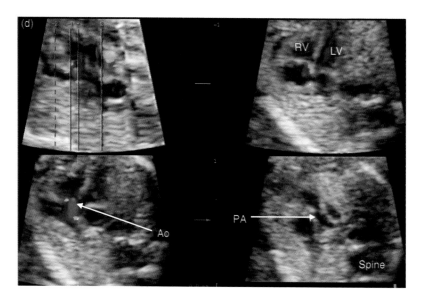

Fig. 3.26.(d). Three tomographic images are shown of tetralogy of Fallot. A fairly normal four-chamber view as expected (upper right), the aorta displaced anteriorly and arising astride an outlet ventricular septal defect (bottom left) and a small pulmonary artery with confluent branches (bottom right), crossing over the aorta in a normal fashion. Note the discrepancy in the size of the great arteries, with the aorta larger than the pulmonary artery which is always abnormal.

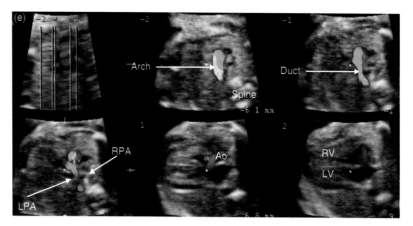

Fig. 3.26.(e). These five tomographic images are obtained from a volume set in a fetus with classic tetralogy of Fallot. The four-chamber view is fairly normal (bottom right), although the apex is a little to the left. The aorta arises astride the ventricular septal defect (middle of bottom row). The pulmonary artery is smaller than normal (lower left image). The duct is smaller than normal (upper right) in comparison with the size of the aortic arch (upper middle). Small confluent branch pulmonary arteries could be seen (lower left) receiving forward flow from the right ventricle.

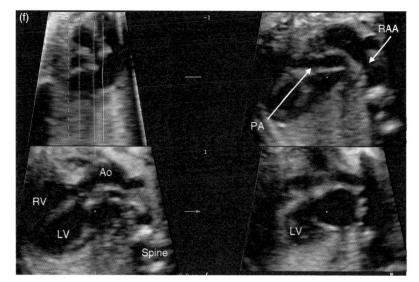

Fig. 3.26.(f). Contd. The tomographic images are taken from an acquired cardiac volume in a case of tetralogy of Fallot. The image on the top right is the most cranial section. In it the aorta stays to the right of the midline and forms a right aortic arch (RAA). The pulmonary artery in this section is seen to be smaller than the aorta, which is seen best on the lower left image. In this section, the aorta is seen to arise astride the crest of the ventricular septum.

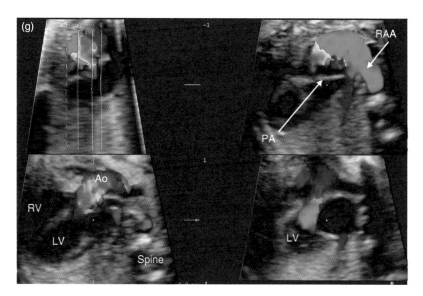

Fig. 3.26.(g). Adding color imformation to the same frame as Fig. 3.26(c), illustrates aortic override more clearly in both frames in the lower panel.

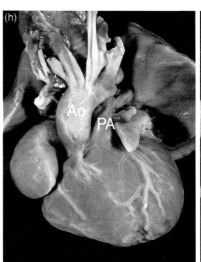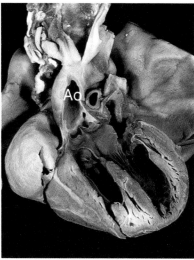

Fig. 3.26.(h). An example of a fetal specimen with tetralogy of Fallot is shown. The left-hand panel shows the exterior of the intact specimen, showing the characteristic hypoplasia of the pulmonary trunk and an enlarged aorta. On the right-hand panel, the heart has been sectioned to show the left ventricular outflow tract and the small pulmonary trunk in cross section. There is lack of continuity between the anterior wall of the aorta and the ventricular septum due to a large ventricular septal defect. As a consequence, the aortic valve overrides the crest of the ventricular septum. There is still continuity more posteriorly between the aortic and mitral valves.

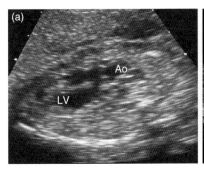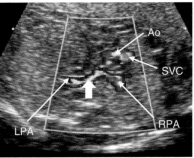

Fig. 3.27.(a). The aorta appears larger than normal, displaced anteriorly and arising astride the crest of the ventricular septum. No main pulmonary artery was seen, nor forward flow into the pulmonary trunk. With this anatomy, a remnant of main pulmonary artery can often be identified pathologically as a fibrous strand, with no lumen, leading back from the confluence of the pulmonary arteries to the right ventricle and the ventriculo-arterial connection is thus concordant. There was reverse flow in the arterial duct (arrowhead), which is seen in the left pulmonary artery in the right-hand panel in this case of tetralogy of Fallot with pulmonary atresia.

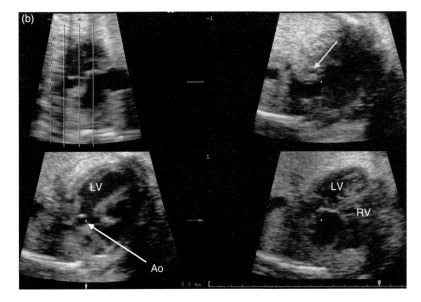

Fig. 3.27.(b). The tomographic images are taken from an acquired volume set. A normal four-chamber view is seen (bottom right). Aortic override is seen just above the level of the four-chamber view. Only a tiny remnant of a pulmonary artery was seen in its expected position (yellow arrow), on searching back and forward through the volume between the ascending aorta and the aortic arch, where the pulmonary artery would be found in the normal heart.

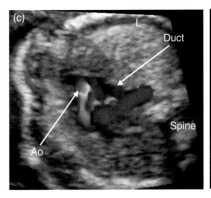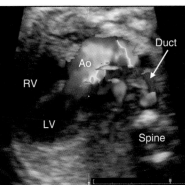

Fig. 3.27.(c). Both panels show examples of pulmonary atresia. In both fetuses the spine is at about 4 o'clock position, but the fetus on the left lies with the head behind the screen (HB) and the fetus on the right with the head in front of the screen (HF). In the left-hand panel, there is a left arch and reverse flow seen in a small left-sided arterial duct, whereas on the right-hand panel, there is reverse flow seen in a small right-sided arterial duct. The fetus in the latter case, had tetralogy of Fallot with a right-sided aortic arch.

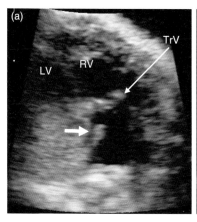
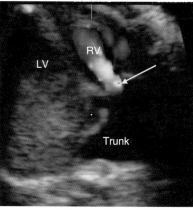

Fig. 3.28.(a). On the left-hand panel, the only great artery seen arising from the heart was astride an outlet ventricular septal defect and arose predominantly from the right ventricle. It gave rise to both the aorta and aortic arch, and the pulmonary artery (broad arrow). This is a common arterial trunk. Note the thickened truncal valve (TrV). On the right-hand panel, in the same frame with color information added, the arterial valve is seen to be regurgitant (yellow arrow) on color flow mapping.

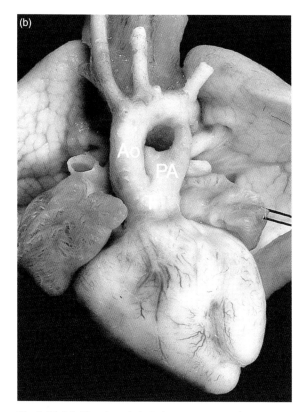

Fig. 3.28.(b). There is a relatively short common trunk arising from the ventricular mass which then divides into separate aortic and pulmonary pathways. The trunk gives rise to both the pulmonary arteries, the head and neck arteries as well as the much smaller coronary arteries.

The appearance of arterial override will occur in a **common arterial trunk** where there is only one great artery arising from the heart but it gives rise to both the aorta and the pulmonary artery (Figs. 3.28(a)–(c), 3.29). The arterial (truncal) valve is often abnormal, thickened, and dysplastic, a finding which can help to differentiate this diagnosis from tetralogy of Fallot with pulmonary atresia. The velocity of blood flow across a truncal valve is generally modestly increased above the normal range, a velocity of up to 150 cm/s being not unusual. However, it will be higher than this if there is significant stenosis of the truncal valve, which can occur. In addition, if the valve is dysplastic, it may be regurgitant on pulsed Doppler or color flow mapping (Fig. 3.28(a)).

If the great artery astride the septum is the pulmonary artery (recognized by its branching pattern), this is nearly always associated with the aorta anterior, in the setting of **double outlet right ventricle** (Fig. 3.30).

Transposition (ventriculo-arterial discordance)

This refers to the situation where the aorta arises solely from the right ventricle and the pulmonary artery entirely or mainly from the left ventricle. Most

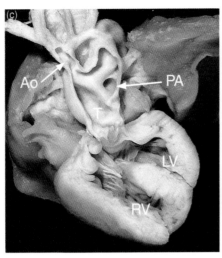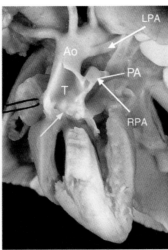

Fig. 3.28.(c). Contd. The heart in the left panel has been sectioned in a left ventricular outflow view to show the ventricular septal defect and the truncal valve overriding the crest of the ventricular septum. Again, the trunk divides more distally into aortic and ductal paths but in this fetus the aortic arch is much smaller than the arterial duct and there is coarctation. The specimen in the right-hand panel is again sectioned to show the left ventricular outflow tract. Although the ventricular septal defect is small in this fetus, there is lack of continuity between the anterior wall of the great artery and the ventricular septum. The truncal valve is dysplastic (yellow arrow). This example is unusual in that the right pulmonary artery arises anteriorly and the left pulmonary artery arises from the underside of the aortic arch via a duct. This can be easily confused echocardiographically with tetralogy of Fallot with pulmonary atresia.

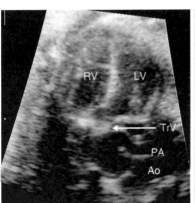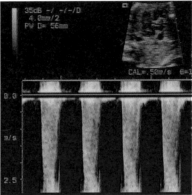

Fig. 3.29. The truncal valve (TrV) was thickened (left-hand panel) and restricted in motion in the moving image. The single vessel arising from the heart divided into the aortic arch and the main pulmonary artery. The left pulmonary artery and arch are seen here. The velocity of flow in the single great artery was increased at over 2.5 m/s due to truncal valve stenosis (right-hand panel).

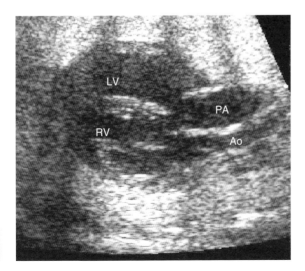

Fig. 3.30. The great artery seen astride the crest of the ventricular septum proves to be the pulmonary artery, but the aorta arises anterior to it, from the right ventricle. This is double outlet right ventricle. Note also that the aorta is significantly smaller than the pulmonary artery indicating a possible associated coarctation of the aorta.

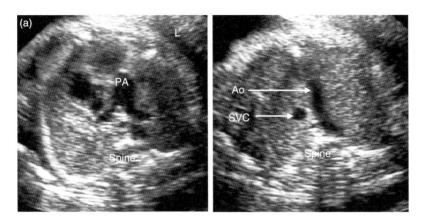

Fig. 3.31.(a). Moving cranially from a normal four-chamber view, the first great artery formed branches soon after the valve, indicating it is the pulmonary artery (left-hand panel). Above this level, the aortic arch is seen arising more anteriorly than normal, from the right ventricle. This is simple transposition of the great arteries. Note that it is not possible to obtain a normal three-vessel view, because the pulmonary artery lies entirely below the level of the aorta.

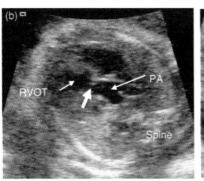
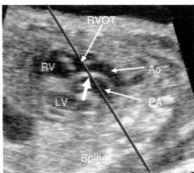

Fig. 3.31.(b). The image in the left-hand panel, corresponding to a level between the planes of the two images shown in Fig. 3.31(a), gives the false initial impression that the pulmonary artery arises from the right ventricle. However, this is because of the close proximity of the right ventricular outflow (RVOT) to the pulmonary artery arising directly behind it from the left ventricle. The structure indicated by the bold arrow is not in fact the pulmonary valve, which lies below this section, but the adjacent walls of the right ventricular outflow and pulmonary artery. The right-hand panel shows a sagittal plane through the same fetus. The dense line indicates the approximate plane of section of the image on the left.

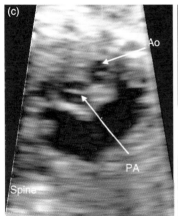
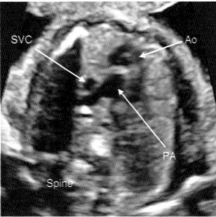

Fig. 3.31.(c). In the left-hand image, the great arteries are imaged just above the four-chamber view, where a normal three-vessel view is expected. However, here there are two circular valve rings seen in the same section, instead of seeing the aorta first and the pulmonary artery above it with the normal "tube" shape of the pulmonary artery and duct and circular cut of the ascending aorta. (Compare with Figs. 3.2 or 3.4.) Following each great artery from this section demonstrates that the anterior great artery arising from the right ventricle gives rise to the aortic arch, whereas the posterior artery arises from the left ventricle and branches laterally. These findings indicate that the anterior valve ring seen here is the aorta and the posterior one is the pulmonary artery and that this is transposition of the great arteries. The usual positional relationship of the great arteries in transposition are clearly seen here, with the aorta anterior and to the right of the pulmonary artery. The right hand panel is a similar, slightly more cranial cut in transposition, where the branching great artery (the pulmonary artery) is seen in the middle of the thorax. The aortic valve ring lies anterior to it. Note the differences here from the appearance of the normal three-vessel view.

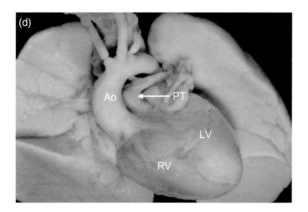

Fig. 3.31.(d). Contd. The typical arrangement of the great arteries in transposition is shown as seen from the exterior view of the anatomical specimen. The two great arteries are parallel to one another with the aorta to the right, anterior and more cranial than the pulmonary valve. The aorta arises from the right ventricle and pulmonary trunk from the left ventricle. Compare this arrangement of the great arteries to the normal, as shown in Fig. 3.2(f).

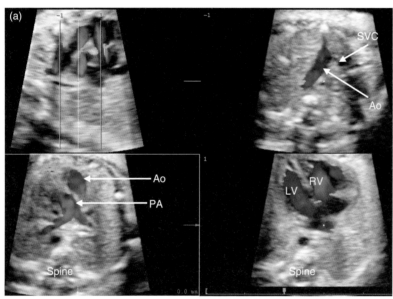

Fig. 3.32.(a). Three cuts of the heart are displayed from a volume set. The four-chamber view is normal in the bottom right image, the first artery seen above this level, (bottom left) branches laterally, with the aorta anterior to it. This is a three-vessel view but it is clearly abnormal with the aorta completely anterior to the pulmonary artery (compare with normal three-vessel views, such as in Fig. 3.2). The aortic arch (top right) could be followed and was seen to connect to the anterior right ventricle.

commonly by far, this occurs in association with a concordant (normal) atrioventricular connection. However, less commonly it may occur with a discordant atrioventricular connection. It is important to distinguish the two situations as, although the appearances are superficially similar, the physiology and consequences are very different.

Transposition with atrioventricular concordance

In this condition, the four-chamber view will usually be normal. The pulmonary artery arises from the left ventricle and the aorta from the right (transposition of the great arteries). Therefore, the first great artery to be found above the level of the four-chamber view is the branching pulmonary artery (Figs. 3.31(a)–(d), 3.32(a) and (b)) with the aortic valve (connected to the arch) above this level. Because of the close proximity of the

right ventricular outflow (giving rise to the aorta) and the pulmonary artery behind it in combination with the acute backwards angulation of the pulmonary artery, images may give the false impression that the pulmonary artery is arising from the right ventricle (Fig. 3.31(b)). However, the normal "crossover" appearance of the great arteries is not found and the normal three-vessel view is not seen (Fig. 3.31(c)) because the pulmonary artery and duct lie below the aorta and aortic arch. This contrasts to the situation in the normal heart, where the aorta is the first great artery seen in an upward sweep from the four chamber plane and the ascending aorta, pulmonary valve, and pulmonary branches together with the superior vena cava are seen together at the slightly higher level in the three-vessel plane. As a result of their abnormal connection, the great arteries arise in parallel orientation (Fig. 3.31(d)),

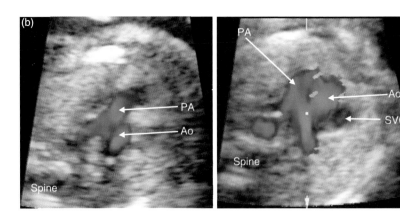

Fig. 3.32.(b). On the left-hand panel, a normal three-vessel view is seen. Note that the pulmonary artery extends much more anteriorly than the aorta, which normally arises in the middle of the chest. On the right-hand panel is a case of transposition of the great arteries, where the clue on the three-vessel view was that the aorta arose slightly anterior to the pulmonary artery. This was a difficult case to diagnose, with a rather unusual arrangement of the great arteries, but close analysis of the three-vessel view was clearly abnormal.

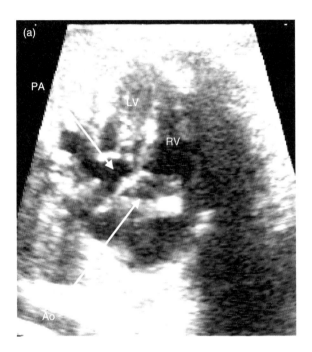

with the aortic valve anterior and (usually) to the right of the pulmonary artery (Figs. 3.31–3.33). The diagnosis of transposition can be made or suspected in transverse views but the parallel arrangement of the vessels is easier to recognize in long-axis views of the heart (see Chapter 4). These views should be used to confirm a suspected diagnosis of transposition. In simple transposition, there are no other abnormal findings in the heart except for the transposed great arteries and this is the most common form of transposition. Complex transposition is when there are additional findings such as pulmonary stenosis, a ventricular septal defect (Fig. 3.33(a)–(c)) or tricuspid atresia (Fig. 3.33(d)). Extracardiac abnormalities are not common in transposition, so the case illustrated in Fig. 3.33(c) is unusual.

Transposition with atrioventricular discordance

The appearance of this condition in the four-chamber plane is described in Chapter 2. The great artery views

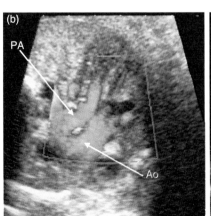
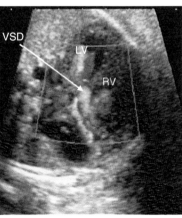

Fig. 3.33.(a). The great artery arising from the left ventricle is branching, therefore is the pulmonary artery. The anterior great artery does not cross over the other one but two great arteries arise in parallel arrangement with the aorta anterior and to the right of the pulmonary artery. Note also the pulmonary artery is slightly smaller than the aorta, indicating a degree of pulmonary stenosis. Just below the level of the great arteries, there was a moderate-sized ventricular septal defect with entirely left-to-right shunting (Fig. 3.33(b)), confirming a degree of pulmonary stenosis, which was more marked later in pregnancy.

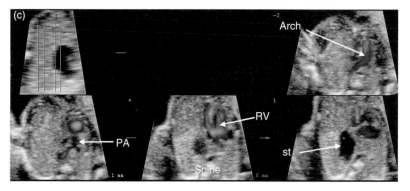

Fig. 3.33.(c). Contd. In the four-chamber view of a volume set (bottom right) the stomach (st) can be seen in the left chest and the heart is displaced to the right. The left ventricle is much smaller than the right, on this and the central image. A small branching pulmonary artery is seen just above the level of the four-chamber view on the bottom left image. It arose from the left ventricle. The aorta arose very anteriorly (top right image) from the right ventricle and formed the arch. This was transposition, with a ventricular septal defect and pulmonary stenosis in a fetus with a diaphragmatic hernia.

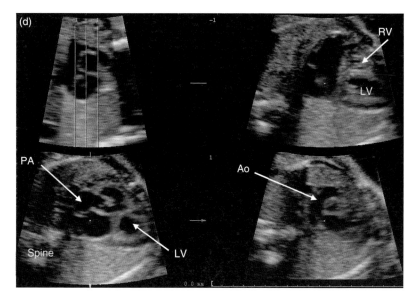

Fig. 3.33.(d). These views are obtained from a volume set. On the top right is the four-chamber view, showing a small right ventricle and in the moving image the tricuspid valve was atretic. On the lower left image, a great artery is seen arising from the left ventricle. The ventricular septal defect allowing blood flow from the left ventricle to the small rudimentary right ventricle is well seen in this section. On the plane immediately above this slice (bottom right image), the great artery arising from the small right ventricle forms the aortic arch. This therefore is the aorta. The great artery which arises from the left ventricle, shows early branching, therefore is the pulmonary artery. This is tricuspid atresia with transposed great arteries.

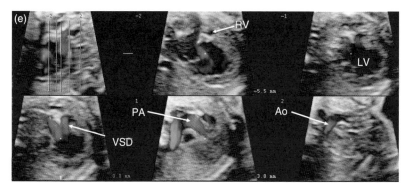

Fig. 3.33.(e). In a similar example, with color information added, there is flow into the left ventricle in the four-chamber view but none visible into the small right ventricle (upper middle image). As the beam moves cranially, a ventricular septal defect (VSD) is seen supplying some blood flow to the right ventricle (upper right and lower left images). The pulmonary artery is seen arising from the left ventricle (lower middle) and the aorta from the small right ventricle (bottom right).

will also be abnormal, as the great arteries are also transposed, thus "correcting" the physiology of the circulation. In anatomical terms, the left atrium connects to the right ventricle, which is in turn connected to the aorta and the right atrium connects to the left ventricle, which connects to the pulmonary artery. Thus, the pulmonary venous blood reaches the aorta and the systemic blood the pulmonary artery as in the normal circulation, albeit through the morphologically inappropriate ventricle. This condition is therefore known as congenitally corrected transposition, or as double discordance, as both the atrioventricular and ventriculo-arterial connections are discordant. The great arteries arise in parallel orientation with the aortic valve anterior but to the left of the pulmonary valve (Fig. 3.34(a) and (b)). Contrast this with transposition of the great arteries with concordant atrioventricular connections, where the aorta usually lies anterior and to the right of the pulmonary artery.

Double outlet right ventricle

Double outlet right ventricle refers to a group of disparate conditions in which both great arteries arise predominantly from the right ventricle.

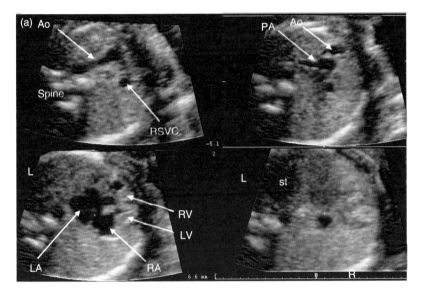

Fig. 3.34.(a). A volume set shows a complete picture in this fetus, which is typical (although not invariable) for double discordance. The bottom right image shows the stomach and normal arrangement of the aorta and inferior vena cava in the abdomen. In the bottom left image, the apex points mainly to the right, with the morphological left ventricle to the right of the right ventricle, whereas the left atrium lies, as normal, to the left of the right atrium. In the upper right panel, a branching great artery (which therefore must be the pulmonary artery) arises in the middle of the chest from the left ventricle. A second great artery arises anterior and to the left of the pulmonary artery and gives rise to the transverse aortic arch (upper left frame). Note that a normal three-vessel view cannot be obtained.

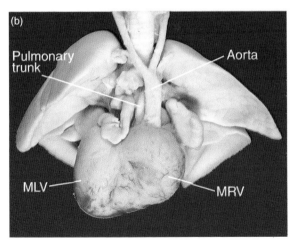

Fig. 3.34.(b). The anatomical specimen here is very similar to that shown on the echocardiogram in Fig. 3.34(a). The direction of the apex is to the right. The morphological right ventricle (MRV) lay to the left of the morphological left ventricle (MLV). The aorta is positioned anterior, cranial and to the left of the pulmonary trunk.

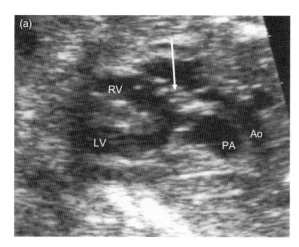

Fig. 3.35.(a). The great arteries arise in parallel orientation with the aorta anterior to the pulmonary artery. The pulmonary artery arises astride the ventricular septum but mainly from the right ventricle. There is anterior deviation of the septum (arrow) between the great arteries (the conal septum), which narrows the outflow to the aorta.

If the aorta is anterior to the pulmonary artery this is "transposition-like," and the designation double outlet indicates that the ventricular septal defect is subpulmonary but the pulmonary artery arises more than 50% from the right ventricle (Fig. 3.35.(a)–(g)). On the other hand, if the pulmonary artery overrides less than 50%, the correct designation is transposition with subpulmonary ventricular septal defect rather than double outlet, although the surgical implications are similar. In the "transposition" type of double outlet right ventricle, the great arteries arise in parallel orientation as in transposition.

Double outlet right ventricle can be used to describe a situation where the aorta is posterior to the pulmonary artery and overriding the septum but it arises more than 50% from the right ventricle. This is "tetralogy of Fallot-like" double outlet right ventricle (Fig. 3.36). In this setting, the great arteries would show a normal crossover pattern.

More unusually, double outlet right ventricle may occur with both great arteries arising exclusively from

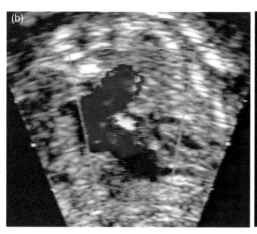

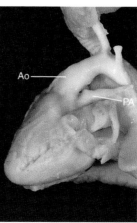

Fig. 3.35.(b). Both great arteries arise from the anterior right ventricle, with the aorta anterior to the pulmonary artery. There is aliased color flow in the small posterior pulmonary artery, implying pulmonary stenosis. The pathological specimen on the right-hand panel is similar to the echocardiographic example. The two great arteries arise in parallel with the pulmonary artery smaller and posterior to the aorta.

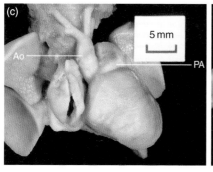

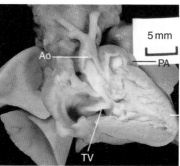

Fig. 3.35.(c). In this example of double outlet, there is a more side-by-side arrangement of the great arteries with the aorta to the right. Nevertheless, both great arteries originated from the right ventricle (right-hand panel). There was a small subaortic ventricular septal defect in this fetus and associated mitral atresia.

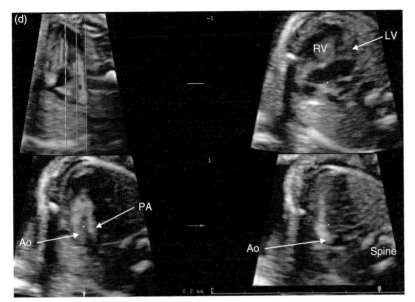

Fig. 3.35.(d). Contd. Double outlet right ventricle is the most common arterial connection in right atrial isomerism. On the top right image, there is a common atrioventricular valve to a dominant right ventricle. On the bottom left, both great arteries were seen arising as parallel tubes above the right ventricle, with the pulmonary artery behind and smaller than the aorta. On the bottom right image, the anterior great artery could be followed to the aortic arch confirming this vessel as the aorta.

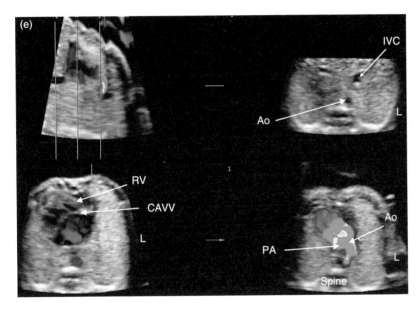

Fig. 3.35.(e). In this fetus, also with right atrial isomerism, the abdominal vessels in the top right image are typical for this condition with the aorta and the inferior vena cava lying on the same side of the abdomen, in this case both on the left side. The fetus lies HB. On the bottom left image, in the four-chamber view, the apex pointed to the right, there was a dominant right ventricle and a common atrioventricular valve (CAVV). The two great arteries arose from the anterior right ventricle in parallel orientation, with the pulmonary artery posterior to the aorta.

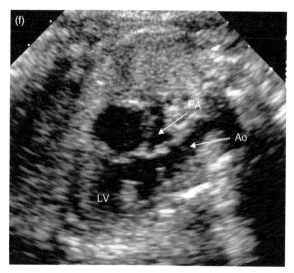

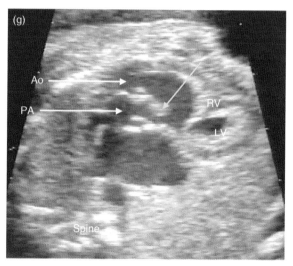

Fig. 3.35.(f). Contd. Double outlet right ventricle is the most common arterial connection in so-called upstairs/downstairs arrangement of the ventricles (see Chapter 2). The left ventricle lies inferior to the right ventricle, instead of their usual side-by-side position in a four-chamber view. There is a large ventricular septal defect. The right ventricle gives rise to both great arteries with the aorta anterior to the pulmonary artery. There was severe pulmonary stenosis in this case.

Fig. 3.35.(g). As the beam was moved superiorly from the four-chamber view, both great arteries were seen arising predominantly from the right ventricle, with the aorta anterior to the pulmonary artery. Note here the subpulmonary narrowing also, due to posterior deviation of the outlet septum (yellow arrow).

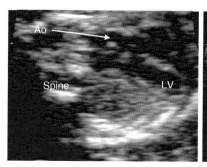

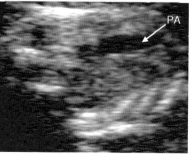

Fig. 3.36. On the left-hand panel, the aorta can be seen arising above a ventricular septal defect but predominantly from the right ventricle. Further cranially, the pulmonary artery arises more anteriorly and crosses over the aortic origin. Thus, this is double outlet right ventricle but of a "tetralogy of Fallot-like" arrangement.

the right ventricle, without override and with the VSD remote from either vessel. This is double outlet right ventricle with an uncommitted VSD and has important implications in surgical terms. Commonly in double outlet right ventricle, there is pulmonary stenosis or even complete pulmonary atresia. The pulmonary artery therefore will be smaller than the aorta. Alternatively, there may be associated coarctation of the aorta, in which case the aorta will be small relative to the pulmonary artery. Double outlet right ventricle is the typical arterial connection in right atrial isomerism (Fig. 3.35(d)–(g)) (see also Chapter 4).

Dysplastic aortic or pulmonary valve

The aortic valve will be thickened and dysplastic in **aortic stenosis**, which will usually lead to a smaller than normal aorta as we have seen earlier in the chapter, but may occasionally be associated with a post-stenotic dilation of the aorta. In addition, the valve can be dysplastic in an **aorto-left ventricular tunnel** in which the aorta is generally larger than normal. The pulmonary valve can be dysplastic in **pulmonary stenosis**, especially when this diagnosis is associated with Noonan's syndrome. In pulmonary stenosis, the pulmonary artery will be smaller than normal. The pulmonary valve is dysplastic in the **absent pulmonary valve syndrome** as described earlier. In trisomy 18, **polyvalvar dysplasia** is

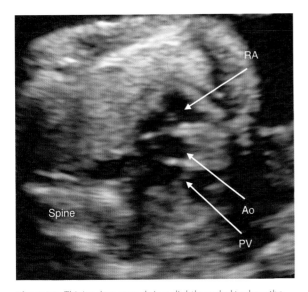

Fig. 3.37. This is a three-vessel view, slightly angled to show the morphology of the abnormal pulmonary valve. The pulmonary valve was thickened and dysplastic, and doming on the moving image. This type of dysplasia, especially when it is polyvalvar, is a marker of trisomy 18.

common, often affecting both arterial valves and/or the atrioventricular valves (Fig. 3.37).

Persistent left superior caval vein

This is not strictly speaking a great artery abnormality, but it is an abnormality which is seen in the great artery views. As described in the four-chamber section, a persistent left superior caval vein is a fairly common normal variant, which causes dilatation of the coronary sinus. The distal section of the left superior vena cava is seen indenting the left atrium in the four-chamber view (Fig. 2.52) and the proximal portion is seen in the three vessel view, where four vessels are seen instead of three (Fig. 3.38(a) and (b)). Note that the right superior vena cava is usually smaller than normal when there is a persistent left vein taking some of the venous return.

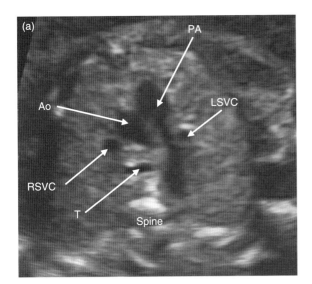

Fig. 3.38.(a). Four vessels are seen in the three-vessel view. The right superior vena cava (RSVC) is often smaller than normal as some of the blood flow in the head, neck and arms returns to the heart via the persistent left superior caval vein (LSVC), which is seen in its short axis lying to the left of the pulmonary artery.

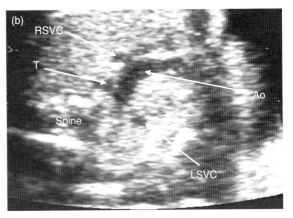

Fig. 3.38.(b). This view shows three vessels but it does not resemble a normal three-vessel view. The aorta arose from close to the front of the chest, from the right ventricle. There is no visible pulmonary artery in this section as it lay below the plane of the aorta. The right superior vena cava (RSVC) is in the normal relationship to the right of the aorta and the persistent left (LSVC) to the left of the aortic arch. This was double outlet right ventricle with bilateral superior caval veins.

Abnormalities of the aortic arch

Coarctation of the aorta

Coarctation of the aorta is a discrete narrowing of the aortic arch in the juxtaductal region of the distal arch. Identification of the coarctation shelf itself in the long-axis view of the arch is not usual in the fetus, although sometimes an abnormal angle of attachment of the aortic arch to the duct and descending aorta can be appreciated (see Fig. 3.40(e)). The diagnosis is inferred from secondary findings of ventricular and great artery disproportion, with the right-sided structures dilated relative to the left-sided structures and these signs are usually the first clue to the diagnosis. Note, however, that if there is a ventricular septal defect of moderate size, which is not necessarily immediately obvious, there may not be ventricular disproportion and the first sign will be a size discrepancy in the great arteries. A ventricular septal defect in association with a coarctation is not uncommon. The findings in coarctation may come about because of a diminution of the right-to-left shunt at the atrial septum, as a result of the increased afterload of the left ventricle, caused by the narrowing of the aorta. The decrease in the normal volume of right-to-left shunt at the atrial level, leads to a relative fall in left heart blood flow and rise in right heart flow. Comparison of the transverse arch with the arterial duct will show arch hypoplasia, also caused by the arch receiving less blood flow than normal, and this is the most reliable indicator of coarctation prenatally (Figs. 3.39, 3.40). Arch hypoplasia is a usual feature of the neonatal type of coarctation, but the degree of hypoplasia varies. In contrast to the situation post-natally, the Doppler velocity across the coarctation site itself is not increased in the fetus, where the arterial duct is always open. There is no clear distinction between ventricular and great artery disproportion occurring as a normal variant, especially in late pregnancy, and the findings indicating underlying coarctation. In general, the more marked the discrepancy in size between right and left heart structures, the more likely there is to be coarctation, or other left heart disease, causing it. However, quite striking size differences are compatible with a normal outcome and conversely, coarctation may be present with only mild disproportion. A fetal diagnosis of coarctation will generally be a provisional one, which must be either confirmed or refuted after birth as the arterial duct closes, as a false positive diagnosis of coarctation is not uncommon in fetal life, even by experienced observers.

Interruption of the aorta

Interruption of the aortic arch is complete atresia of a portion of the aortic arch, often with that portion of the arch being completely absent. By convention, the term "aortic atresia" refers to atresia at the level of the aortic valve rather than obstruction within the aortic arch, which is termed interruption. The most common site of interruption is between the second and third aortic arch vessels, so-called type B. Thus, the left carotid artery arises from the ascending aorta and the left subclavian artery from the descending aorta (Fig. 3.19(a)). A less common type is type A where the site of interruption is at the isthmus, which is that portion of the transverse arch between the origin of the left subclavian artery and the descending aorta. This latter type is difficult to differentiate from a severe coarctation. In aortic arch interruption, there is almost always a ventricular septal defect, usually a large defect and, as a result, the ventricles are usually equal in size, in contrast to coarctation where the ventricles are usually disproportionate unless there is a large ventricular

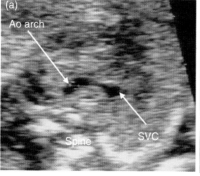
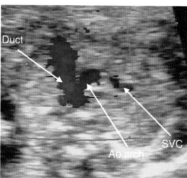

Fig. 3.39.(a). On the left-hand panel, the transverse arch can be seen to be very small. When the duct and arch sizes are compared on color flow mapping on the right, the arch is confirmed to be small. Arch hypoplasia is the most reliable indicator of coarctation of the aorta in the fetus.

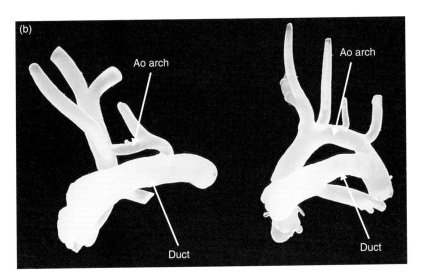

Fig. 3.39.(b). Contd. Two specimens of arch casts are seen, with a fairly typical arch found in fetal coarctation shown on the left, and a normal arch on the right. Note the normal smooth junction between the arch and duct in comparison with the angled junction, which is a common feature of coarctation in the fetus and neonate.

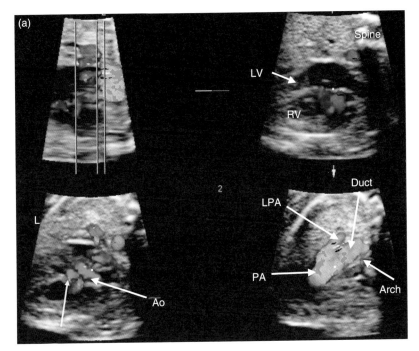

Fig. 3.40.(a). A series of images obtained from a volume set are shown. In the upper right panel, the four-chamber view shows ventricular disproportion. In the lower left panel, the aorta appears small and there is a ventricular septal defect (yellow arrow), which showed mainly left-to-right flow. The pulmonary artery, seen on the lower right image, is much larger than the aorta. Also in this image, the duct is much larger than the transverse arch.

septal defect. The ascending aorta is usually very small in interrupted aortic arch (Fig. 3.13(a)) and, in type B interruption, the ascending aorta forms a typical "two-pronged fork" appearance in longitudinal views (Fig. 4.39(a) and (b)).

Right aortic arch

This can occur in isolation in an otherwise normal fetus, or it can be part of complex heart disease, particularly tetralogy of Fallot or common arterial trunk. Instead of the aorta crossing the midline in front of the trachea and descending on the left, it stays on the right of the trachea. By the time it reaches the level of the four-chamber plane, the aorta may have returned to the left of the spine or it may remain to the right. The duct is usually left sided and connects with the descending aorta behind the trachea (Fig. 3.41(a) and (b)), forming a "U" appearance in the upper thorax. This is much the most common pattern.

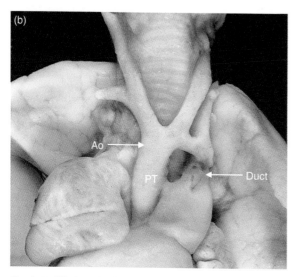

Fig. 3.40.(b). Contd. The anatomical specimen from a fetus with coarctation of the aorta, shows relatively mild hypoplasia of the transverse arch in comparison with the arterial duct.

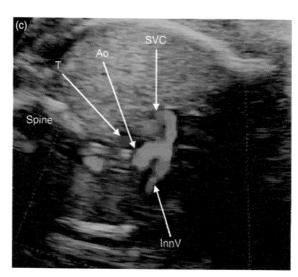

Fig. 3.40.(c). A small tortuous arch is seen in a transverse view in this case of severe coarctation of the aorta. It was only detectable on color flow mapping. The vessel, which lies above and anterior to the arch, is the innominate vein (InnV), which crosses the middle of the upper thorax to drain to the superior vena cava.

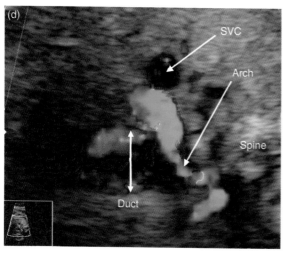

Fig. 3.40.(d). The transverse arch is imaged just above the three-vessel view. The aorta tapers dramatically across the transverse portion of the arch. Compare the distal arch with the size of the superior vena cava and the duct, marked by the double-headed arrow.

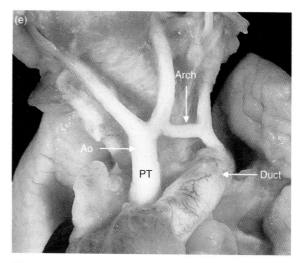

Fig. 3.40.(e). The anatomical specimen is similar to the echocardiographic examples shown in Figs. 3.40(c) and (d), with severe hypoplasia and tortuosity of the transverse arch in comparison with the size of the arterial duct lying just below it.

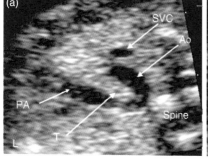
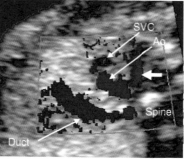

Fig. 3.41.(a). Instead of crossing the midline in front of the trachea as usual, the aorta stays on the right of the trachea and descends, at least initially, on the right side of the thorax. (Compare with Figs. 3.3(c) or 3.5, for example.) The duct passes behind the trachea to connect to the descending aorta. The vessels in the upper thorax, instead of forming a "V" shape as usual, form a "U", with tissue separating the vessels (compare with Fig. 3.8). There is also an aberrant left subclavian artery (arrowhead), which arises from ductal tissue which passes behind the trachea.

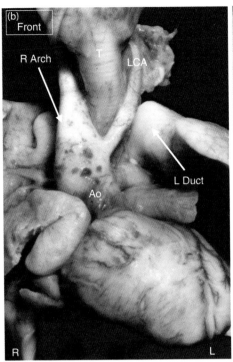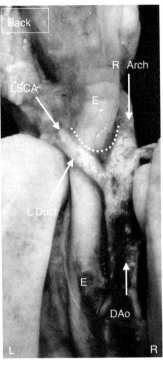

Fig. 3.41.(b). Contd. This fetus has the same anatomy as that seen in Fig. 3.41(a). From the front of the specimen in the left-hand panel, the aortic arch cannot be seen as it descends to the right of the trachea behind the ascending aorta (compare with the normal course of the arch in earlier anatomical images). From the back, however (right-hand panel), the right-sided descending aorta (DAo) can be seen. A small left duct was seen passing behind the esophagus (E) and trachea and joining the right-sided arch posteriorly, forming a "U" behind the esophagus. The first branch of the aorta is the left carotid artery (LCA). The left subclavian (LSCA) arises aberrantly from the left duct, as in the echocardiogram in Fig. 3.41(a).

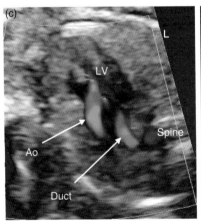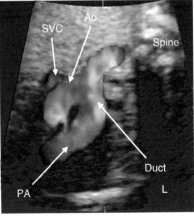

Fig. 3.41.(c). The arch and duct formed an unusual pattern in the upper thorax, which was first identified at 11 weeks of gestation. In the left-hand panel, at 20 weeks, with the spine down, the aorta could be seen arising from the left ventricle towards the right but staying on the right side to form the arch. Underneath the arch, the arterial duct could be seen also on the right side. At 28 weeks, the fetus lay with the spine anterior but the abnormal pattern of the arch vessels could again be seen.

However, if the duct is also right sided, a different pattern is seen (Fig. 3.41(c)). The branching pattern of a right aortic arch is usually a mirror image of that of a normal left arch. The first branch is a left brachiocephalic artery, giving rise to both the left common carotid and left subclavian arteries, and the right common carotid and right subclavian arteries arise from the arch separately and distally. In the usual case where the aorta forms a right arch, the left brachiocephalic artery will cross in front of the trachea above the level of the aortic arch. The left subclavian artery can arise aberrantly behind the trachea (Fig. 3.41(a) and (b)).

A right aortic arch may also be formed by the aorta in complete "mirror image" dextrocardia. In this case, the aorta ascends towards the left side, then crosses the midline to descend on the right. The overall appearance will resemble a complete mirror image of the normal, rather than the more common type of appearance of a left arch in dextrocardia, which mimics that of a right arch in the upper thorax (Fig. 3.41(d)).

Double aortic arch

Double aortic arch describes the situation where both right and left embryonic aortic arches persist, forming a complete vascular ring around the trachea and

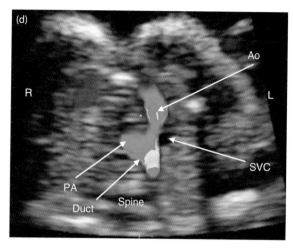

Fig. 3.41.(d). Contd. At first glance, the vessels are difficult to understand and somewhat similar to Fig. 3.41(c). The fetus lies HB, therefore this fetus had a right apex, with the aorta arising from the anterior right ventricle. There was a left arch and left duct. Note that the superior caval vein lay on the left side in this fetus with right atrial isomerism.

esophagus, with a resultant potential for upper airways compression. This may occur with approximately symmetrical arches of similar size, each giving rise to a separate common carotid and subclavian artery to the corresponding side. However, it is more usual for the arches to be asymmetrical, and it is usually the right arch which is the dominant one. In this variety of double aortic arch, where the right arch is dominant and the left small, the appearance is a very similar to an uncomplicated right arch and therefore difficult to distinguish from it. However, in a double arch, there is a branch of the ascending aorta crossing in front of the trachea, usually with a more caudal and horizontal course than the left brachiocephalic artery. It attaches posteriorly to the descending aorta, potentially forming a ring, which can compress the trachea and esophagus in postnatal life (Fig. 3.42(a)). A posterior (aberrant) origin of the left subclavian artery in the setting of an otherwise apparently uncomplicated right sided aortic arch usually

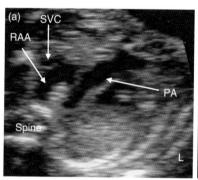

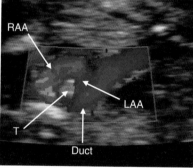

Fig. 3.42.(a). The transverse aorta divides into the left arch (LAA), which passes in front of the trachea, and the right arch (RAA), which stays on the right. This forms an "O" shape and has the potential for tracheal and esophageal compression postnatally. Although the trachea (T) is not well seen, it lies within the circle of the "O".

indicates the presence of a fibrous remnant completing an additional left arch (Fig. 3.42(a)) and therefore indicates the possibility of a vascular ring syndrome. The branching pattern of a right arch is not always easy to interpret, either before or after birth, in terms of its likelihood to cause symptoms. The fetus illustrated in Fig. 3.42(b) appears to have the characteristics of a double arch but the infant appears to be asymptomatic and therefore has not been subjected to magnetic resonance imaging which is the most reliable way of discerning the arch anatomy. It is possible that the "ring" is not complete between the left carotid and the left subclavian arteries.

Aorto-pulmonary window

This is a rare defect, which is difficult to identify in prenatal life. It is a direct communication between the

ascending aorta and the pulmonary artery just above the level of the pulmonary valve (Fig. 3.43). It is particularly important to exclude an associated abnormality of the aortic arch, such as coarctation or interruption, which are quite common associated features, and will have important implications for postnatal symptoms, management and outcome.

Constriction of the arterial duct

This is an uncommon lesion, which I have rarely seen and have no example of. It can occur with no apparent underlying cause in late gestation, although usually it will be secondary to maternal ingestion of non-steroidal anti-inflammatory medication. Indomethacin for polyhydramnios or for tocolysis is now rarely prescribed for this reason. The duct will appear narrow for

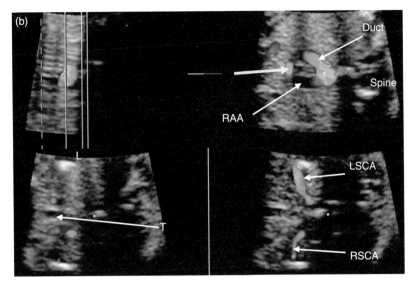

Fig. 3.42.(b). Tomographic planes are ideal to try to understand the branching pattern of an abnormal arch. In the top right-hand image, a right arch (RAA) is seen at the level of the duct. The first branch of the aorta (yellow arrow) passes in front of the trachea at this level towards the left. Just above this level, two arteries are seen arising symmetrically on each side of the trachea (bottom left image), the pattern which would be expected in a double arch. The anterior vessels should be the left and right carotid arteries and the posterior the left and right subclavian arteries. The most cranial section is seen on the lower right image, where it can be confirmed that the posterior vessels are the left (LSCA) and right subclavian arteries (RSCA).

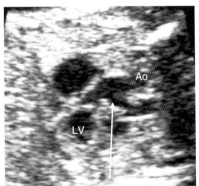
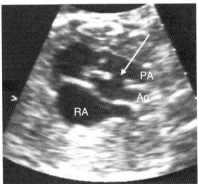

Fig. 3.43. The images in this condition can be confusing. On the left-hand panel, the great artery that arises from the left ventricle appears to be branching (arrow) – could it be transposition? But the vessel continues and gives rise to the aortic arch, excluding this possibility. Could it be a form of arterial trunk then? But the right-hand panel clearly shows two arterial valves and the septum is intact in other views, excluding this diagnosis. The defect is clearly shown in the right-hand panel, a "punched-out" hole (arrow) in the wall between the aorta and the pulmonary artery. This is a typical appearance of this unusual defect, an aorto-pulmonary window. The aorta falsely appears to "branch" through the aorto-pulmonary window.

the gestational age with an aliased color flow signal and increased Doppler velocity through it. It can lead to complete premature closure of the duct. Tricuspid regurgitation and poor right ventricular function will develop if ductal constriction is prolonged.

Absence of the arterial duct

This typically occurs in association with the absent pulmonary valve syndrome although it is not an invariable feature (Fig. 3.23). It is also a frequent finding with a common arterial trunk, except when there is associated aortic arch interruption.

Abnormal position of the arterial duct

A small, tortuous, abnormally positioned duct can be a feature of severe cases of tetralogy of Fallot with pulmonary atresia, particularly with non-confluent pulmonary arteries. Instead of connecting to the descending aorta as usual, the duct can arise from the undersurface of the aortic arch (Fig. 4.37) or even from the head, neck or arm vessels.

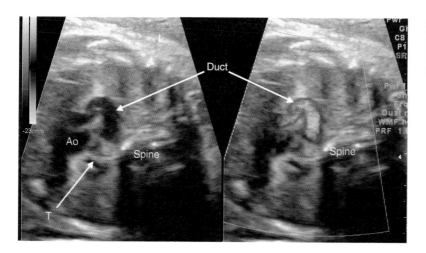

Fig. 3.44. In views of the upper thorax in late pregnancy, the duct often appears tortuous instead of its usual straight course in the earlier fetus (compare with Figs. 3.5, 3.8).

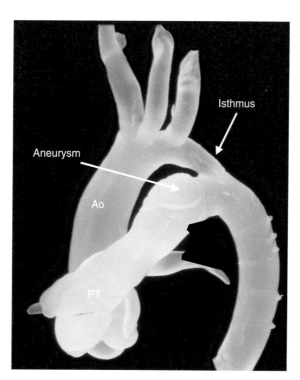

Fig. 3.45. A cast of the great arteries of a third trimester fetus is shown. There is a small aneurysm of the arterial duct present. In addition, despite the aortic isthmus being less than half the size of the ascending aorta, there was no discrete coarctation found.

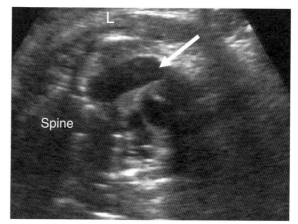

Fig. 3.46. Scanning in the upper thorax, in the three-vessel view, there appears to be a large cystic structure within the left upper chest (arrow). Color flow mapping showed it to be vascular and it could be connected to the main pulmonary artery and to the descending aorta. This is an aneurysm of the arterial duct, not an uncommon finding in the last weeks of pregnancy.

Tortuosity of the arterial duct

As gestation advances, the ductal connection between the pulmonary artery and the descending aorta becomes less straight and more tortuous (Fig. 3.44). It has been suggested that this can cause restriction to ductal flow, but this is probably not true and it is simply a normal variant in the mature fetus.

Ductal aneurysm

At the end of gestation, a bulbous, dilated duct is not an uncommon normal finding (Fig. 3.45). Sometimes this can be large enough to give the appearance of a cyst in the left chest (Fig. 3.46). However, color flow mapping will show it to be a vascular structure, connecting between the pulmonary artery and the descending aorta. A ductal aneurysm usually involutes after delivery without symptoms, although rarely it has been reported to rupture.

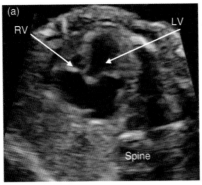
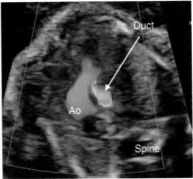

Fig. 3.47.(a). The four-chamber view on the left-hand panel shows a small right ventricle. On the color flow map of the great arteries, there is reverse flow in a small arterial duct. This is pulmonary atresia with intact ventricular septum.

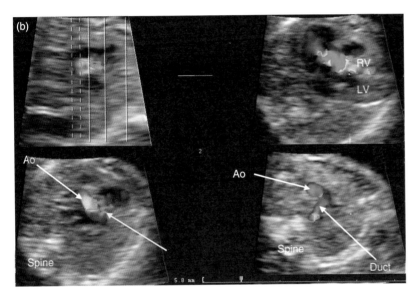

Fig. 3.47.(b). In the four-chamber view (upper right image), the heart is enlarged due to moderately severe tricuspid regurgitation seen on color flow mapping. This was due to Ebstein's malformation of the tricuspid valve. The bottom left image shows the origin of the aorta and a tiny ventricular septal defect (yellow arrow). On the bottom right image, in the three-vessel view, there is reverse flow seen in a small arterial duct. There was no forward flow across the pulmonary valve. This is pulmonary atresia in the setting of severe Ebstein's anomaly.

Abnormalities of great artery function

Valve atresia

The arterial valve will not open in **valvar atresia** and there will be **no flow** across the valve on color flow mapping or pulsed Doppler. The diagnosis will be confirmed by finding **reversed flow** in the **aortic arch** in aortic atresia (Fig. 3.17(a) and (b)) or **reverse flow** in the **arterial duct** in **pulmonary atresia** (Fig. 3.47).

Valve stenosis

An **arterial valve will not open** freely if it is stenosed and the valve cusps may be visible throughout the cardiac cycle (Fig. 3.48(a)), in contrast to the normal valve (Figs. 3.8 and 3.11). This will usually be combined with an **increased velocity of flow** across the narrowed valve, which is highlighted by aliasing of the color flow signal across the valve (Fig. 3.11). The Doppler velocity across a stenosed valve will generally be less than that associated with a similar degree of stenosis postnatally, because of the lower pressures in the fetal system and the capacity to divert flow through the non-obstructed side of the heart. The increase in Doppler velocity of flow will reflect the severity of valvar obstruction up to the point until ventricular function becomes compromised, at which time the velocity will then decrease. If

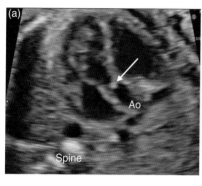 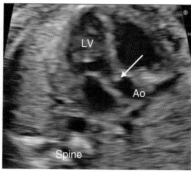

Fig. 3.48.(a). Throughout the cardiac cycle, the aortic valve could be seen, in contrast to the normal aortic valve. The left-hand panel is a diastolic frame and the right-hand panel a systolic frame, when the aortic valve cusps should open and "disappear" as they flatten against the arterial walls. This indicates aortic stenosis. Unusually, the aorta is of fairly normal size. The mitral valve does not open very much in diastole (left-hand panel), as there is a high pressure in the left ventricle, as a result of aortic stenosis.

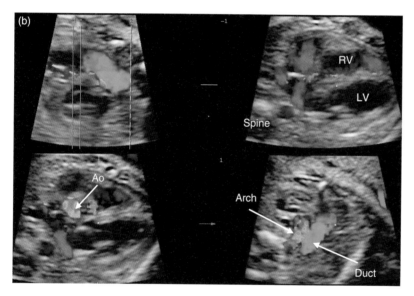

Fig. 3.48.(b). Three tomographic images are shown in aortic stenosis. In the four-chamber view (upper right), there is little filling of the left ventricle in comparison with the right. The shunt at the atrial septum is predominantly left to right. Despite the poor filling of the left ventricle, there is a jet of forward flow across the aortic valve (bottom left). However, there is reverse flow in the transverse aortic arch indicating severe aortic valve obstruction. Rather unusually here, the ascending aorta and transverse arch are of a good size.

the valvar obstruction is severe, there will be reversed flow in the aortic arch in aortic stenosis (Fig. 3.48(b)), or reverse flow in the arterial duct in pulmonary stenosis.

A modestly increased velocity of flow above the normal range, up to about 150 cm/s, may occur in the aorta in tetralogy of Fallot or in pulmonary atresia. The velocity of flow is increased to a similar extent in a common arterial trunk, or to higher values if the truncal valve is stenosed.

Valve regurgitation

Rarely, mild aortic regurgitation is seen in the fetus (Fig. 5.36) and has no pathological implication, but follow-up is recommended to exclude subsequent development of aortic valve disease. Severe aortic regurgitation is seen in the rare condition of aorto-left ventricular tunnel, when the regurgitant jet is around the valve rather than through it, via an abnormal tunnel-like communication between the ascending aorta and the left ventricle. Rarely, mild pulmonary

regurgitation is seen as a transitory finding in utero and it seems to have no pathological significance. Moderate or severe pulmonary regurgitation is characteristic of the absent pulmonary valve syndrome, a variant of the tetralogy of Fallot. We have now seen three cases of typical tetralogy of Fallot, with pulmonary regurgitation as an additional feature in early pregnancy (Fig. 3.49). One developed dilated branch pulmonary arteries later in pregnancy and behaved like a (relatively mild) case of absent pulmonary valve syndrome in postnatal life. In the two other cases, regurgitation became much less later in gestation and they behaved like the usual form of tetralogy after birth.

A truncal valve often shows regurgitation, which is usually mild, but can be moderate to severe if the valve is dysplastic (Fig. 3.28(a)).

Abnormal arch flow

Reverse flow in the aortic arch or arterial duct will confirm severe **obstruction to the left or right ventricular**

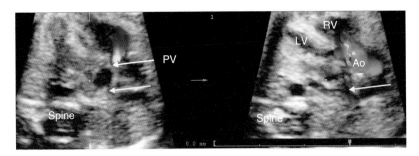

Fig. 3.49. Two tomographic images are displayed from a volume set obtained at 23 weeks of gestation. In the right image, in the left ventricular outflow tract view, the aorta arises astride the crest of the ventricular septum. The slice above the aorta (left-hand panel) shows the pulmonary artery. There is fairly marked pulmonary regurgitation from a thickened pulmonary valve (PV). The branch pulmonary arteries (yellow arrows) are actually a little smaller than normal, typical of the usual form of tetralogy of Fallot, in contrast to examples of the absent pulmonary valve syndrome (see Fig. 3.23).

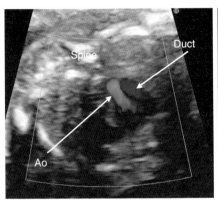
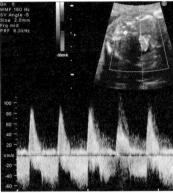

Fig. 3.50. The color flow map of the transverse arch and duct shows reverse flow in the arch in this 23-week fetus. This was confirmed on pulsed Doppler in the right-hand panel. The aortic valve was normal with forward flow across it, excluding left ventricular outflow tract obstruction as the cause, and the fetus was normal in size for the gestational age, also excluding growth retardation as the diagnosis. This finding was due to an arteriovenous malformation in the head.

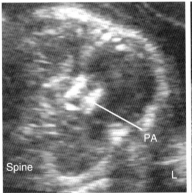
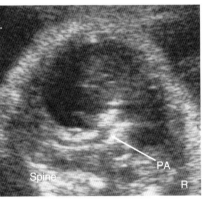

Fig. 3.51. Two cases are shown of increased echogenicity in the arterial walls. The fetus on the left-hand panel had severe late untreated twin–twin transfusion syndrome and subsequently died. The fetus on the right-hand panel had a large pericardial effusion and ascites with excess calcification of other vessels due to idiopathic arterial calcification of infancy (see also Fig. 4.46).

outflow tracts, respectively. Alternatively, reverse flow in the arch can indicate **severe growth retardation** or an **arteriovenous fistula in the brain** (Fig. 3.50).

Bidirectional flow in either the aortic arch or the pulmonary artery and arterial duct can be seen in the early (11–14-week) fetus associated with trisomy 18 or 13. It may indicate dysplasia or even absence of the arterial valve cusps (see Chapter 6).

In **arterial duct constriction**, the color flow map will show aliasing and the Doppler velocity within it will be increased above the normal range.

Miscellaneous rarities

Figure 3.51 illustrates an unusual finding in the great arteries where the vessel walls appear abnormally echogenic. This can occur in the recipient twin in severe twin-to-twin transfusion syndrome or the autosomal recessive condition idiopathic arterial calcification of infancy. Idiopathic arterial calcification becomes apparent only beyond about 26 weeks of gestation and is characterized by extensive calcification of the large arteries and coronary arteries, pericardial effusion and polyhydramnios.

Summary

There are only a limited number of abnormalities of the great arteries. These are:

Aortic atresia, stenosis or dysplasia

Aorto-left ventricular tunnel

Pulmonary atresia, stenosis or dysplasia

Arterial valve override

Aortic valve overriding

Tetralogy of Fallot with pulmonary stenosis or atresia

"Shared" arterial valve overriding

Common arterial trunk

Pulmonary valve overriding

Pulmonary override in double outlet right ventricle or transposition

Transposition of the great arteries

With AV concordance

With AV discordance (corrected transposition)

Double outlet right ventricle

Arch anomalies

Right aortic arch

Double aortic arch

Aberrant right subclavian artery

Coarctation

Interruption of the aorta

Aorto-pulmonary window

Abnormalities of the arterial duct

Small

Constricted

Absent

Abnormally positioned

Tortuous

Aneurysmal

Abnormalities of the superior vena cava

Small (or, rarely, absent) in persistent left superior vena cava

Dilated in intracranial AV malformation or supracardiac total anomalous pulmonary venous drainage

Arterial wall calcification

Additional views: normal and abnormal

In Chapters 2 and 3, the focus has been on the standard, most important views of the fetal heart and how their appearance may deviate from the normal. In my opinion, the most important and useful views are the four-chamber view and the transverse sweep of the great arteries, up to the arch and duct. However, there are other views of the fetal heart or its vascular connections, which are important to recognize and understand, as they may be useful if the transverse views are difficult to obtain, or they may contribute additional information to the diagnosis in an abnormal heart. The method of obtaining all the views has been described in Chapter 1.

Transverse section of upper abdomen

Normally, very early in the development of the embryo, the fetus develops a left and a right side. Although many parts of the body are mirror images of the other side, for example, the limbs, some of the thoracic and abdominal organs are different on each side, that is, they demonstrate laterality. The main structures that demonstrate laterality are the bronchi, the pectinate muscles of the atria or intra-atrial "trabeculations," the atrial appendages, the liver, intestines, spleen, and the inferior vena cava (Fig. 4.1). The atria and bronchi and lungs are paired structures, with one to each side, but have an intrinsically different form in their right and left types. For example, a normal right lung has a three-lobed form and a left lung has two lobes. Generally, the structures on the same side of the body will share the same form when there is an abnormality of laterality. Thus, if the right-sided bronchus has left type form it is

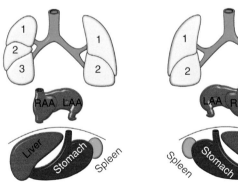
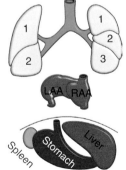

Normal situs

Usual

Mirror image or situs inversus

Mirror image

Fig. 4.1. Laterality is illustrated in cartoon form. In the normal, the lungs, bronchi, atrial appendages, liver and spleen are not identical on both sides, but instead show laterality. There is a longer bronchus on the left than the right and the left lung is bilobed, the right trilobed. The right atrial appendage has a broad junction with the atrium, whereas the left has a narrow junction. The liver lies on the right, the stomach and spleen on the left. Note that the arrangement in situs inversus (right-hand panel) is a mirror image of the normal, with the normal right-sided structures on the left and vice versa.

likely that the right-sided atrium will also have left type form, but there are exceptions to this.

There are **three possibilities for abnormality of laterality**. The first is **situs inversus, or mirror image** arrangement (Fig. 4.1). Here structures on each side are different, but the left side of the body will have the form normally associated with a right-sided position, whereas the structures on the right side of the body will have the form associated with the left-sided position. There are also cases when both sides of the body have organs of identical form, either both of left type or both of right type. These are referred to as **left and right isomerism**, respectively (Fig. 4.2), or collectively as **situs ambiguus**. An individual case will show some or all of the organs affected but the most reliable aspect is the atrial anatomy. There is normally a broad,

blunt atrial appendage, with a broad junction to the atrial mass on the right and a pointed atrial appendage, with a narrow junction, on the left (Fig. 4.3(a)), which sometimes can be appreciated echocardiographically in various non-standard views (Fig. 4.3(b)). There are some features, which can only be seen in the anatomical specimen, which are more definitive determinants of laterality, unlike the echocardiographic features, which can be inconsistent. In the opened atria, the pectinate muscles reach the crux in the right, but not in the left atrium (Fig. 4.4(a) and (b)). Bilateral left-type atrial appendages and bronchi, a central liver, malrotation of the intestines, an interrupted inferior caval vein and polysplenia are typical, but not all invariably present, features of left isomerism. Bilateral right-type atrial appendages and bronchi, a central liver, malrotation of

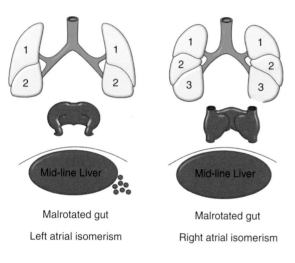

Left atrial isomerism

Right atrial isomerism

Fig. 4.2. In heterotaxy syndromes or situs ambiguus, there are either two left-type sides or two right-type sides, in left or right isomerism, respectively, affecting the bronchi, lungs and atrial appendages. In both syndromes, the liver is midline and there is a high incidence of malrotation of the gut. In left isomerism, there tend to be multiple small spleens, whereas in right isomerism, there is usually asplenia.

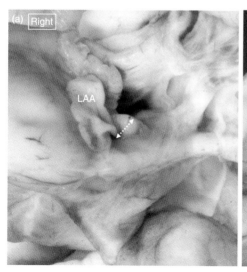
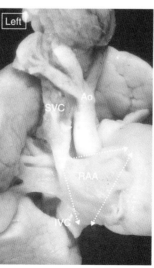

Fig. 4.3.(a). The shape of the atrial appendages are seen in a close-up view. Note the broad shape to the right appendage (left-hand image) as compared to the narrow, hooked shape of the left (right-hand image). The right appendage has a broad junction to the right atrium (left-hand panel) whereas the left has a narrow junction (right-hand panel).

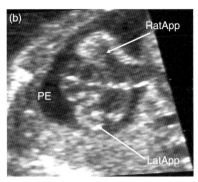

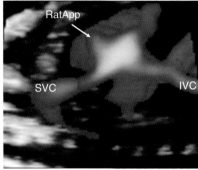

Fig. 4.3.(b). Contd. The atrial appendages are not usually well seen echocardiographically in the normal heart, except when they are outlined with fluid in a pericardial effusion (PE), as in the left-hand panel. The right appendage (RatApp) is broad and blunt in comparison with the narrower pointed left appendage (LatApp). In a power Doppler, glassbody-rendered long-axis view of the inferior and superior vena caval junction (right-hand panel), the right appendage (RatApp) is well seen. Note its particular shape. The left atrial appendage unfortunately cannot be as readily seen for comparison with the right with this type of imaging.

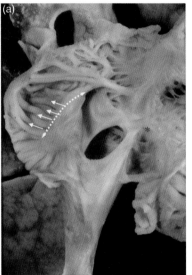

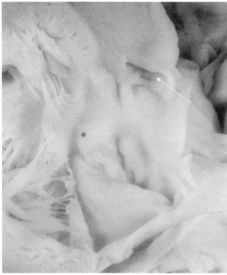

Fig. 4.4.(a). On the right side of the heart (left-hand panel), the right atrium is opened to show that the pectinate muscles (yellow arrows) reach to the crux of the heart, marked by the red star. On the left side of the heart (right panel), with the left atrium open, the pectinate muscles (arrow) are confined to the atrial appendage, resulting in a smooth surface on the left atrial side of the crux (red star).

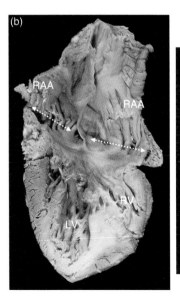

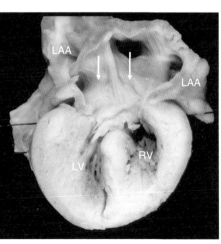

Fig. 4.4.(b). On the left-hand image, the heart is cut in a four-chamber view. Both atria show pectinate muscles reaching the crux of the heart and therefore are morphologically right atria on both sides. On the right-hand image, both atrial appendages are narrow and pointed with smooth surfaces (arrows) reaching to the crux of the heart. This is left atrial isomerism. Note that both hearts also show a common atrioventricular junction, the most common mode of connection in laterality syndromes. Also, that the ventricles are the mirror image of normal. The anatomically right ventricle, which is therefore left sided, is also hypoplastic in both examples of isomerism illustrated here.

the intestines and asplenia are typical but not invariably found in right isomerism (Figs. 4.5 and 4.6). There is asplenia in about 75% of cases of right isomerism, whereas polysplenia occurs in about 95% of cases of left isomerism. Malrotation of the gut occurs in over 50% of both conditions. The stomach and heart are discordant for side (on opposite sides, whether the heart is left or right sided) in over 50% of cases, slightly more frequently in right than in left isomerism.

The importance of laterality abnormalities to fetal echocardiography is that they are frequently associated with intracardiac defects of characteristic types. Although most of the features indicating laterality can only be seen in the anatomical specimen, the relative arrangement of the inferior caval vein and aorta in the upper abdomen (the abdominal situs) can be used echocardiographically to identify laterality, mostly, though not always completely, reliably.

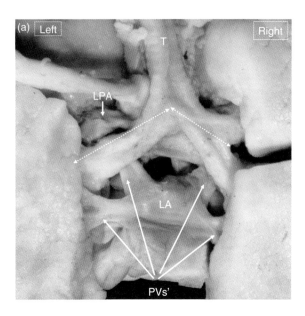

Fig. 4.5.(a). The bronchi are seen from the back in the normal fetus. On the right side, the bronchus branches after a short distance from the trachea (T), whereas the left bronchus appears longer. Note the position of the four pulmonary veins joining the left atrium, and the left pulmonary artery (LPA) above the left bronchus.

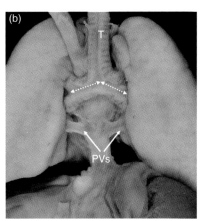
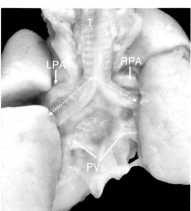

Fig. 4.5.(b). On the left-hand panel, the two bronchi appear the same from the back and are both short, like right bronchi. This is right atrial isomerism. On the right-hand panel, the two bronchi are long, like left bronchi. This is left atrial isomerism.

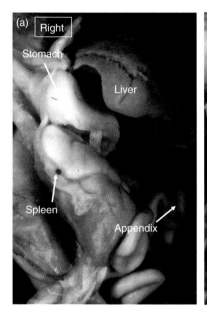 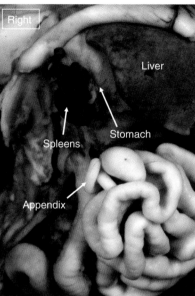

Fig. 4.6.(a). The organs in the abdomen are seen in a case of right atrial isomerism on the left-hand panel and left isomerism on the right-hand panel. There is only a tiny knob representing the spleen in right isomerism and multiple spleens in left isomerism. Note here the central liver, abnormal gut position and that the stomach is right-sided in both examples.

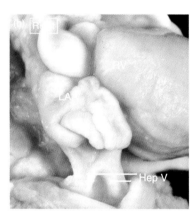 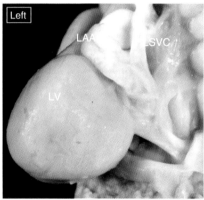

Fig. 4.6.(b). There are narrow hooked appendages to both atrial appendages, in this example of left atrial isomerism.

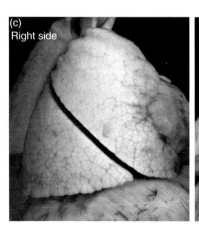 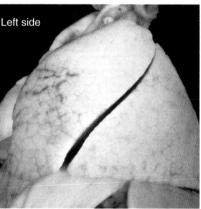

Fig. 4.6.(c). Both lungs are bi-lobed (like left lungs) in this case of left atrial isomerism.

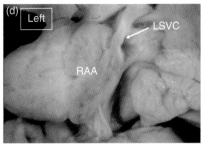
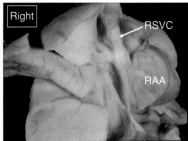

Fig. 4.6.(d). Contd. The atria on both sides of the heart are broad and blunt in this case of right atrial isomerism.

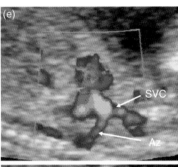
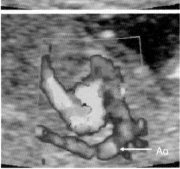
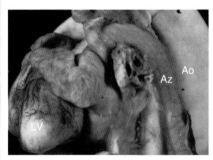

Fig. 4.6.(e). A typical feature of left atrial isomerism is that the inferior caval vein is interrupted in the abdomen. The blood returning to the heart finds an alternative route in the azygous vein (Az), which becomes dilated. The azygous vein drains to the superior vena cava just below the level of the aortic arch. This can be appreciated in the echocardiographic images on the left-hand panels, which are obtained from the same cineloop of the same patient, to illustrate the aortic arch in a slightly different plane of section, just above the azygous vein.

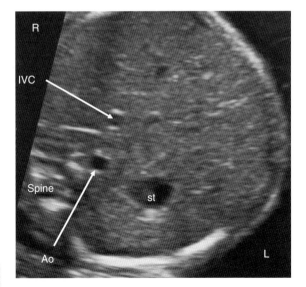

Fig. 4.7. A cross-section through the upper abdomen shows the stomach (st) lying to the left, in its typical position with the inferior vena cava anterior and to the right of it. The relative position of the descending aorta and inferior vena cava are a relatively reliable predictor of atrial situs. The fetus lies HB.

Normal appearance

The aorta lies posteriorly in the upper abdomen, just to the left of the spine, whereas the inferior vena cava lies more anteriorly and to the right of the aorta (Fig. 4.7). This pattern reflects normal situs or **situs solitus**.

Possible deviations from normal

(1) The stomach and aorta lie to the right with the inferior vena cava to the left in inverted situs or **situs inversus** (Fig. 4.8). This is the mirror image of normal. This can occur with the apex also on the right (complete situs inversus) or less commonly with the apex on the left (inverted abdominal

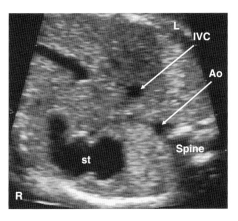

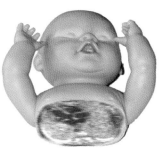

Fig. 4.8. At first glance, the left-hand panel appears to show normal atrial situs, as the stomach (st), aorta and inferior caval vein are in a normal relationship to one another, and the apex was on the same side of the fetus as the stomach. Only by working out the fetal position could it be seen that both the stomach and the heart lay on the right side of the fetus. The head of the fetus here was found to be behind the screen (HB), not in front of it as expected.

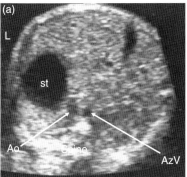

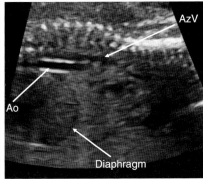

Fig. 4.9.(a). In the left-hand panel, the abdominal vessels are seen in left atrial isomerism in a transverse section. Note the aorta lying to the left with the azygous vein (AzV) alongside it. In the long-axis view in the right-hand panel, two vessels of approximately equal size are seen in the abdomen and crossing the diaphragm into the thorax.

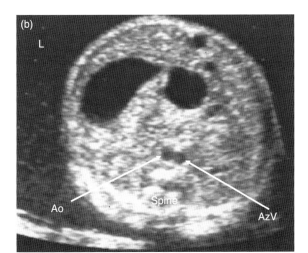

Fig. 4.9.(b). The characteristic arrangement of two vessels, the aorta and the azygous vein, in the posterior abdomen is seen. There is a "double bubble" appearance of the stomach. This is not due to duodenal atresia but to bowel obstruction from gastrointestinal malrotation in left atrial isomerism. Malrotation is common in isomerism syndromes although it does not usually present until after birth.

situs). Note that the pattern of the relationship between the stomach, aorta and inferior vena cava appears normal but if the operator has worked out the left–right orientation as explained in Chapter 1, he/she will know that the stomach lies on the right side of the fetus instead of the left.

(2) There is no detectable inferior vena cava in its usual position, but there is a dilated azygous vein lying behind or to the right of the aorta (Fig. 4.9(a) and (b)). This (nearly always) indicates that the inferior vena cava is interrupted or atretic at the level of the kidneys. This usually, though not always, indicates **left atrial isomerism** (or two left sides). An interrupted inferior vena cava occurs in 90% of left atrial isomerism. The blood from the lower body then drains to the heart using an alternative route, the azygous vein, which is normally present though small (Fig. 4.10(a)), but which dilates and becomes more readily visible when this extra volume of blood is delivered to it because of interruption of the inferior vena cava.

121

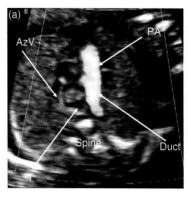
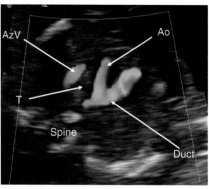

Fig. 4.10.(a). The normal azygous vein (AzV), seen on the left-hand panel, can often be seen in views of the upper thorax when imaging the transverse arch and arterial duct, but usually only on color flow mapping. It drains to the superior vena cava, which lies to the right of the ascending aorta. The trachea (T) lies between the azygous vein and the transverse portion of the aortic arch. On the right-hand panel, the azygous vein can be seen in the transverse views to be dilated, because of interruption of the interior vena cava in left atrial isomerism.

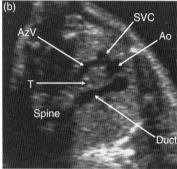
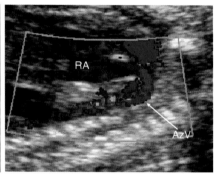

Fig. 4.10.(b). The transverse view of a dilated azygous connection is seen on the left-hand panel on 2D, and the long axis view of the azygous connection to the superior vena cava on color flow on the right-hand panel, in left isomerism.

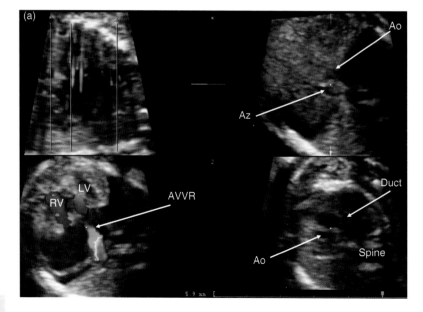

Fig. 4.11.(a). In the abdomen, the aorta and azygous veins are seen lying side-by-side posteriorly (upper right image). In the four-chamber view, there is marked cardiomegaly. There was a partial atrioventricular septal defect and moderately severe atrioventricular valve regurgitation (AVVR). In the three-vessel view, the aorta was very small as a result of coarctation.

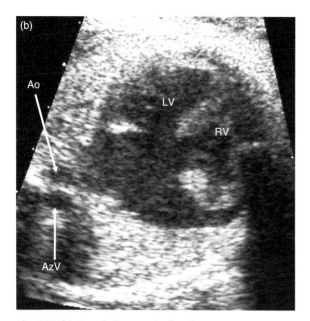

Fig. 4.11.(b). Contd. Two vessels of similar size are seen in cross-section behind the four-chamber view. These are the descending aorta and azygous vein. The azygous vein lies slightly posterior and to the right of the aorta, although its position relative to the aorta can vary. Note that the four-chamber view also demonstrates a complete atrioventricular septal defect.

The azygous vein lies in a variable position beside the aorta, travels up through the diaphragm and connects to the superior vena cava just below the aortic arch and can be seen on transverse as well as longitudinal views of the upper mediastinum (Fig. 4.10(b)). The intracardiac findings in left atrial isomerism are variable. There is most commonly an atrioventricular septal defect, but a simple ventricular septal defect or normal intracardiac anatomy is possible. The great arteries are usually normally connected but double outlet right ventricle, pulmonary or aortic stenosis or coarctation can all be found. Cardiomegaly, especially in the setting of complete heart block is common (Fig. 4.11(a)). Two vessels (instead of one), the aorta and the azygous vein, are seen in short axis behind the heart on a four-chamber projection (Fig. 4.11(b)). Note that the esophagus can sometimes be seen behind a four-chamber view, lying between the aorta and the left atrium (Fig. 4.11(c)), but this is in a different position from the azygous vein. This structure does not fill on color flow mapping indicating that it is not vascular in nature (Fig. 4.11(d)).

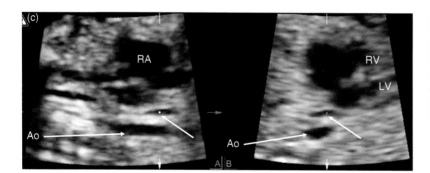

Fig. 4.11.(c). In the long-axis view on the left-hand panel, there is a tubular structure passing through the diaphragm anterior to the aorta. Positioning the dot (arrowhead) in the structure allows its relationship to the four-chamber view to be seen in the right-hand panel. It lies in the midline (unlike the azygous vein) between the aorta and the left atrium.

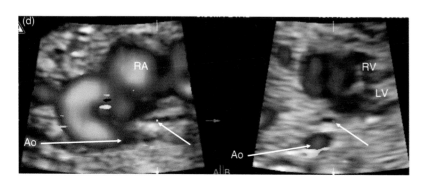

Fig. 4.11.(d). The color flow map shows that this structure is not vascular, so it must be the esophagus, which should not be confused with the azygous vein. The esophagus is not usually seen, but can be if image quality is good or if it is dilated in upper bowel obstruction.

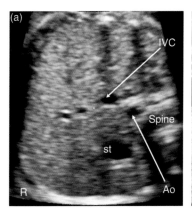
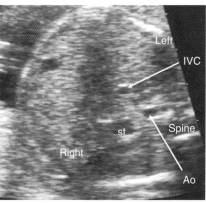

Fig. 4.12.(a). In both these abdominal cross-sectional views, the stomach lies on the right but in the four-chamber view, the apex lay on the left side. The aorta and inferior vena cava both lie on the left, close to each other in an abnormal positional relationship (compare with Fig. 4.7). This is suggestive of right atrial isomerism.

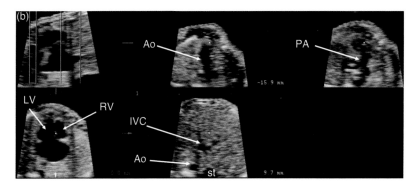

Fig. 4.12.(b). In the abdomen, the aorta and inferior vena cava lay on the same side of the fetus, on the opposite side to the stomach, which lay on the left side (lower middle image). There was a complete atrioventricular septal defect in the four-chamber view (lower left image). The pulmonary artery (upper right) arose from the right ventricle below the level of the aorta (upper middle), which also arose from the right ventricle. The pulmonary artery was smaller than the aorta indicating pulmonary stenosis. This combination of findings are typical for right atrial isomerism.

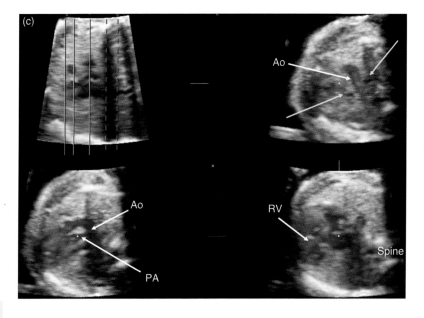

Fig. 4.12.(c). In the four-chamber view (lower right), there was only flow across the right-sided atrioventricular component of a common valve. Both great arteries arose from the right ventricle, with the aorta anterior to and larger than the pulmonary artery, indicating double outlet right ventricle with pulmonary stenosis. Bilateral superior caval veins (yellow arrows) can be seen in the view of the aortic arch. These findings are all common features in right isomerism.

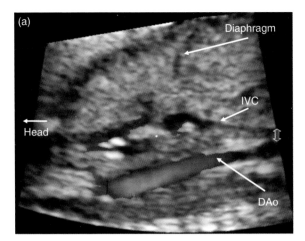

Fig. 4.13.(a). The descending aorta (DAo) and inferior vena cava (IVC) are seen in long-axis views to lie close together in the lower abdomen (double-headed red arrow) and separate as they approach the diaphragm, with the aorta passing behind the heart to the upper thorax and the inferior vena cava connecting to the right atrium at the base of the heart.

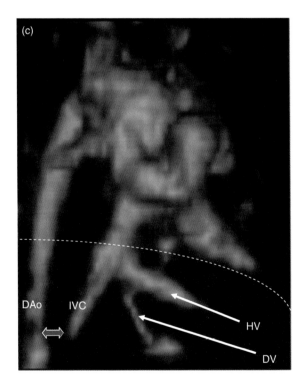

Fig. 4.13.(c). In the rendered image, the "funnel" shape of the ductus venosus is seen below the heart, joining the hepatic vein, just at its junction with the inferior vena cava. Note how the aorta and inferior vena cava are close together in the lower abdomen (red double-headed arrow) and separate as they approach the diaphragm, represented by the dotted line.

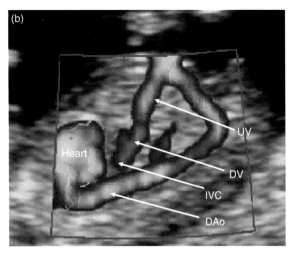

Fig. 4.13.(b). The ductus venosus is seen in a long-axis view of the abdomen connecting the umbilical vein to the inferior vena cava.

(3) The aorta and inferior vena cava lie on the same side of the fetus (either to the right or left of the midline), closer together than normal. This usually indicates **right atrial isomerism** (Fig. 4.12(a)). This is usually a clue to the presence of a complex cardiac malformation (Fig. 4.12(b) and (c)).

(4) If an area of accelerated **high velocity flow** is seen **in the abdomen** (as there was in the case illustrated in the left-hand panel in Fig. 4.15) this can indicate the point of junction of a descending vein draining a pulmonary venous confluence in **infracardiac total anomalous pulmonary venous drainage** or can be due to **turbulence in the ductus venosus**.

Long-axis view of the abdominal vessels

This view is necessary for obtaining the Doppler flow profile in the ductus venosus.

Normal appearance

The aorta and inferior vena cava have a particular pattern of relationship in the long-axis view of the abdomen, with the vessels close together in the lower abdomen but separating as they course towards the diaphragm (Fig. 4.13(a)). The aorta remains posterior to pass behind the heart, whereas the inferior vena cava is joined by the ductus venosus and the hepatic veins, and is directed anteriorly to pass through the diaphragm to its connection to the base of the right atrium (Fig. 4.13(b) and (c)).

125

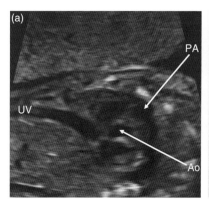
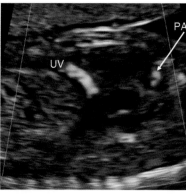

Fig. 4.14.(a). A dilated vessel is seen in the abdomen, which connects directly between the umbilical vein (UV) and the inferior vena cava at its junction with the right atrium. This is due to an absent ductus venosus.

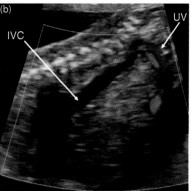
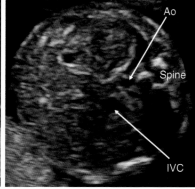

Fig. 4.14.(b). The inferior vena cava was dilated in longitudinal (left-hand panel) and transverse (right-hand panel) views, due to direct drainage of the umbilical vein (UV) into one of the iliac veins in the pelvis.

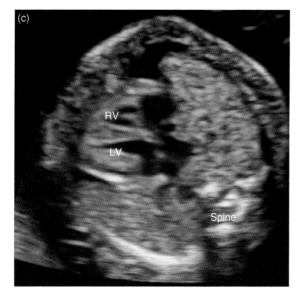

Possible deviations from normal

Absence of the ductus venosus

This is a fairly uncommon anomaly where the umbilical vein connects directly to the right atrium or other vein without the restriction of flow which occurs in the normal venous duct (Fig. 4.14(a)). If the umbilical vein drains directly to it, the inferior vena cava is dilated (Fig. 4.14(b)). This leads to mild right atrial and ventricular dilatation, which can sometimes progress to cause fetal hydrops (Fig. 4.14(c)). Apart from some volume overload, it is usually benign from the cardiac point of view, but has implications for lung or hepatic function postnatally.

Fig. 4.14.(c). There is mild skin edema and small pleural effusions as a result of absence of the ductus venosus.

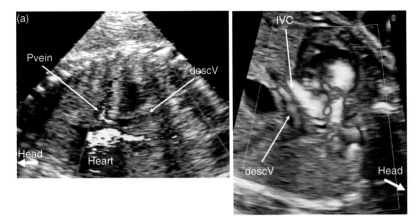

Fig. 4.15.(a). On the left-hand panel, there is an additional vessel seen in the abdomen, which drained to the portal system in the liver. This is a descending vein (desc V) draining a confluence of the pulmonary veins (Pvein), which does not connect to the left atrium. On the right-hand panel, there is a vein passing through the diaphragm connecting a pulmonary venous confluence, which lay behind the heart (see Fig. 2.51(c)), with the portal system. Both fetuses had right atrial isomerism with infracardiac drainage of all the pulmonary veins.

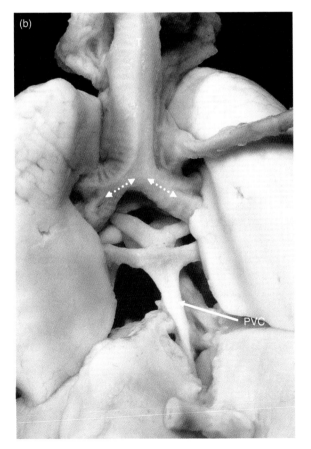

Fig. 4.15.(b). In this pathological specimen, the bronchi are symmetrically "short," like right bronchi (dotted arrows). The pulmonary veins form a confluence (PVC) behind the heart, do not connect to the left atrium but drained via a descending vessel below the diaphragm to the portal system. This is right isomerism with infracardiac total anomalous pulmonary venous drainage. Compare this with the normal in the same projection in Fig. 4.5(a).

Infradiaphragmatic drainage of totally anomalous pulmonary veins

When the pulmonary veins drain to a confluence, which then drains below the diaphragm, there is an additional vessel passing through the diaphragm with caudal flow in it (Fig. 4.15(a)), therefore flow in the same direction as the aorta, although it is venous flow on the Doppler pattern. It usually drains into the portal system or directly to the inferior vena cava (Fig. 4.15(b)). The junction site is usually partially obstructed leading to an area of high velocity flow within the liver.

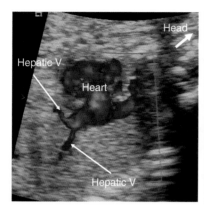
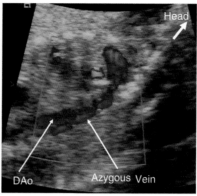

Fig. 4.16. Searching the base of the right atrium in a long-axis view, no inferior vena cava could be found. However, hepatic veins could be seen draining directly into the atrial chambers (left-hand panel). In a different plane of section in the same patient (right-hand panel), the dilated azygous vein could be seen lying behind the descending aorta in this case of left atrial isomerism.

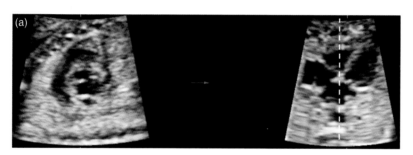

Fig. 4.17.(a). On the left side, the left ventricle is seen in its short axis, just below the aortic origin, with the right ventricular outflow tract arching over the front of it. The section at right angles to this view shows the cut through the four-chamber projection necessary to obtain this view. The beam cuts through the right ventricle anteriorly and the left in short axis posteriorly.

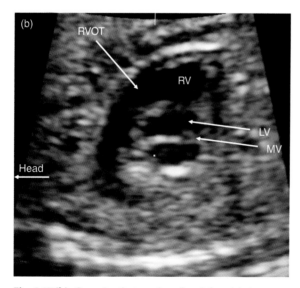

Fig. 4.17.(b). Sweeping the transducer from left to right in a sagittal section shows the left ventricle from the apex to the mitral valve ring in short-axis views. This particular section is at the level of the mitral valve in the left ventricle and also cuts through the right ventricular outflow tract anteriorly.

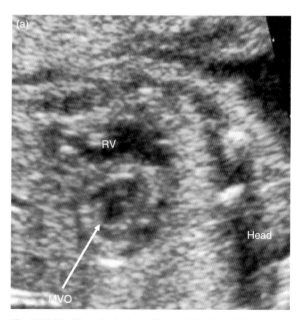

Fig. 4.18.(a). The mitral valve orifice (MVO) has been likened to a fish-mouth as it opens. In the normal heart, it fills most of the left ventricular cavity when open, as here.

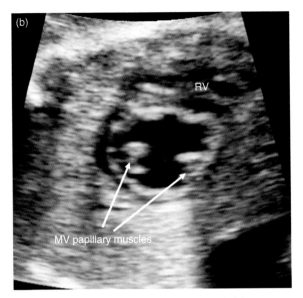

Fig. 4.18.(b). Contd. When the beam is moved slightly more apically from Fig. 4.18(a), the papillary muscles, which support the mitral valve leaflets via the chordae, are seen in the free wall of the left ventricle.

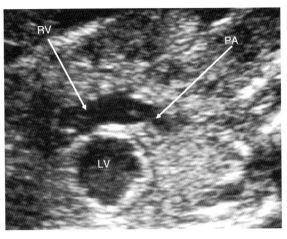

Fig. 4.19. In this case of critical aortic stenosis, the left ventricle was a tense circular structure with very little contraction in the moving image, whereas the right ventricle contracted normally anterior to the left.

Interrupted inferior vena cava

No inferior vena cava is seen in the usual position (Fig. 4.16) and in other views two vessels are seen posteriorly which pass through the diaphragm behind the heart (see also Fig. 4.9). As indicated above, this is a common feature of left atrial isomerism. In the more posterior vessel, flow is cranial, in the opposite direction to the aorta, which is usually the more anterior vessel of the two. The posterior vessel is the azygous continuation of the inferior vena cava, which is interrupted at about the level of the renal vessels. The hepatic veins, which usually join the inferior vena cava before it passes through the diaphragm, thus drain directly to the floor of the atrial mass.

Short-axis view of the left ventricle

This is not an essential view to obtain during routine scanning but can be useful in specific situations. It should be readily obtainable and recognizable to the experienced scanner. Figure 4.17(a) shows that it is obtained in a sagittal plane, slightly to the left of the midline.

Normal appearance

The right ventricle is "banana-shaped" in this section and lies anterior to the left ventricle, which is circular in shape (Fig. 4.17(b)). The operator should become familiar with the normal size relationship of the ventricles in this view, with the width of the right ventricle similar to the width of the left, although this is better appreciated in other views. The contraction of the left ventricle in particular can be readily assessed visually in this view. There is a valve in both ventricles, which are separated from each other by the interventricular septum, which should be intact. The mitral valve has a "fish-mouth" appearance on opening (Fig. 4.18(a)). Sweeping more apically, there are two papillary muscles (supporting the mitral valve) seen in the body of the left ventricle positioned around the circumference (Fig. 4.18(b)).

Possible deviations from normal

An **abnormal size relationship** of the ventricles is usually better seen in other views, particularly the four-chamber view, but hypoplasia of the left or right ventricle can also be noted in this view. Causes of abnormal ventricular sizes are detailed in Chapter 2. **Diminished contraction** of the ventricles, especially of the left can be well appreciated in this view (Fig. 4.19). Causes of diminished contraction of the ventricles are detailed

129

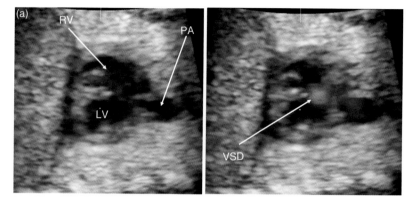

Fig. 4.20.(a). In the short-axis view of the left ventricle, the right ventricle and pulmonary artery are seen anteriorly. There is a defect in the muscular part of the ventricular septum, which was seen best on color flow mapping in the systolic frame on the right-hand panel. All the blood flow was from left to right, indicating some form of associated left ventricular outflow obstruction, in this case, coarctation.

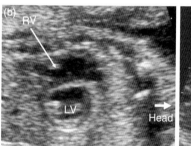
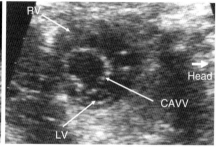

Fig. 4.20.(b). The fetuses shown in both panels lie in the same position with the head to the right and the abdomen to the left. Note the difference between the normal short-axis view of the left ventricle on the left-hand panel and an atrioventricular septal defect on the right. The mitral valve lies completely in the left ventricle in the normal, whereas the leaflets of the common valve (CAVV) are shared between both ventricles across the ventricular septal defect.

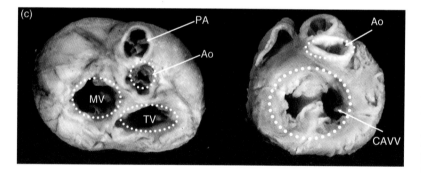

Fig. 4.20.(c). The atria are removed and the pathological specimens are viewed from the atria, looking towards the apex. In the normal heart on the left, there are two discrete valve orifices. The common valve (CAVV) on the right, has one valve ring and opens across the line of the ventricular septum as the valve leaflets are shared between the two ventricles. Note that the normal wedging of the aortic valve between, and closely related to, the two atrioventricular valves is lost in an atrioventricular septal defect, as it is displaced above the common valve ring.

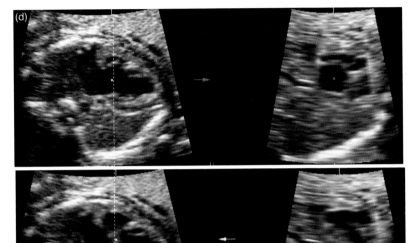

Fig. 4.20.(d). Contd. There is a common atrioventricular valve, seen open in the upper left-hand panel on the four-chamber view. The view obtained through the line indicated on the left-sided images are shown on the right. Note the common valve opening to both ventricles. The common valve is closed in the lower panels. This is an unbalanced atrioventricular septal defect to a dominant right ventricle.

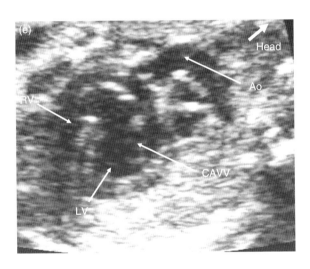

Fig. 4.20.(e). The heart is viewed in a short-axis view of the left ventricle. The common atrioventricular valve can be seen shared between the two ventricles (CAVV). The aorta overrides the ventricular septum at its origin. This is an atrioventricular septal defect with tetralogy of Fallot.

in Chapter 2. **Muscular ventricular septal defects** can sometimes be confirmed in this view (Fig. 4.20(a)), although they will usually be seen initially on the four-chamber view. In an **atrioventricular septal defect**, the valve ring can be seen "en face" in this view, allowing recognition of the shared nature of this valve across both ventricles (Fig. 4.20(b)–(d)). An atrioventricular septal defect can occur with tetralogy of Fallot, which will be associated with trisomy 21 in over 50% of cases (Fig. 4.20(e)).

In some cases of **mitral stenosis**, the papillary muscles can be seen lying closer together than normal, or even fused, and the limited opening of the valve can be appreciated (Fig. 4.21(a)). The pulmonary valve can often be well seen in this section. In Fig. 4.21(b), the **pulmonary valve** is seen to be **thickened and dysplastic** in this view. It was restricted in opening in the moving image, with an increased velocity of flow on pulsed Doppler. In Fig. 4.21(c), the infundibulum (the muscular sleeve of tissue below the pulmonary valve) was patent and the pulmonary artery was a good size but the valve did not open throughout the whole cardiac cycle. The color flow map (Fig. 4.21(d)) confirmed **pulmonary atresia**.

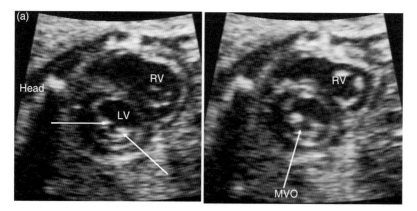

Fig. 4.21.(a). In the left-hand panel, the papillary muscles of the mitral valve are seen as they attach to the wall of the left ventricle (arrows). Here they are slightly closer together than normal. As the beam moves slightly higher in the left ventricle, the orifice of the mitral valve (MVO) is seen, opening less than normal (compare with Fig. 4.18 (a)). This is due to moderate mitral stenosis.

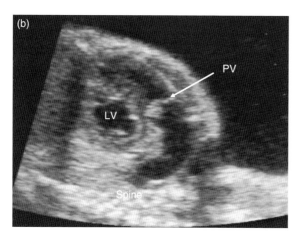

Fig. 4.21.(b). In the short-axis view of the left ventricle, the pulmonary valve can often be well seen, as it is here. In this fetus, the valve is thickened and dysplastic in a case of trisomy 18.

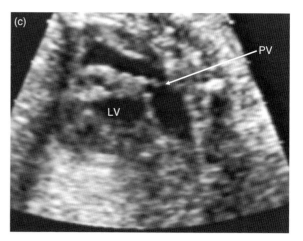

Fig. 4.21.(c). In the short-axis view of the left ventricle, the infundibulum of the right ventricle was patent but the pulmonary valve (PV) did not "disappear" during systole, as it normally does when the valve opens.

Long-axis view of the left ventricle

This is similar to the view of the aortic origin obtained in a transverse sweep but the transducer is slightly more tilted (see Chapter 1) in order to "open out" the left ventricular outflow tract (Fig. 4.22).

Normal appearance

The continuity of the ventricular septum with the anterior wall of the aorta is seen more clearly than in the straight transverse view of the aortic origin (compare Fig. 4.22 with Fig. 3.6, for example). In addition, there is continuity of the anterior leaflet of the mitral valve with the posterior wall of the aorta. Although the coronary arteries arise from the aorta just above its origin from the left ventricle, these are usually too small to be seen. However, in late pregnancy, after about 35 weeks gestation (or earlier if the fetus is growth retarded and

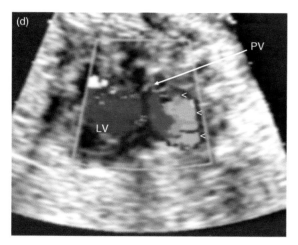

Fig. 4.21.(d). The color flow map showed reverse flow coming into the main pulmonary artery from the arterial duct (arrowheads), being reflected off the atretic pulmonary valve and then flowing forward (in blue) to reach the branch pulmonary arteries. This fetus had pulmonary atresia with intact ventricular septum.

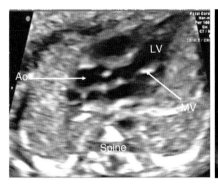
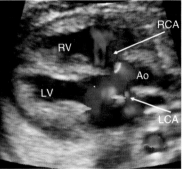

Fig. 4.22. The transducer has been angled slightly on the aortic origin in order to see a longer length of aorta as it arises. On the left-hand panel, this shows more clearly the continuity of the ventricular septum with the anterior wall of the aorta. There is also continuity of the posterior wall of the aorta with the anterior leaflet of the mitral valve (MV). Usually there are no early branches visible to the vessel arising from the left ventricle, thus designating it the aorta. However, in late pregnancy (after about 35 weeks) the coronary arteries can sometimes be seen on color flow mapping when imaging is ideal (right-hand panel). They arise from the aorta just above the aortic valve.

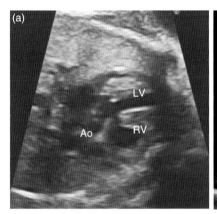
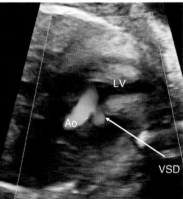

Fig. 4.23.(a). There is a ventricular septal defect seen in the long-axis view of the aorta. The aorta, however, still arises wholly from the left ventricle (compare with Fig. 4.23(b)). There is a left-to-right shunt across the defect on color flow mapping in the right-hand panel. This is a perimembranous defect.

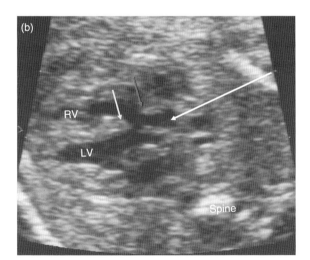

Fig. 4.23.(b). There is no continuity between the ventricular septum (yellow arrow) and the anterior wall (red arrow) of the great artery (white arrow) arising from the heart. Note the anterior displacement on the anterior vessel wall. By opening out the vessel to look for early branches or by following it cranially and determining whether it connects to the arch or duct, the artery can be identified.

the coronaries are dilated), the coronary arteries can sometimes be seen if the image quality and fetal position are favorable (Fig. 4.22). In this view, normally only the aorta arising from the left ventricle is seen, as the pulmonary artery lies above this level and will cross over cranial to this plane.

Possible deviations from normal

There is a break in continuity between the ventricular septum and the anterior wall of the vessel arising from the left outflow, indicating a **ventricular septal defect** situated either in the **perimembranous** region (Fig. 4.23(a)) or in the **outlet** portion of the septum. Frequently, in association with an outlet VSD, the great artery that arises in the center of the heart arises astride the crest of the ventricular septum (Fig. 4.23(b)). The branching pattern and connection of this artery will allow identification of which great artery it is astride the septum. Most commonly, the artery astride is the aorta and the underlying diagnosis is **tetralogy of Fallot**. If, on the other hand, the

133

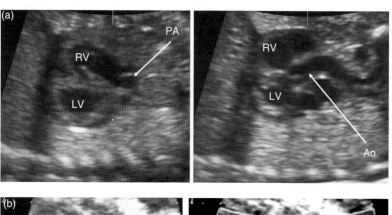

Fig. 4.24.(a). The crossover of the great arteries can also be appreciated in a long-axis projection of the fetus, but because of their respective orientation, only one great artery can be seen at a time in the normal fetus. On the left-hand panel, the origin of the pulmonary artery is seen in a view of the short axis of the left ventricle. Angling the transducer from this view allows the aortic origin to be seen.

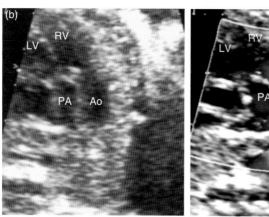
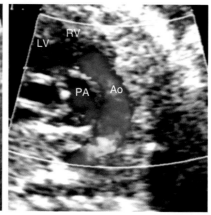

Fig. 4.24.(b). In transposition, angling the transducer to view the left ventricular outflow tract shows two vessels arising in parallel orientation in contrast to Fig. 4.24(a). Following the vessels out of the heart shows that the vessel arising from the left ventricle branches laterally, therefore is the pulmonary artery. The great artery arising from the anterior right ventricle on the other hand forms the aortic arch, therefore is the aorta. This is simple transposition of the great arteries.

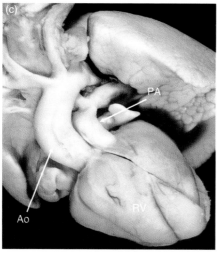
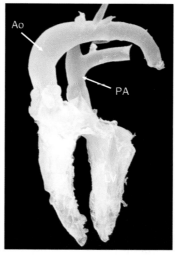

Fig. 4.24.(c). Both anatomical specimens demonstrate the abnormal parallel arrangement of the great arteries as they arise from the heart in fetal transposition. On the right is a cast of the chambers and vessels.

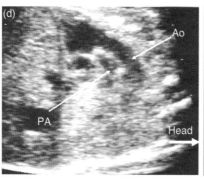
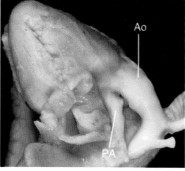

Fig. 4.24.(d). In the echocardiogram on the left-hand panel, the great arteries arise in parallel arrangement, both from the anterior right ventricle. The pathological specimen, turned to the same orientation, is very similar. The aorta is anterior to, and larger than, the pulmonary artery indicating a degree of pulmonary stenosis, a common feature in double outlet right ventricle.

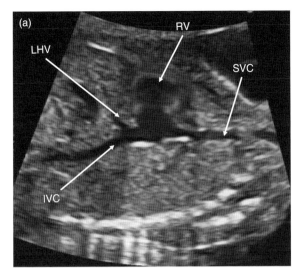

Fig. 4.25.(a). In a sagittal section just to the right of the midline, the superior and inferior caval veins can be seen connecting to the heart. The left hepatic vein (LHV) joins the inferior vena cava just before it crosses the diaphragm.

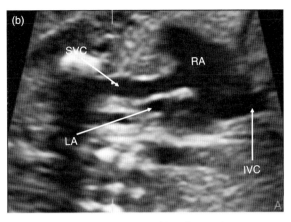

Fig. 4.25.(b). In this sagittal view of the inferior and superior caval veins, the ultrasound beam is aimed more leftwards and cuts through the left atrium posterior to the right. Note the broad shape of the right atrial appendage anteriorly.

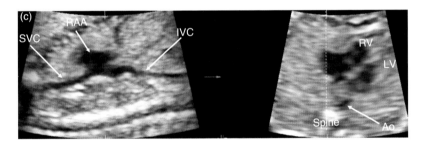

Fig. 4.25.(c). These images are taken from a volume set. The section shown on the right-hand panel is that obtained by cutting along the dotted line on the left-hand panel. On the left-hand section, the inferior and superior vena cava are illustrated, in a long-axis projection. On the right-hand panel, the section at right angles is shown at the level of the four-chamber view. The beam (dotted line) cuts through the right atrial appendage (RAA) anteriorly and catches the great veins, which lie in a plane just to the right of the descending aorta.

artery forms early lateral branches, it is a pulmonary artery and the underlying diagnosis will be **transposition**. If there is discontinuity between the great artery and the mitral valve, and the vessel arises more than 50% from the right ventricle, it is **double outlet right ventricle**. Alternatively, there can be a single great artery astride the ventricular septum, giving rise to both the aorta and aortic arch and the pulmonary arteries in **common arterial trunk**. Each of these conditions are illustrated in Chapter 3.

Normally, in sagittal views, the transducer can be tilted slightly from a long-axis view of the left ventricle, to demonstrate the crossover of the pulmonary artery (Fig. 4.24(a)). If, however, when the transducer is tilted to open out the left ventricular outflow tract, two vessels are seen in the same plane, lying in parallel

arrangement, this is transposition (Fig. 4.24(b) and (c)). A **parallel arrangement of the great arteries** occurs in simple or complex **transposition**, most cases of double outlet right ventricle (Fig. 4.24(d)) and in **corrected transposition**.

Long-axis view of the superior and inferior caval vein

Normal appearance

In this view, the inferior vena cava connects to the floor of the right atrium and the superior vena cava drains opposite to it, into the roof of the right atrium (Fig. 4.25(a)–(c)). The two veins are similar in size and both lie to the right of the midline.

135

Possible deviations from normal

The inferior vena cava can be **interrupted** and therefore not found in this section. This abnormality has been described above. The inferior vena cava can drain to the left side of the atrial mass, which is exceedingly rare with normal atrial appendages, but can occur in atrial isomerism. The inferior vena cava can appear **dilated** when there is a direct connection of the umbilical vein to the inferior vena cava, usually associated with absence of the ductus venosus (Fig. 4.14(a)). The umbilical vein and right heart will also be dilated in this anomaly.

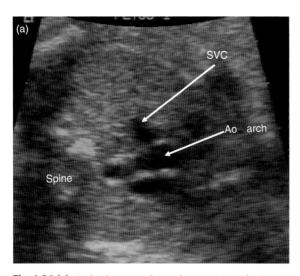

Fig. 4.26.(a). In the three-vessel view, the superior caval vein appeared slightly larger than normal compared to the aorta and arterial duct. This fetus had total anomalous pulmonary venous drainage to the innominate vein, which was therefore delivering more blood than normal to the superior vena cava.

The connection of the **superior vena cava** to the right atrium is rarely abnormal but can be **atretic** in the presence of a left superior caval vein. The superior vena cava can appear **dilated** when it is receiving more blood than usual. This can occur in **total anomalous pulmonary venous drainage** when the drainage channel is superior (Fig. 4.26(a)) or in upper body **arteriovenous malformations** such a vein of Galen malformation in the head (Fig. 4.26(b) and (c)). The superior vena cava sometimes can look a little **smaller** than normal in the setting of a persistent **left superior caval vein**, but this is easier to appreciate in a three-vessel view (Fig. 4.27(a)). It can also very rarely appear to be **displaced** further from the aorta than normal (Fig. 4.27(b)).

Long-axis view of the arterial duct

Normal appearance

This view is also known in pediatric practise as the short-axis view of the great arteries, and is a complex view to understand initially. It demonstrates the normal right heart structures "wrapping around" the origin of the aorta in the center of the scan plane and displays the ductal connection to the descending aorta in a sagittal view (Fig. 4.28 (a) and (b)). Familiarity with this view will allow it to be used to confirm abnormalities, which are suspected in other views. The inferior vena cava is often seen connecting to the floor of the right atrium. The normal size relationships of the atria and also the great arteries can be noted. Forward flow can be verified through the right heart and in the pulmonary artery and duct. It is a good view to position the Doppler sample volume in the pulmonary artery, as the flow is in line with the ultrasound beam. The cusps of the aortic valve

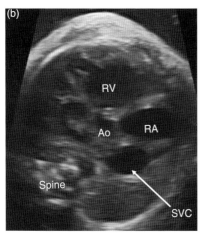

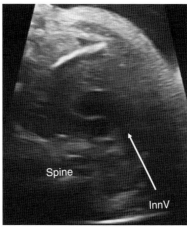

Fig. 4.26.(b). In the three-vessel view on the left-hand panel, the superior vena cava is seen to be very dilated. Moving superiorly, the innominate vein (InnV) was also seen to be very dilated in the right-hand panel. This implies excessive blood flow in the region drained by these vessels, particularly the head. This fetus had a vein of Galen arteriovenous malformation in the brain.

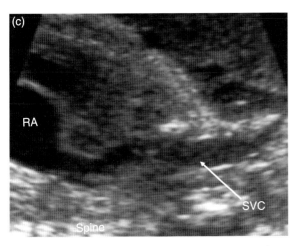

Fig. 4.26.(c). Contd. In a long-axis view of the superior caval vein, the vessel is seen to be dilated right up into the neck. This was due to a vein of Galen malformation in the brain.

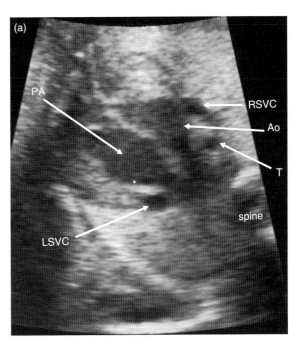

Fig. 4.27.(a). The right-sided superior caval vein (RSVC) is smaller than normal because some of the upper body venous return is carried in a persistent left superior caval vein (LSVC).

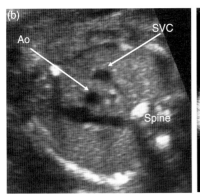
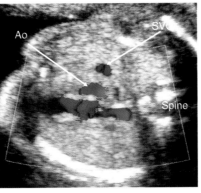

Fig. 4.27.(b). Contd. The superior vena cava seems to be displaced further rightwards in the chest than normal, separated from the ascending aorta by tissue (compare with Fig. 3.2–3.4). This seems to have had no pathological significance.

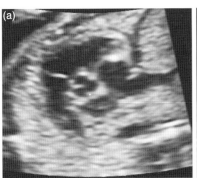
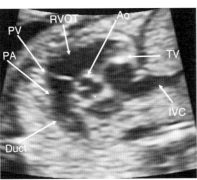

Fig. 4.28.(a). The arterial duct is seen in a long-axis view. This view demonstrates the right heart connections, from the inferior vena cava and right atrium through the tricuspid valve, right ventricular outflow tract, pulmonary artery and duct. The left-hand panel is the same view unobstructed by labeling.

137

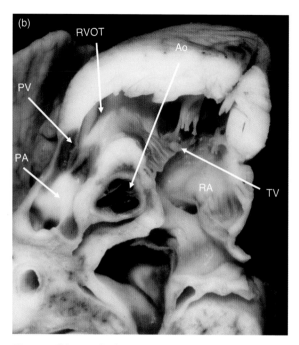

Fig. 4.28.(b). Contd. The anatomical specimen is oriented to match the echocardiographic section in Fig. 4.28(a) and similarly shows the right heart structures wrapping around the central aorta.

(normally an evenly divided trifoliate structure) can also be examined in later pregnancy if image quality is good. In the sweep between the short-axis view of the left ventricle and this view, the perimembranous part of the septum is displayed just below the aortic valve.

Possible deviations from normal

Where the right heart structures do not wrap around the left in the normal way, this view demonstrates a **parallel arrangement** of the great arteries (Fig. 4.29(a) and (b)). A parallel arrangement of the great vessels is seen when trying to obtain either a long-axis view of the aorta or a long-axis view of the arterial duct. This occurs classically in **transposition** of the great arteries, but also in **double outlet right ventricle** or **corrected transposition**. This therefore is a useful view to confirm the suspicion of an abnormality of great artery connection. When the **inferior vena cava** is **interrupted**, it will not be found

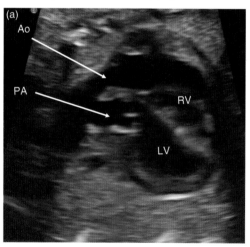

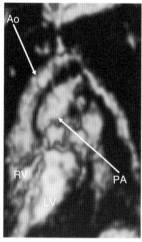

Fig. 4.29.(a). In a sagittal view of the fetus, the great arteries are seen in parallel orientation at their origin. In a rendered view, shown in the right-hand panel, the parallel arrangement of the vessels can also be appreciated.

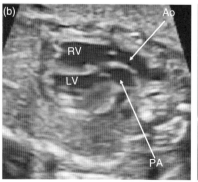

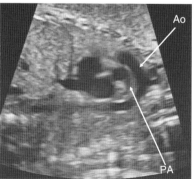

Fig. 4.29.(b). On the left-hand panel, two great arteries are seen arising from the heart, one from each ventricle. They arise as parallel tubes. This must mean that the aorta is anterior to the pulmonary artery, but moving the beam slightly leftwards (right-hand panel) proves it, by showing the head vessels arising from the anterior vessel, which in turn arises from the anterior right ventricle.

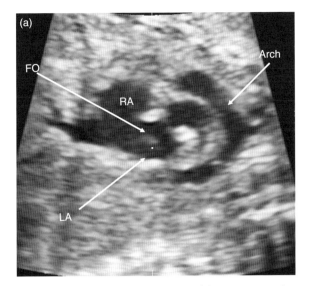

in its normal position in this projection (Fig. 4.16). Dilatation of one or other atrium can be confirmed in this section. The **foramen ovale** defect can be confirmed as **intact** or **restrictive** in the setting of left heart disease or in transposition of the great arteries (Fig. 4.30 (a) and (b)). **Any disturbance to right heart flow** such as tricuspid regurgitation or atresia, pulmonary stenosis or atresia, ductal constriction or reverse flow in the arterial duct can be verified in this view (Fig. 4.31(a)).

Fig. 4.30.(a). In this case of transposition of the great arteries, the foramen ovale (FO) appeared widely patent throughout gestation, with the flap valve in the body of the left atrium.

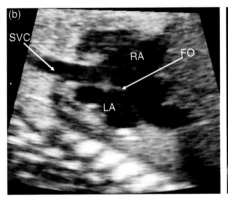

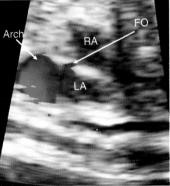

Fig. 4.30.(b). In this case of transposition, the foramen flap (FO) remained close to the atrial septum throughout the cardiac cycle, in contrast to the normal foramen flap which has a wide excursion as in Fig. 4.30(a). On the color flow map, only a small right-to-left shunt through the foramen could be seen. This suggested that the atrial septum would prove to be restrictive after birth, which did occur in this fetus.

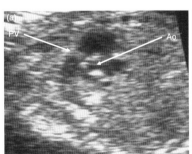

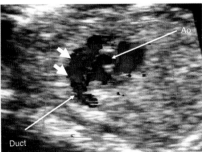

Fig. 4.31.(a). In the long-axis view of the arterial duct, the pulmonary valve cusps appeared thicker than normal and they were seen throughout the cardiac cycle, indicating a restriction in their excursion. On the color flow map, there was aliasing (arrowheads) of flow through the pulmonary valve indicating an increased velocity, due to pulmonary stenosis.

A small pulmonary artery or aorta relative to the other great artery, which will usually suspected be in other views, can be confirmed in this view (Fig. 4.31(b)). The aortic valve in short axis has a trileaflet appearance which is readily appreciated postnatally but imaging is not commonly adequate to see this accurately prenatally. However, a **bicuspid aortic valve** (a common, usually fairly benign abnormality)can be seen sometimes in late pregnancy, especially if looked for in the setting of coarctation of the aorta.

Long-axis view of persistent left superior caval vein

In the early embryo, there are paired superior caval veins but the left sided vein involutes and disappears, leaving only a right-sided vein draining the upper body and connecting to the upper pole of the right atrium. About 1/300 people, however, have persistence of the left-sided vein in addition to the right. This vessel drains the left side of the upper body, usually has a connection to the right-sided system via a transverse vein in the upper thorax (the innominate vein), and descends on the left side of the mediastinum. The left superior caval vein connects to the coronary sinus (which is the venous drainage of the heart), which in turn drains into the right atrium. The left superior caval vein can be seen in transverse views of the great arteries and has been described in these views in Chapter 3. It can also be seen in long axis views descending on the left side of the thorax to the diaphragmatic surface of the heart to connect to the coronary sinus in the left sided atrioventricular groove (Fig. 4.32(a) and (b)).

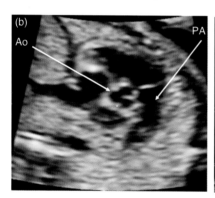
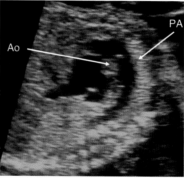

Fig. 4.31.(b). Contd. On the left-hand panel, the great arteries are normally related to each other in size. On the right-hand panel, the aorta can hardly be seen, whereas the pulmonary artery is a good size, in this example of aortic atresia.

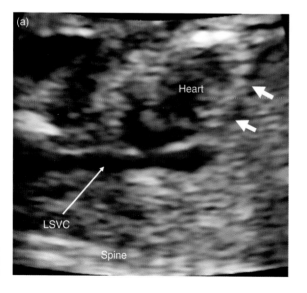

Fig. 4.32.(a). A persistent left superior caval vein drains the head and arm on the left side and runs on the left side of the mediastinum to drain to the coronary sinus on the left border of the heart in the atrioventricular groove. This image is obtained on the left side of the fetus in a long-axis view. The broad arrows indicate the diaphragm. Note that the left superior vena cava joins the coronary sinus below the heart itself, on its diaphragmatic surface.

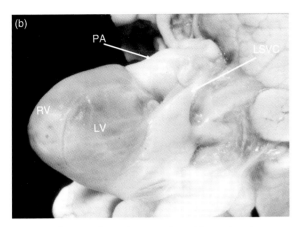

Fig. 4.32.(b). Contd. The heart is reflected forwards and seen from the left side to show the course of a left superior vena cava (LSVC) as it travels within the mediastinum to the left of the pulmonary artery to connect to the coronary sinus, which lies below the mitral valve ring in the atrioventricular groove.

Tricuspid-pulmonary view

Normal appearance

This is a common view to "find" on sagittal imaging of the fetus (Fig. 4.33), as it is imaged by cutting the fetus in front of the left shoulder to just behind the right shoulder, a common fetal position relative to the transducer, cutting just in front of the ventricular septum. However, it is not a very useful view in fetal echocardiography. It does show the tricuspid valve, right ventricular outflow tract and pulmonary valve, with the aorta coming into this view as it sweeps anteriorly out of the left ventricle, which lies behind this view. The normal size and positional relationships of the aorta and pulmonary artery can be noted.

Possible deviations from normal

Any condition which affects the relative **size** of the great arteries can be confirmed in this view, such as pulmonary stenosis or atresia, aortic stenosis or atresia or coarctation. When the great arteries are not normally connected, the parallel arrangement of their origin will also be seen in this view.

Long-axis view of the aortic arch

Normal appearance

The aorta arises in the middle of the thorax and is directed superiorly before turning in a tight hook shape to form the aortic arch (Fig. 4.34(a) and (b)). The

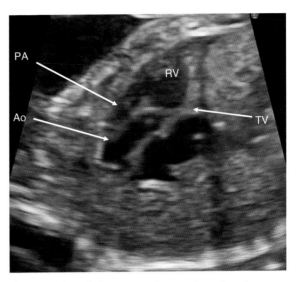

Fig. 4.33. The right heart connections are shown, from the right atrium through the tricuspid valve to the pulmonary artery. This view is obtained by cutting from the apex just anterior to the ventricular septum. The aorta appears in this view as it sweeps anteriorly out of the left ventricle, which lies behind the plane of section.

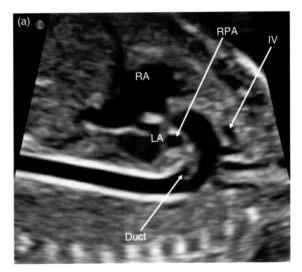

Fig. 4.34.(a). This view shows the aortic arch in a long-axis view. Three branches are seen arising from the superior aspect of the vessel to supply the head, neck, and arms. Note the relative positions of the two atria, the junction of the duct, right pulmonary artery, and innominate vein (IV) with the aortic arch, as seen in this view.

right pulmonary artery and left atrium lie within the "hook," behind the ascending aorta and in front of the descending aorta. Three head, neck and arm vessels arise from the superior aspect of the aortic arch. There is normally only forward flow in the arch. Although this view is standard in pediatric echocardiography,

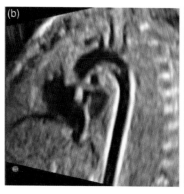 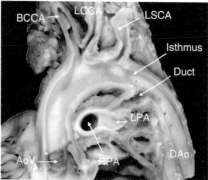

Fig. 4.34.(b). The aortic arch view is turned to match the orientation of the pathological section. They are almost a perfect match and demonstrate the three arch branches, the brachiocephalic (BCCA), the left common carotid (LCCA), the left subclavian artery (LSCA), the site of the isthmus, and the junction of the arterial duct to the descending aorta (DAo).

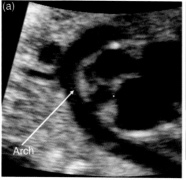 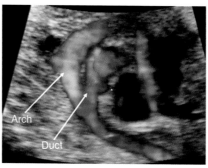

Fig. 4.35.(a). The aortic arch is wider in shape than normal (compare with Fig. 4.34) as it arises close to the chest wall from the anterior right ventricle in transposition of the great arteries. This vessel can be identified as the arch because of the branch arising from its superior aspect. The color flow map shows the relationship of the arch to the main pulmonary artery and duct, which in transposition lie below the level of the aorta and arch.

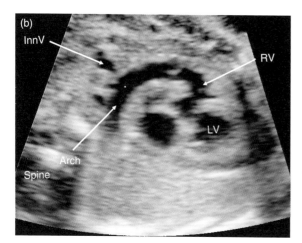

Fig. 4.35.(b). In this fetus, the anterior great artery gave rise to superior branches and formed the most cranial "arch," therefore must be the aorta. The aorta arose from a small right ventricle, which communicated with the left ventricle via a ventricular septal defect. This was a complex form of transposition with tricuspid atresia. Note the position of the normal innominate vein (InnV) which lies above, and anterior to, the aortic arch. (See also Fig. 4.41.)

and is "pretty" to obtain prenatally, it is of limited value in fetal echocardiography and can even be misleading.

Possible deviations from normal

A "splayed" arch, or a **wider shape** to the hook, is seen when the aorta arises from the anterior ventricle, as in transposition or double outlet right ventricle (Fig. 4.35(a)). In a 4D volume set, the aortic arch can be "followed" to the right ventricle, confirming a discordant ventriculo-arterial connection (Fig. 4.35(b)). **Reverse flow** can be seen in the arch in severe obstruction to aortic flow, such as aortic atresia (Fig. 4.36(a)–(c)). **Reverse flow** is sometimes seen in the distal arch in conditions where the cerebral blood flow is abnormal, such as in severe growth retardation or vein of Galen malformation (see Fig. 3.50). **Reverse flow in the arterial duct** can be seen in the long-axis view of the arch in **pulmonary atresia** (Fig. 4.37).

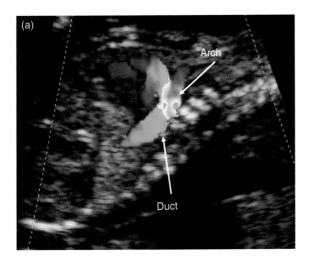

Fig. 4.36.(a). In a sagittal view of the fetus, there is forward flow in the arterial duct but reverse flow above this vessel, therefore in the aortic arch, in aortic atresia.

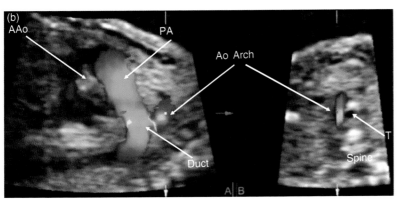

Fig. 4.36.(b). An acquired volume illustrates the relationship between the long-axis view (left-hand panel) and the transverse view of the aortic arch (right-hand panel), which lie at right angles to each other. The "dot" of the volume set is positioned in the transverse arch in each panel. Reverse flow in the aortic arch is seen in both views in this case of aortic atresia. The tiny atretic ascending aorta (AAo) can be seen lying arising in the center of the heart behind the pulmonary artery in the sagittal view. The trachea (T) can be seen lying in front of the spine behind the small aortic arch in the transverse view.

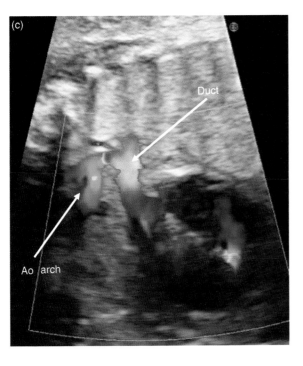

Fig. 4.36.(c). Usually the aortic arch lies directly on top of the arterial duct, but in this fetus with aortic atresia, the arch, showing flow reversal was a little higher in the thorax than usual, so that at first it was difficult to find on transverse views. The long-axis view clearly showed the relationship of the arches, allowing confirmation of the expected reverse flow in this fetus with the hypoplastic left heart syndrome.

143

The long-axis view of the aortic arch is **rarely useful in the diagnosis of coarctation of the aorta**, as the "shelf" of the coarctation itself cannot be seen (Fig. 4.38(a)) and the commonly associated hypoplasia of the transverse arch is more difficult to appreciate than it is in transverse views. Hypoplasia of the transverse arch can be readily recognized in transverse views as the size of the arch can be directly compared to the ductal arch in the same section. Normally the junction between the arch and duct is smooth. In addition, some views of the arch can be misleading (Fig. 4.38(b)). Only very occasionally tortuosity of the arch in a long-axis view can serve to add weight to a possible diagnosis of coarctation, suspected from other views (Fig. 4.38(c)). The acceleration of flow around the arch, which is seen in postnatal life in coarctation, is not seen in fetal life when the arterial duct is open. In **interruption of the aorta type B**, the normal hook of the aortic arch cannot be demonstrated. Instead the ascending aorta forms a typical "two-pronged fork" appearance in longitudinal views (Fig. 4.39(a) and (b)).

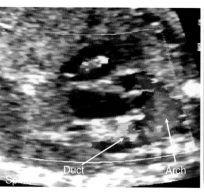 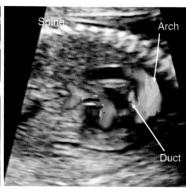

Fig. 4.37. In the long-axis view of the arch, reverse flow is seen underneath the arch in the arterial duct, in two cases of pulmonary artresia. In the left-hand panel, the fetus lies with the spine down. This is a case of pulmonary atresia with intact septum where the arterial duct usually lies in a normal position connecting to the descending aorta. In contrast in the right-hand panel, the fetus lies spine up. The arterial duct in this case of tetralogy of Fallot with pulmonary atresia was very small and tortuous, arising from the undersurface of the transverse arch.

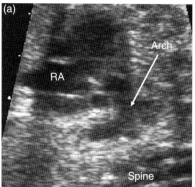 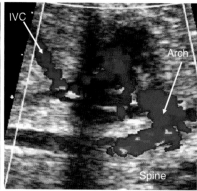

Fig. 4.38.(a). This fetus had coarctation, inferred from other views, but the long-axis views of the arch, both on cross-sectional and color flow imaging, are misleadingly normal in appearance.

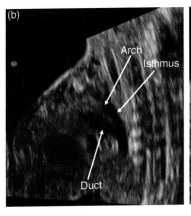
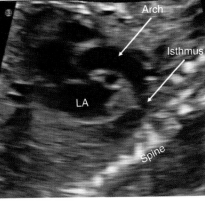

Fig. 4.38.(b). Contd. On the left-hand panel, the normal smooth junction of the arch and duct is well seen (compare with Fig. 4.38(c)). On the right-hand panel, this is a normal aortic arch but the isthmal region appears narrowed in this slice and the anterior "shelf" where the duct joins is prominent. This normal appearance must not be mistaken for a true coarctation shelf, which always lies in the posterior aspect of the arch.

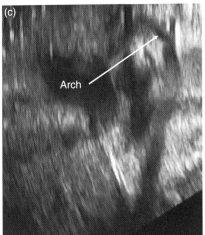
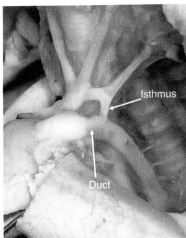

Fig. 4.38.(c). In the left-hand panel, the long-axis view of the arch in this fetus with coarctation appears abnormal, rather narrow in its transverse portion and not making a smooth join with the descending aorta (compare with the normal arch in Fig. 4.34 and the normal "join" in 4.38(b)). The right-hand panel shows a similar specimen, with a small arch and an angle formed by the junction of the isthmus with the duct and descending aorta.

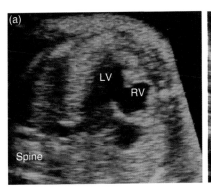
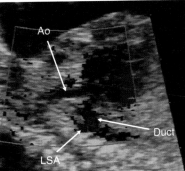

Fig. 4.39.(a). The left-hand panel shows rather an oblique view demonstrating a ventricular septal defect. The ventricular septal defect in interrupted aortic arch is usually large but found in a rather unusual orientation as here, which is neither a four-chamber view nor a long-axis view of the left ventricle. In the right-hand panel, in a sagittal view, the small aorta does not form an arch but branches superiorly into two head and neck vessels (only one is shown here). The left subclavian artery (LSA) is seen here arising from the descending aorta, after the junction of the arterial duct. This indicates interruption of the aorta type B.

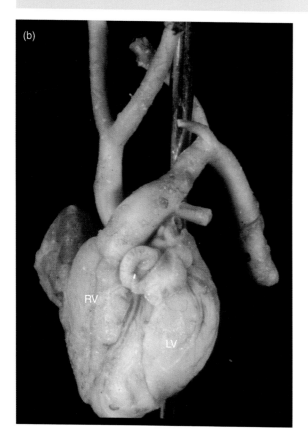

A long-axis view of the arch can demonstrate **collateral arteries** arising from the descending portion of the aorta to supply the lungs in tetralogy of Fallot with pulmonary atresia (Fig. 4.40).

Vessels seen above the aortic arch

In transverse views, immediately cranial to the aortic arch, the innominate vein is normally seen crossing the midline to drain to the superior vena cava (Fig. 4.41(a)). Above the level of the aortic arch, the three head, neck and arm branches of the aorta can sometimes be seen cut in short axis (Fig. 4.41(b)). Immediately above this level, both subclavian arteries are seen passing to each arm (Fig. 4.42(a)–(f)). The internal mammary arteries

Fig. 4.39.(b). Contd. The fetal heart is seen viewed from the left side. The course of the pulmonary artery, duct and descending aorta is well seen. The aorta is smaller than normal in relation to the pulmonary artery and does not form an arch to join the duct, but divides into two head and neck vessels superiorly. This is interrupted aortic arch type B.

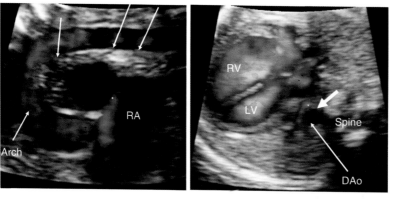

Fig. 4.40. In the left-hand panel in the long-axis view of the arch, in this case of tetralogy of Fallot with pulmonary atresia, multiple collateral arteries were seen arising from the descending aorta to supply the lungs in the absence of confluent central pulmonary arteries. Three are labeled on this still frame (arrows) but in other views, at least two more could be seen. On the right-hand panel, the most caudal collateral seen on the left is shown in a transverse view. It arose from the right anterior side (thicker arrow) of the descending aorta (DAo) and coursed around the front of the aorta to supply the left lung.

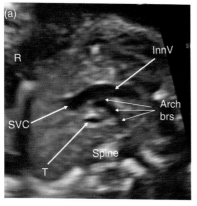
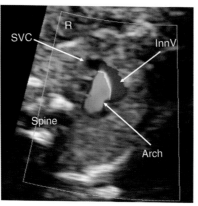

Fig. 4.41.(a). Moving cranially from the aortic arch, the innominate vein can be seen crossing the midline from left to right to drain to the superior caval vein. Either the aortic arch (right-hand panel) or, a little higher, the three branches (arch brs) of the arch in cross-section (left-hand panel) can be visualized, lying behind, and at an angle to, the innominate vein. Note the normal position of this vessel within the chest.

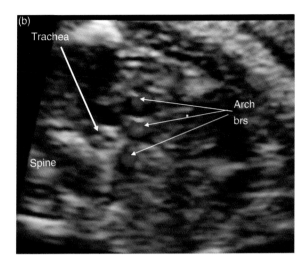

Fig. 4.41.(b). Contd. Just above the level of the innominate vein, the three branches of the aorta can sometimes be seen in their short axis on color flow mapping.

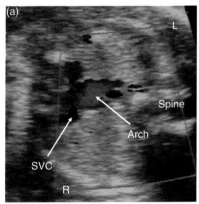 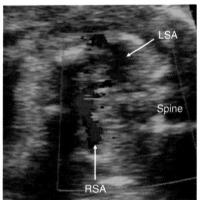

Fig. 4.42.(a). On the left-hand panel, the aortic arch passes from right to left in front of the trachea and spine. Just above this level of the aortic arch in the same patient, the right and left subclavian arteries are seen in their normal position on color flow mapping on the right-hand panel. In order to distinguish the arteries from the arm veins, which run close to each other, the color map must be as expected, with flow away from the aortic arch in both arteries. Also, a long course of vessel extending outside the confines of the thorax must be seen, which will ensure differentiation from the branch pulmonary arteries, which lie just below the level of the arch.

Fig. 4.42.(b). In this slightly oblique view in the upper thorax, the course of the normal left subclavian artery (LSA) is seen. It arises from the distal aortic arch at its junction with the arterial duct and runs leftwards to the arm. The innominate vein (InnV) is seen anteriorly, draining to the superior vena cava.

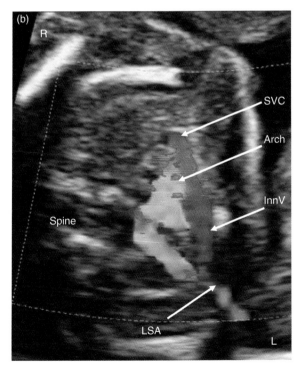

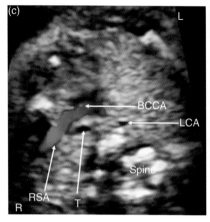

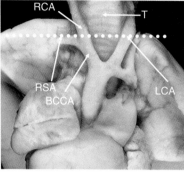

Fig. 4.42.(c). Contd. The echocardiographic section on the left-hand panel is taken above the level of the aortic arch. The right subclavian artery (RSA) arises from the brachiocephalic artery (BCCA), which in turn has taken origin from the most right-sided part of the transverse portion of the aortic arch. The right subclavian artery lies a little more leftwards than usual in this example and passes in front of the trachea, which lies in front and slightly to the right of the spine. Note that the beam cuts the left carotid artery (LCA) in short axis, lying to the left of the trachea. On the right-hand panel, the position of the section is shown on the anatomical specimen, with the cut at the junction of the right carotid and right subclavian where they arise from the brachiocephalic artery. RCA = right carotid artery.

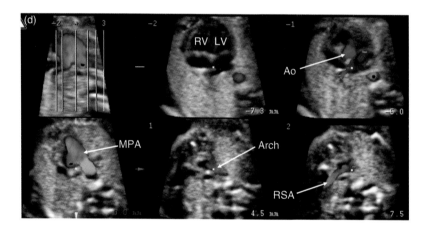

Fig. 4.42.(d). This series of views illustrates successively from the middle upper row to the lower middle image, the four-chamber view, the aortic origin, the pulmonary artery and duct and the transverse arch. In this 20-week fetus, the normal right subclavian artery (bottom row, right) lies 3 mm above the aortic arch (lower image, middle row) and 14.8 mm above the four-chamber view.

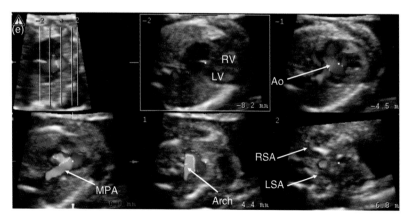

Fig. 4.42.(e). This series of tomographic images shows the four-chamber view, the origin of the aorta, the pulmonary artery and duct, the transverse arch and the subclavian arteries sequentially from the upper middle image to the bottom right. Again, the relationship of the subclavian arteries to the other views, in terms of distance, is shown. The subclavian arteries usually have a tortuous course as seen here.

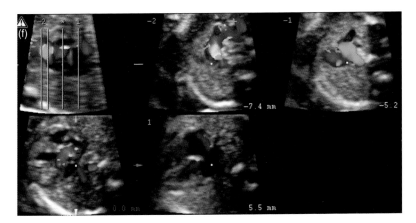

Fig. 4.42.(f). Contd. The tomographic images are from the four-chamber view (lower middle image) to the origin of the aorta (lower left) through the arch and arterial duct (upper right), to the normal course of the right subclavian artery. Note the typical tortuosity of the right subclavian and that it lies 12.9 mm above the level of the four-chamber view.

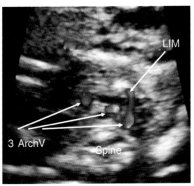
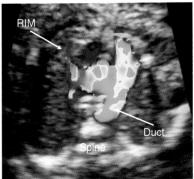

Fig. 4.43. On the left-hand panel, the three head and neck vessels (3 archV) can be seen in short axis having arisen from the aortic arch which lies just below this plane of section. Arising from the left subclavian artery near its origin, is the left internal mammary artery (LIM). On the right-hand panel, the right internal mammary artery can be seen (RIM). This vessel arises from the base of the right subclavian artery and passes forward towards the front of the chest. This cut is slightly oblique so that the pulmonary artery and the duct are seen on the left side of the chest.

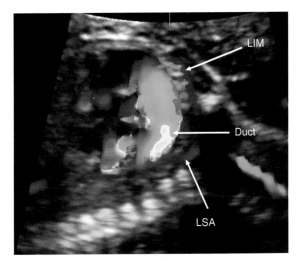

Fig. 4.44. In a long-axis view, the pulmonary artery arising from the right ventricle and the arterial duct are seen. The left subclavian artery (LSA) arises from the aortic arch at its junction with the arterial duct. The left subclavian gives off the left internal mammary artery (LIM) close to its origin. This vessel runs down the inside of the anterior chest wall.

are sometimes seen in transverse or long-axis views. These arise from the base of the subclavian arteries on each side (Fig. 4.43) and pass anteriorly to travel down the front of the thorax (Fig. 4.44).

Possible deviations from normal

The **innominate vein** can be **dilated** if it receives drainage of **anomalous pulmonary veins** or in the setting of an **arteriovenous malformation** in the upper body (Fig. 4.26(b), right-hand panel). The right subclavian artery usually arises from the right brachiocephalic artery, which is the first branch of the aorta, coming off the proximal aortic arch. It arises significantly above the aortic arch and can usually be readily seen in the upper mediastinum with color flow mapping (Fig. 4.42). Occasionally, it arises from the descending aorta after its junction with the arterial duct and it courses behind the trachea and esophagus (Fig. 4.45(a)–(f)). This is termed an **aberrant right subclavian artery** and occurs in about 1%–2% of normal people. It is increased in incidence in Down's syndrome to between 10% and 20%, so is an important marker for this condition.

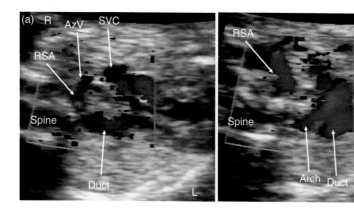

Fig. 4.45.(a). An aberrant right subclavian artery arises from the descending aorta, behind the trachea and below the level of the aortic arch at the level of the duct, in contrast to the normal right subclavian which arises above the arch (Fig 4.42). On the left-hand panel a vessel is seen arising from the descending aorta at the level of the duct, and heading to the right. Following this vessel on color flow mapping as it courses cranially, it can be seen passing rightwards towards the right arm in the right-hand panel. Note the close proximity of the azygous vein (AzV), which can be distinguished by its venous flow profile on pulsed wave Doppler, heading towards the superior vena cava.

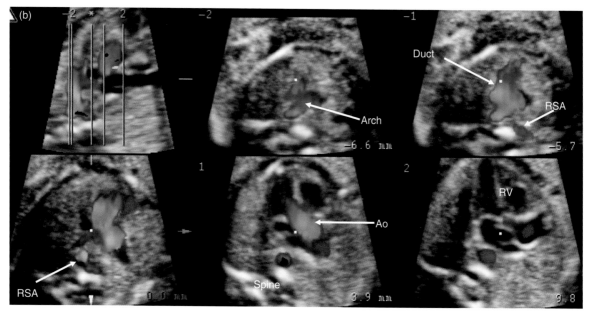

Fig. 4.45.(b). The tomographic images show a four-chamber view (lower right image), origin of the aorta (lower middle), origin of the pulmonary artery (lower left), duct and transverse arch (upper right) and transverse arch alone (upper middle). There is an aberrant right subclavian artery seen arising in the lower left and upper right images. Note that the aberrant right sublcavian arises below (here 6.6 mm) the level of the arch, in contrast to the normal RSA which arises substantially above the arch. The vessel then courses upwards and rightwards to the arm.

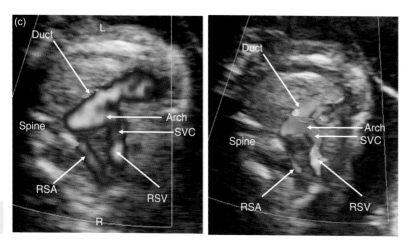

Fig. 4.45.(c). In the power Doppler image on the left hand panel, there is clearly a vessel arising from the aorta at the level of the arterial duct and passing behind the trachea, which should not be there. There is also a vessel apparently in the correct position for the right subclavian artery. However, the color Doppler frame in the right-hand panel shows that in the posterior vessel the direction of flow is towards the arm, whereas flow in the more anterior vessel comes from the arm. This latter vessel is venous and drains to the superior caval vein, just to the right of the aortic arch, therefore is the right subclavian vein (RSV). The posterior vessel is arterial, which was confirmed on pulsed Doppler, and is an aberrant right subclavian artery.

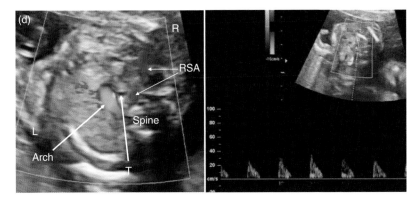

Fig. 4.45.(d). Contd. On the left-hand panel, the transverse arch is seen crossing the midline from right to left. A vessel is seen behind the trachea (T) coursing towards the right arm. The whole course of the vessel is not seen because of its tortuous nature. Pulsed Doppler of the vessel (right-hand panel) confirms that this vessel is arterial. This is an aberrant right subclavian artery.

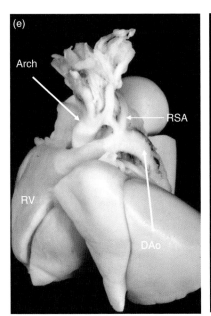
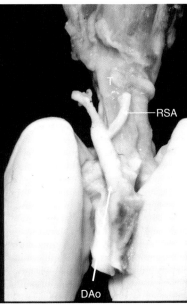

Fig. 4.45.(e). On the left-hand panel, the aortic arch is seen viewed from the left side. A fourth artery arises from the arch at the junction of the isthmus and duct and is directed rightwards. On the right-hand panel, the course of this artery is seen from behind. It passes behind the trachea and courses up and right towards the right arm.

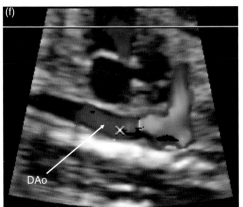
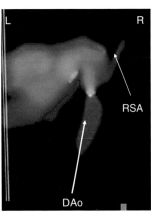

Fig. 4.45.(f). The image in the right-hand panel is rendered from the sagittal view of the aortic arch seen on the left. The arch is seen from behind, matching the view seen in the right-hand panel of Fig. 4.45(e). There is an aberrant right subclavian artery (RSA) arising from the distal arch and coursing rightwards. Note that this vessel is not seen in a standard long-axis view of the arch.

Idiopathic calcification of the arteries

This is a rare condition but one which can present in fetal life. It usually presents with fetal hydrops in the third trimester. As it is caused by a recessive gene, there may be a history of loss of a previous child or pregnancy. The ascending aorta and pulmonary artery can show calcification at their origins (see Fig. 3.51) but the most striking finding is marked echogenicity of the arterial walls of the descending aorta and iliac vessels (Fig. 4.46).

3D/4D volumes

Acquisition of 3D/4D volumes can allow the relationships of the normal intrathoracic structures outside the heart to be demonstrated. For example, Fig. 4.47(a) shows the normal position of the esophagus and trachea in the chest and the situation of these structures relative to the heart and central vessels. Exploration of acquired volume sets (Fig. 4.47(b)–(c)) is very useful to further the understanding of all the intrathoracic anatomy, in both the normal and the abnormal setting and also the how each view is obtained relative to another.

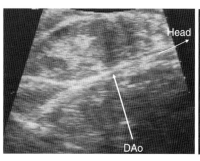 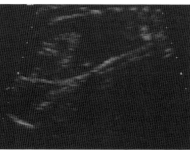

Fig. 4.46. On the left-hand panel, the trunk of the fetus is seen with the head to the right. The walls of the descending aorta and iliac branches are brightly echogenic due to abnormal calcium deposition within them. On the right-hand panel, the gain is turned right down so that only the most dense structures of the fetal anatomy (mostly bone) are still seen. Because of the abnormal calcium in the arterial walls, the aorta remains visible.

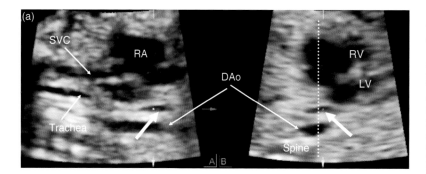

Fig. 4.47.(a). The acquired volume, in the left-hand panel, shows a sagittal view of the heart on the right side of the chest but directed towards the descending aorta on the left (indicated by the dotted line on the right-hand panel). The "dot" (thick arrow) is positioned in an unidentified structure, which can be seen in the four-chamber view (right-hand panel) to lie between the left atrium and the descending aorta. This is the esophagus. Note that the trachea is seen in the upper thorax in its long axis in the left-hand panel. As expected, the trachea ends in the mid-thorax behind the heart and just above the atria, when it branches into the two bronchi, the right coming towards us, the left going away from us in this plane.

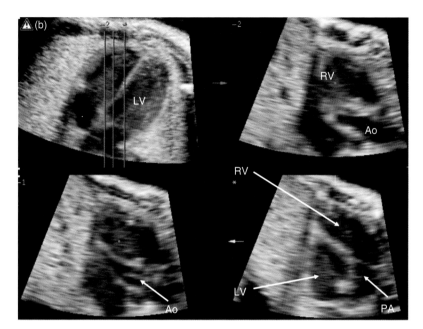

Fig. 4.47.(b). Contd. Three cuts are made across the four-chamber view in a sagittal plane. The view obtained by each cut is shown. The most leftward cut on the upper left image generates a view of the ascending aorta, the middle cut generates a view of the aortic origin with the aortic valve, whereas the most rightward section shows the right ventricular outflow tract and the left ventricle in short axis.

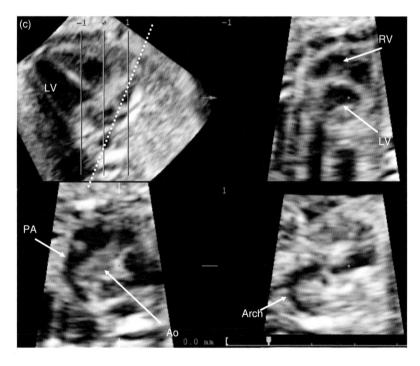

Fig. 4.47.(c). The three cuts made across the four-chamber view in a sagittal plane in this series are wider apart than those in Fig. 4.47(b). The left ventricle in short axis, the right ventricular outflow tract and the aortic arch are seen successively from top right to bottom left. In order to achieve a perfect aortic arch view, the 1 plane (the right-hand section on the upper left image) would need to be angled towards the left as indicated by the dotted line or by turning the four-chamber view in the volume set as in Fig. 4.47(d).

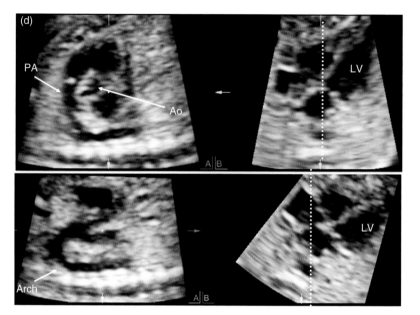

Fig. 4.47.(d). Contd. In the upper panels, the long-axis view of the arterial duct is seen in the left-hand image. The cut across the four-chamber view in order to achieve this image is shown in the right-hand panel. Similarly, in the lower panels, the complete aortic arch is seen with the correlative four-chamber view. Note that the four-chamber view has been rotated from the position necessary for the duct, in order to produce the aortic arch.

Summary

The additional views are not essential during a routine normal fetal heart evaluation but it is important to be able to obtain and recognize them if necessary. There are situations where they can add useful extra information to the understanding of an abnormality. It is also important to be able to recognize normal vascular structures within the thorax even if they are not particularly useful in cardiac diagnosis, like the internal mammary arteries, for example.

Chapter 5

Color and pulsed Doppler, M-mode and rendering

Color flow mapping

Introduction

In the early years of fetal echocardiography, around 1980, the structure of the normal and abnormal heart could be identified with a high degree of accuracy without color flow mapping. However, the color facility, which became generally available in the mid-1980s, considerably adds to the speed and accuracy of cardiac analysis. Color flow mapping is now essential for detailed fetal cardiac evaluation, and it is extremely useful, once it is understood, in routine fetal cardiac assessment. It can be used in the quick confirmation of normal flow, or alternatively in displaying or confirming an abnormality of flow. It is particularly useful to identify a structure as vascular or to help search for very small vessels, either because the vessel under study is abnormally small in a cardiac malformation, or in the early fetus. Color flow mapping is also used to help position the Doppler sample volume accurately for obtaining pulsed Doppler. Although there is no evidence that any form of diagnostic ultrasound exposes the fetus to any risk, the use of color reduces the exposure time to pulsed Doppler. Power Doppler is a form of color modality, which does not indicate flow direction, but which can be useful for defining vessels with low velocity flow, such as the pulmonary venous connections, and for small vessels. Newer modes of color mapping, such as high definition or convergence color, incorporate elements of power Doppler and normal color to give some directional information and to improve vessel filling.

Uses of color flow mapping

(1) To confirm normal patent connections throughout the heart with blood flow in the expected direction.
(2) To ascertain the direction of flow at the atrial septum.
(3) To ensure that there is no flow across the ventricular septum.

(4) To rule out valve regurgitation.
(5) To highlight areas of turbulence if present.
(6) To "find" or confirm the presence of small vessels (either when the vessel under study is anatomically small or when the vessel is abnormally small or when examining the large vessels in a small fetus).

Normal color flow mapping

The fetal heart normally lies between 5 and 10 cm from the ultrasound transducer. At this depth, with carrier frequencies of 3–7 MHz, which are most commonly in use for fetal echocardiography, unaliased color Doppler displays can usually be achieved with normal intracardiac velocities. Aliasing is the display of multiple colors in the center of the color flow image (Fig. 5.1(a) and (b)), which indicates that the velocity of flow at that point is above the velocity measurable with the current color settings. (This is known as the Nyquist limit.) If aliasing occurs, the examiner should check that the color scale is maximized for the transducer frequency in use and, if it is, change to a lower frequency transducer. If aliasing persists, pulsed or continuous wave Doppler must be used to obtain the absolute velocity at the site of aliasing for comparison with normal values. Observing an aliased pattern on color flow mapping thus has the ability to instantly "highlight" an unusually or abnormally high velocity (Fig. 5.1b).

Color evaluation of the heart should take place in a sequential fashion from the venous to the arterial poles. In order to achieve good color images, the flow in the vessel or chamber under study should be as close as possible to parallel to the direction of the ultrasound beam. Conventionally, most ultrasound machines are set to demonstrate flow towards the transducer color coded in red, and flow away from the transducer in blue.

A sequential approach to assessing the heart should be employed in the color examination as in the rest of the fetal echocardiogram, following the course of the circulation from the venous to the arterial poles of the heart. In a long-axis or sagittal view of the fetus,

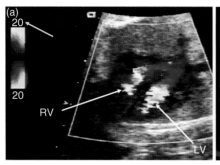
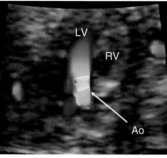

Fig. 5.1.(a). On the left-hand panel, the heart is imaged in the four-chamber view. There is aliasing of color flow (a mosaic of colors in the centre of the flow) across both atrioventricular valves. It can be seen that the color flow settings are very low, with the maximum velocity set at only 20 cm/s (yellow arrow). In mid-gestation, the velocity across the tricuspid valve is of the order of 40–60 cm/s, thus aliasing of the color flow map when the settings are this low is inevitable. If the color flow setting is increased to the highest velocity for this transducer frequency, this appearance will be corrected. In the right-hand panel, the heart is imaged just cranial to the four-chamber view demonstrating the aortic origin. The color flow map shows aliasing in the ascending aorta. This could mean that the velocity across the valve was abnormally high, as would occur in aortic stenosis, or that the velocity was within the normal range, but either that the color settings were too low or that the combination of the depth of the fetus and the transducer frequency was unable to show the color flow map without aliasing. In this instance, the aortic velocity was normal, the settings were as high as possible for this transducer but the far depth and high transducer frequency did not allow unaliased display of the aorta. Use of pulsed Doppler is necessary to exclude aortic stenosis.

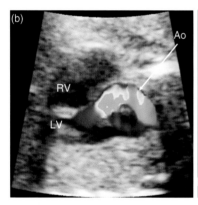
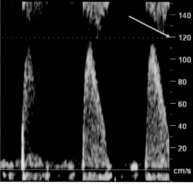

Fig. 5.1.(b). In contrast to the right-hand panel of Fig. 5.1(a), in this fetus, there was aliasing of the color flow map in the aorta, due to an abnormally high velocity of flow, because of aortic valve stenosis. The pulsed Doppler tracing obtained in this 20-week fetus showed a velocity of 120 cm/s (right-hand panel), which is above the normal range.

positioning the color flow map below the diaphragm, the hepatic vein and **ductus venosus** can be identified for pulsed Doppler interrogation (Fig. 5.2(a) and (b)). Color should be used to confirm the inferior and superior vena caval connection to the right atrium again in a long-axis view (Fig. 5.3). Flow in the two main systemic veins is seen connecting to the right atrium in long-axis views of the fetus, the **inferior vena cava** below the diaphragm and the **superior vena cava** above the heart.

The **pulmonary venous connection** to the left atrium should be identified in a four-chamber view (Fig. 5.4(a)) or under the aortic arch in a long-axis view of the arch (Fig. 5.4(b)). Unless flow is documented in color from the pulmonary veins into the left atrium, the pulmonary venous connection has not been positively

defined, as the 2D image can look misleadingly normal. Reducing the color velocity scale can often allow the course of the pulmonary veins from within the lung to be seen more clearly, and using power Doppler is also useful allowing the pulmonary veins to be seen well out into the lung fields even to the branches (Fig. 5.5). Power Doppler is good for low flow vessels, although it is restricted by its lack of directional information. New modalities on modern ultrasound machines can also be useful to confirm the connections, such as the render function, which displays the chambers or vessels as "casts" (Fig. 5.5, right panel).

The **interatrial shunt** can be shown through the foramen ovale, which in the normal fetus is almost exclusively right to left (Fig. 5.6(a) and (b)). However, bidirectional or even what appears to be predominantly

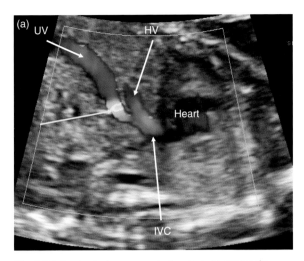

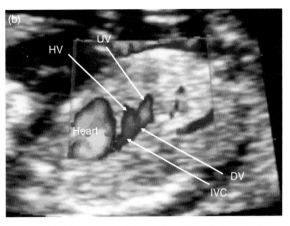

Fig. 5.2.(a). The ductus venosus (yellow arrow) is seen in the abdomen connecting the umbilical vein (UV) with the inferior vena cava (IVC). There is often flow acceleration, which causes aliasing on color, within the ductus venosus as the blood flow stream narrows at this point. The hepatic vein (HV) joins the inferior vena cava before it crosses the diaphragm to connect to the base of the right atrium.

Fig. 5.2.(b). Even at 12 weeks' gestation, when the fetus lies in a favorable position, the color flow map shows the hepatic vein (HV) below the diaphragm with the ductus venosus (DV) lying caudal to it, connecting to the umbilical vein (UV).

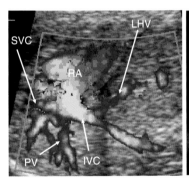

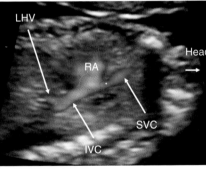

Fig. 5.3. Flow in the two main systemic veins is seen connecting to the right atrium in long-axis views of the fetus, the inferior vena cava (IVC) below the diaphragm and the superior vena cava (SVC) above the heart. On the left-hand panel, the fetus lies with the head to the left whereas in the right-hand panel, the head is to the right. On the left panel, the pulmonary veins (PV) are seen in the lung parenchyma but they connect to the left atrium, which lies behind the right atrium.

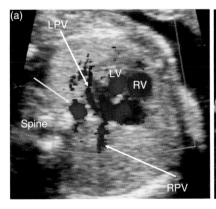

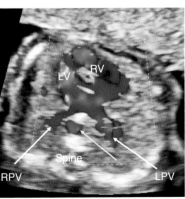

Fig. 5.4.(a). The heart is seen in two four-chamber projections. The color flow map shows flow within the left and right pulmonary veins draining to the left atrium in a normal fashion on either side of the descending aorta. In the left-hand panel because of the orientation of the veins to the transducer, the left pulmonary vein is blue and the right red. In the right-hand panel, both veins are seen in red as the direction of flow in both is towards the transducer in this fetal position. Note the typical relationship of the veins to the descending aorta (yellow arrows).

157

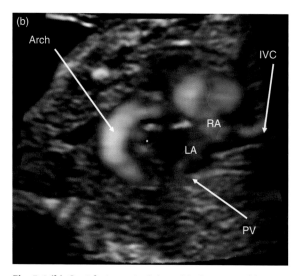

Fig. 5.4.(b). Contd. In a sagittal view of the fetus, part of the aortic arch is seen. One of the left pulmonary veins can be seen underneath the arch, draining to the left atrium.

left-to-right flow can be seen in the normal fetus (Fig. 5.6(c)), although a pathological explanation of this finding, such as left heart disease, should be carefully excluded.

In a four-chamber view, there should be **equal flow** through the **atrioventricular valves** in diastole, with no evidence of regurgitation during systole (Fig. 5.7). It is common to see extension, or smearing, of color across the membranous portion of the ventricular septum in the apical four-chamber view (Fig. 5.8). This does not indicate a ventricular septal defect but is a function of the resolution of the machine and the gain settings, at this thin part of the septum below the atrioventricular valves. If there is uncertainty about a ventricular septal defect in this position, the transducer must be moved around the fetal thorax so that color flow interrogation of a lateral four-chamber view can be performed. Color flow in this projection should not breach the **intact**

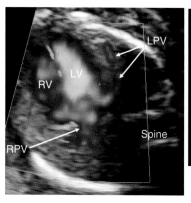

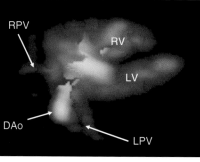

Fig. 5.5. In the left-hand panel, the power Doppler shows pulmonary vein flow very clearly far out into the lungs on the left side and to the first generation branches on the right side. Power Doppler is good for low flow vessels, although it is restricted by its lack of directional information. In the right-hand panel, the chambers have been rendered, showing a cast of the ventricles. Pulmonary veins attaching to the left atrium from each lung are very clearly displayed on either side of the descending aorta (DAo).

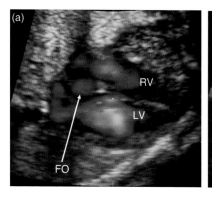

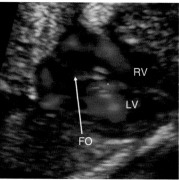

Fig. 5.6.(a). The heart is imaged in a lateral four-chamber view, which is the ideal position for imaging the right-to-left shunt at the foramen ovale. In the left-hand panel, the predominant direction of the shunt can be seen from right to left. In the right-hand panel, a "whiff" of left-to-right shunt is seen at the end of the cycle. This is normal.

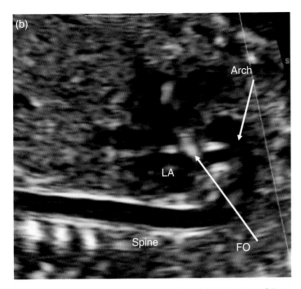

(b)

Fig. 5.6.(b). Contd. The foramen ovale and the direction of the intra-atrial shunt can also be seen under the aortic arch in a long-axis view.

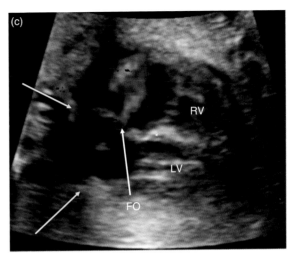

(c)

Fig. 5.6.(c). There was a more prominent jet of left-to-right flow at the atrial septum in this fetus than normal. Careful examination, particularly of the left heart structures, revealed no pathology to account for this. This fetus had had a supraventricular tachycardia which was under control at the time of this image, so it is possible that there was mild left ventricular dysfunction, undetectable by eye or standard Doppler measurements.

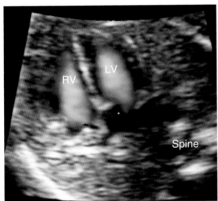

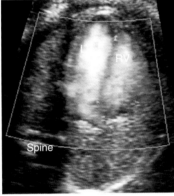

Fig. 5.7. There is equal flow into both ventricles across the atrioventricular valves in diastole. In systole (not shown), there is normally no regurgitation from either atrioventricular valve. Two different types of color flow map are illustrated.

septum (Fig. 5.9(a)). In the absence of outflow obstruction in one or other ventricle, flow across a ventricular septal defect will switch from right to left to left to right during the cardiac cycle (Fig. 5.9(b)). This bidirectionality may help to distinguish color flow artifact from a real defect. Aliasing of color flow across a small ventricular septal defect, which is typical in the postnatal echocardiogram and which immediately highlights it, does not occur prenatally because right and left ventricular pressures in the fetus are similar. Color flow mapping can detect ventricular septal defects which

are so small they are not visible on 2D, and even demonstrate the natural history of ventricular septal defects by showing the defect diminishing in size with advancing gestation (Fig. 5.9(c)).

In the normal fetal heart, there should be **forward flow** from the left ventricle through a **patent aortic valve**, and from the right ventricle through a patent **pulmonary valve**, with **no regurgitation** on color flow mapping (Fig. 5.10(a) and (b)). Flow in the **transverse arch and duct** should be in the **same direction** (Fig. 5.11(a) and (b)). The right and left pulmonary artery branches from

159

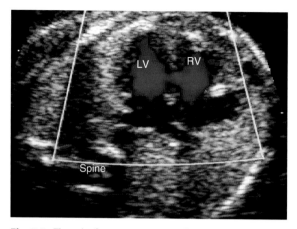

Fig. 5.8. The color flow appears to extend across the ventricular septum just below the crux, raising the question of a defect at this point. This is a common artifactual appearance. When the septum was viewed from a lateral view, no flow across the septum was seen.

the pulmonary trunk can be shown in the transverse views of the thorax (Fig. 5.12), although the left pulmonary artery is directed slightly more cranially than the right so that all three divisions of the main pulmonary artery are not usually seen in the same frame (see also Fig. 3.2(d)). The **pulmonary branches** can be seen on 2D, but often better on color flow mapping. The first branches of the aorta are the **coronary arteries** but these are not usually seen prenatally until after 32–34 weeks of pregnancy and then only if imaging is ideal (Fig. 5.13(a)). The exception to this is in growth retarded fetuses, where the coronary arteries are more prominent earlier in fetal life, or in a coronary artery fistula. A **coronary fistula** can be an isolated malformation with the fistula connecting one of the coronary arteries with either atrium or ventricle, or it can occur in the setting of pulmonary atresia with intact

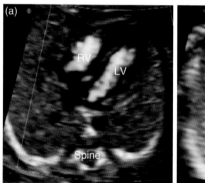
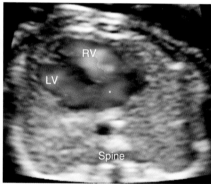

Fig. 5.9.(a). Moving the transducer around the fetus allows the ventricular septum to be seen with the beam more perpendicular to it. This will confirm or refute the presence of a ventricular septal defect at a suspicious point. Note how the color flow map is "held" on each side of the septum in this view.

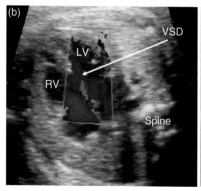
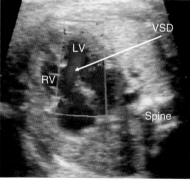

Fig. 5.9.(b). Bidirectional flow is seen across a true ventricular septal defect, left to right in the left-hand panel and right to left in the right-hand panel. This is a small to moderate sized perimembranous muscular defect.

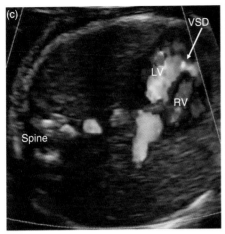

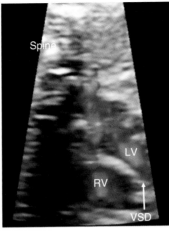

Fig. 5.9.(c). Contd. On the left-hand panel, the apical muscular ventricular septal defect appeared fairly large on color flow mapping at 20 weeks' gestation, but 3 weeks later (right-hand panel) only a tiny defect could be seen. The natural history of ventricular septal defects is for spontaneous closure, especially in muscular defects. Closure can even occur in utero.

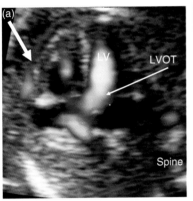

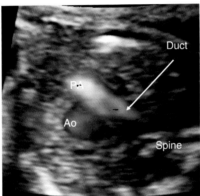

Fig. 5.10.(a). There is laminar flow across the aortic valve out of the left ventricle (left-hand panel) and also across the pulmonary valve out of the right ventricle (right-hand panel). Note that the color flow map is so sensitive it displays the movement of fluid within the pericardial sac (arrowhead) in the left panel. This is an absolutely normal appearance.

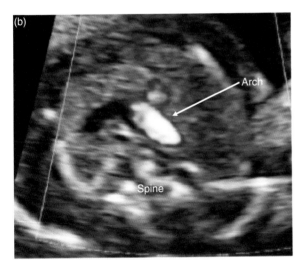

Fig. 5.10.(b). Maintaining a transverse section, immediately cranial to the section in the right-hand panel of Fig. 5.10(a), lies the most superior artery, the transverse aortic arch, arising in the middle of the thorax and crossing the midline from right to left.

ventricular septum (Fig. 5.13(b)–(d)). This subset of pulmonary atresia where there are coronary fistulas, especially if there are areas of stenosis within them (Fig. 5.13(d)), carry a poor prognosis, as evidenced by both fetuses illustrated dying soon after birth, despite treatment. The **head and neck vessels** can be identified arising from the transverse aortic arch when it is imaged in the long axis (Fig. 5.13(c)) and this branching pattern helps to distinguish the aorta from the pulmonary artery. There should be laminar flow in the distal aortic arch. There should be no turbulence to blood flow **at any point** within the normal heart or main vessels.

Abnormal color flow mapping

Abnormal direction of flow can be readily appreciated on color flow mapping from the color code, and aliasing will demonstrate possibly abnormal sites of high velocity or turbulent flow. The color flow findings in specific malformations are described in the relevant chapters.

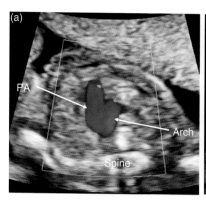 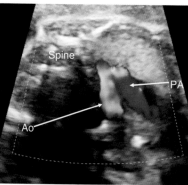

Fig. 5.11.(a). Slight angulation of the transducer in the upper thorax allows both the duct and the transverse arch to be imaged simultaneously. On the left-hand panel, the fetus lies with the back down and there is flow in the same direction, away from the front of the chest, in both the pulmonary artery and duct and the transverse arch. This forms a familiar "V" shape with the pulmonary artery and duct forming a long arm and the transverse arch a shorter arm. Similarly, in the right-hand panel, although the fetus lies with the back up, flow is in the same direction towards the spine in both vessels, the longer arm of the V being the pulmonary artery.

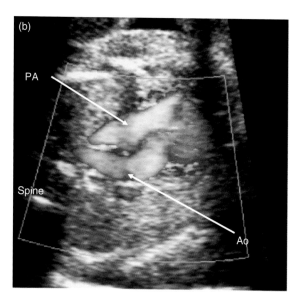

Fig. 5.11.(b). Flow is in the same direction in both vessels here also but because of the position of the fetus, the flow is initially blue in the ascending aorta, but becomes red as the arch turns towards the transducer in its transverse portion.

The use of pulsed Doppler

Normal pulsed Doppler

During a normal fetal echocardiogram, if color flow mapping is used, as it always should be, it is not absolutely necessary to use pulsed wave Doppler if there is unaliased forward flow throughout the heart. However, in some forms of fetal cardiac malformation or fetal compromise, the use of pulsed Doppler may be necessary to complete the evaluation. Thus, it is essential to understand the technique, to be skilled in obtaining tracings correctly, and to be able to recognize normal flow patterns readily. In a normal fetal heart, the highest velocity of flow is in the arterial duct and this may reach up to nearly 2 m/s at term. In most modern ultrasound machines, pulsed Doppler is usually sufficient to record all vascular velocities without aliasing, assuming a range of transducer frequencies from 2.5 MHz upwards is available. Continuous wave Doppler, which is usually only obtainable with specifically cardiac probes, will only be required to estimate abnormally increased velocities which are much higher than the normal range.

Technique

The Doppler sample volume can be positioned at any point within the cardiovascular system. Using color flow mapping often helps to position the pulsed Doppler sample volume precisely, especially in a very small vessel. The transducer should be manipulated on the maternal abdomen in order to align the sample volume with the direction of the blood flow under study. The size of the sample volume gate should usually be as small as possible, but can be adjusted according to the site and size of the vascular structure under consideration. Application of the angle correction bar can be useful to highlight the need to be as close as possible to "in-line" with the flow direction. The angle of flow should ideally always be less than 20°. If evaluating later pregnancy, pulsed Doppler tracings should be recorded during fetal apnea, partly to prevent displacement of the sample volume from its selected position, and partly because the flow characteristics in some sites will be altered by fetal respiration.

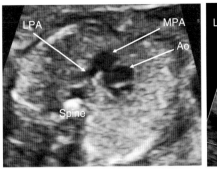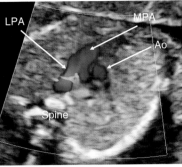

Fig. 5.12. The origin of both branch pulmonary arteries are seen on 2D and color flow mapping.

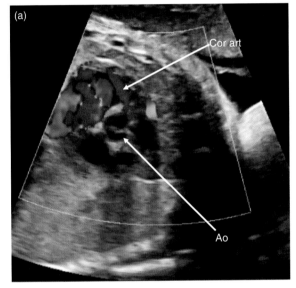

Fig. 5.13.(a). The first branches of the aorta are the coronary arteries (cor art) but these are usually too small to see until late in normal pregnancy and only then if the fetal position and the image quality are ideal. When visible, they can be seen in a long-axis view (see Fig. 4.22) or in a sagittal view of the short axis of the aorta as seen here.

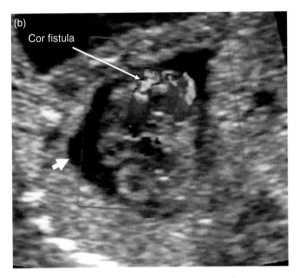

Fig. 5.13.(b). In this fetus with pulmonary atresia with intact ventricular septum, there was a moderate-sized pericardial effusion (arrowhead). A tortuous fistulous connection could be followed from the cavity of the right ventricle to the right coronary artery. There was high velocity bidirectional flow within it on color flow mapping, suggesting stenotic areas within this coronary fistula.

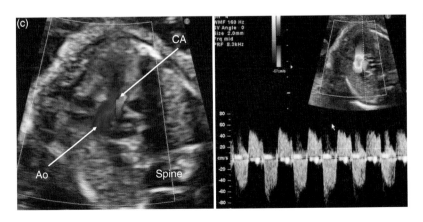

Fig. 5.13.(c). In the long axis view of the left ventricle (left-hand panel), flow was seen in the coronary artery (CA) adjacent to the ascending aorta. There was bidirectional flow in this vessel (right-hand panel).

163

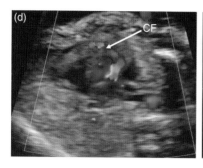

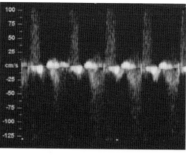

Fig. 5.13.(d). Contd. The coronary artery seen in Fig. 5.13(c) could be followed to the right ventricle (left-hand panel) and communicated with the cavity in this fetus with pulmonary atresia with intact ventricular septum. In a tortuous area of this fistula (CF) the flow was bidirectional with a velocity over 1 m/s in each direction (right-hand panel).

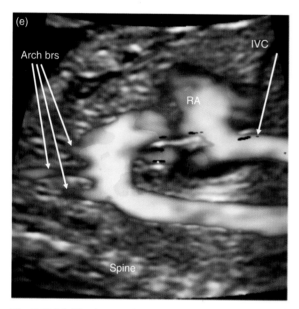

Fig. 5.13.(e). The three arm, head and neck branches (arch brs) are usually the first branches of the aorta to be seen, arising from the superior aspect of the aortic arch in a long-axis view.

There are four aspects of Doppler evaluation to consider:

- Direction of flow, which should be forward through the heart
- Pattern of flow, which will be specific for the site sampled
- Velocity of flow, which will vary according to the site
- Measuring volume flow and function

The direction of flow is most readily seen by color flow mapping, but pulsed Doppler may be useful in confirmation. Some ultrasound machines offer the facility to invert the pulsed Doppler trace, but using this is not recommended in fetal cardiac studies, because it tends to be confusing. The direction of flow in any particular vessel or chamber will of course vary with the fetal position relative to the transducer. The direction of flow as well as its pattern helps to confirm that the signal originates from the intended flow stream rather than from closely adjacent vessels or chambers. The pattern of flow will vary, depending on the site of sampling and can be altered in different pathological states. If absolute velocities are to be estimated, the Doppler sample volume must lie close to parallel to the direction of blood flow. Estimation of a ratio of systolic to diastolic flow is more tolerant of recording at an angle to flow. If the volume of flow is to be calculated, the sample volume should be positioned within a "flat" flow profile (such as the pulmonary artery or ascending aorta) and parallel to the direction of flow, or alternatively, the sample volume should be extended to cover the width of the vessel (Fig. 5.14). A flat flow profile means that the velocity of flow is more or less the same right across the vessel, with only a little "drag" at the walls. This occurs in the great arteries just above the valves. However, further away from the ejection force, for example in the descending aorta, the flow profile is more like a bell-shaped curve, with the higher velocities in the middle of the vessel but decreasing towards the side.

Ductus venosus

A high-velocity stream exits from the ductus venosus into the cephalad portion of the inferior vena cava. The major portion of the jet, which is highly oxygenated, does not mix with the lower velocity flow already in the inferior vena cava and derived from the lower body, but is preferentially streamed across the foramen

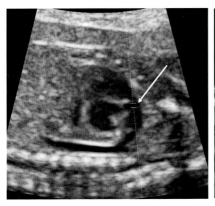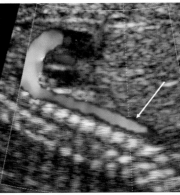

Fig. 5.14. In the left-hand panel, the Doppler sample volume (arrow) is positioned within the pulmonary artery, just above the valve, in the center of the flow in line with the direction of flow (the angle correction line on either side of the sample volume is in line with the direction of flow). The Doppler sample volume can be made as small as possible as the flow profile is essentially "flat" just after it is ejected from the heart. As this is so, the center of flow represents the whole. In contrast, if the descending aorta is to be used to calculate flow, the sample volume must be opened (arrow) to cover the whole vessel, as seen in the right-hand panel.

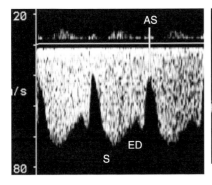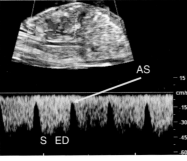

Fig. 5.15. The typical flow profile of the ductus venosus is shown, with almost equal peaks during ventricular systole (S) and early diastole (ED), with a notch in late diastole during atrial systole (AS). On the left-hand panel is a fetus in the mid-trimester of pregnancy with a maximum velocity of about 65 cm/s, and on the right is a fetus at 12 weeks with a maximum velocity of about 40 cm/s.

ovale. The flow profile shows a peak in systole, followed by a peak in early diastole, which are nearly equal in velocity (Fig. 5.15). There is a mild rise in peak velocity from 65 cm/s to 75 cm/s between 18 weeks and term. There is continuous forward flow during atrial contraction, which is represented by a notch in the tracing. The velocity of flow during atrial contraction (at the notch) increases from around 35 cm/s to 45 cm/s between 18 weeks and term. The velocity of flow (or pressure gradient across the ductus venosus) increases during respiration and should be measured during fetal apnea.

Pulmonary veins

The pulsed Doppler sample volume should be positioned parallel to blood flow close to the junction of the pulmonary vein to the left atrium, using color flow mapping to identify the venous channel coursing through the lung parenchyma. The pulmonary venous flow pattern reflects left atrial hemodynamics. There is a peak of forward flow during ventricular

systole representing the "suction" effect of atrial relaxation (Fig. 5.16). This peak is followed by continuous flow as a result of descent of the mitral valve annulus during systole until a second peak in early diastole, which coincides with the mitral valve opening. In late diastole, during atrial contraction, there is cessation of flow in the pulmonary veins or even a small wave of flow reversal. The velocity of flow at the systolic and diastolic peaks is similar. The velocity in both peaks increases with advancing gestation, from around 10 cm/s at 16 weeks to between 30 and 40 cm/s at term. The reversal wave does not exceed 10 cm/s in the normal fetus. The velocity time intervals suggest that about twice the volume of forward flow occurs during ventricular systole compared with diastole. The flow pattern is not affected by respiration or heart rate.

Foramen ovale

The pulsed Doppler sample volume can be positioned in the foramen ovale in order to show the flow profile between the atrial chambers. There is a biphasic pattern

165

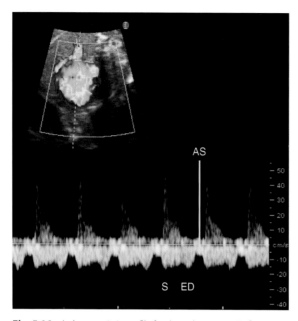

Fig. 5.16. A characteristic profile for the pulmonary vein flow obtained close to the left atrium is shown, with almost equal peaks in systole (S) and early diastole (ED) and absent flow or very little flow during atrial contraction (AS). Note the flow in the opposite direction seen in this particular tracing. This is in the branch pulmonary artery, which lies very close to the vein.

of flow with right-to-left flow occurring in ventricular systole, followed by a diastolic peak corresponding to mitral valve opening and cessation of flow or closure of the foramen ovale flap during atrial contraction (Fig. 5.17). Closure of the septum is said to occupy about 20% of the cycle. There is only a narrow spike of left to right flow at the foramen in a normal heart. The systolic peak velocity is greater than the diastolic peak and increases with gestation from about 10 to 50 cm/s between 16 weeks and term. The velocity of flow in the foramen ovale is influenced by the behavioral state in late pregnancy, suggesting an increase in the right to left shunt during periods of active as opposed to passive sleep.

Mitral valve

The pulsed Doppler sample volume should be positioned on the ventricular side of the mitral valve or across the valve in order to exclude regurgitation, but must be close to parallel to the direction of flow (Fig. 5.18). The mitral valve flow profile shows a biphasic pattern during diastole, representing the passive filling wave (E wave) as the mitral valve opens at the end of systole, and the

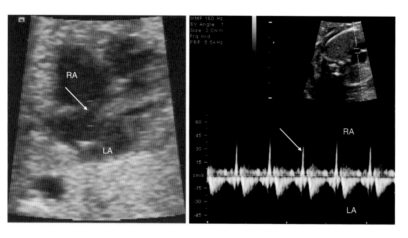

Fig. 5.17. On the left-hand panel, the Doppler sample volume (arrow) is positioned across the foramen ovale defect. On the right-hand panel, it can be seen that most of the flow seen on pulsed Doppler is from right to left (below the baseline) in two main phases of flow, with a narrow jet of left to right flow (arrow) at one point in the cycle.

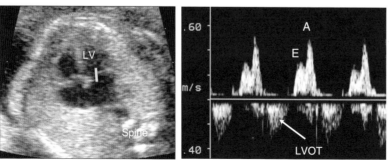

Fig. 5.18. The sample volume is positioned in the left ventricle across the mitral valve leaflets, parallel with the direction of flow. A typical mitral valve tracing for mid-gestation is seen with the E wave less than the A wave. The Doppler sample volume in the mitral valve often partially overlaps the left ventricular outflow tract such that this flow is seen in the opposite direction to the mitral flow. This can be readily distinguished from the flow pattern of mitral regurgitation by its velocity, which is always higher in a regurgitation jet.

active or atrial wave (A wave) reflecting flow through the valve during atrial contraction. There is no flow in systole. If the sample volume is on the ventricular side of the valve, it often overlaps the left ventricular outflow tract, especially in a small heart, and flow in this pathway can be seen during systole, which can be confused with mitral regurgitation. In true mitral regurgitation, however, systolic flow will be seen on the atrial side of the mitral valve and can usually be confirmed by color flow mapping. Mitral regurgitation will only be found by enlarging the Doppler sample to include interrogation of the left atrium as illustrated in the left hand panel of Fig. 5.18. The E wave increases from about 15 cm/s at 12 weeks' gestation to about 50 cm/s at term. The A wave also shows a mild increase during gestation from about 35 to 65 cm/s. The E/A ratio therefore rises with advancing pregnancy from about 0.5 to close to 1 (Fig. 5.20(b)). Thus in early pregnancy, most of the ventricular flow occurs in late diastole. This is in contrast to postnatal life, where the E/A ratio is normally around 1.5, indicating that most of the flow into the ventricle occurs in early diastole. The velocity of the E wave reflects the gradient

between the left atrium and the left ventricle, which is greater with advancing gestation, probably due to maturation in myocardial relaxation properties. The velocity of the A wave reflects left ventricular end-diastolic pressure and is fairly constant between fetal and postnatal life. Mitral valve velocities increase during fetal breathing so Doppler values should be obtained during apnea. A uniphasic pattern where the E and A waves are merged is not uncommon in the fetus and does not usually signify pathology (Fig. 5.19), although ventricular dysfunction as a possible explanation should be looked for before accepting it as within normal.

Tricuspid valve

The sample volume should be positioned on the ventricular side of the tricuspid valve, parallel to the direction of flow (Fig. 5.20(a)). As with the mitral valve, the tricuspid valve flow profile shows a biphasic pattern during diastole, representing the passive filling wave (E wave) as the tricuspid valve opens at the end of systole, and the active or atrial wave (A wave) reflecting flow through the valve during atrial contraction.

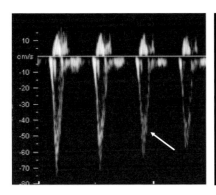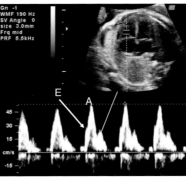

Fig. 5.19. On the left-hand panel, the atrioventricular valve tracing does not show the usual bifid pattern but is uniphasic (arrow). This is not uncommon, particularly in later pregnancy, and does not appear to be of pathological significance, although dysfunction of the ventricle should be looked for. On the right-hand panel, the E wave is almost buried in the A wave. There is an artifact from some other structure producing a spike in the tracing (thin arrow) which could be mistaken for the A wave. If the E wave is then overlooked, this could be wrongly interpreted as an abnormal mid-trimester tracing with the E wave higher than A wave.

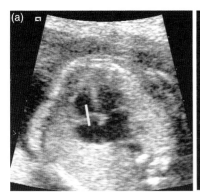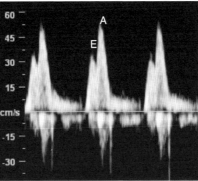

Fig. 5.20.(a). A typical tricuspid valve tracing for mid-gestation is seen with the E wave lower than the A wave. Because the outflow tract of the right ventricle is not close to the tricuspid valve, flow in the other direction is not usually seen on the right side of the heart as it is on the left.

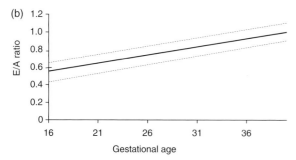

(b)

Fig. 5.20.(b). Contd. The E/A ratio is seen in the atrioventricular valves throughout gestation. Note the gradual change throughout gestation. This is due to progressive increase in the E wave, whereas the A wave stays more or less the same from fetal to adult life.

There is no flow in systole or tricuspid regurgitation in the normal fetal heart. The velocity of flow through the tricuspid valve is usually slightly higher than that through the mitral valve in the same fetus. The E wave increases from about 20 cm/s at 12 weeks' gestation to about 50 cm/s at term. The A wave also shows a mild increase during gestation from about 35 to 60 cm/s. The E/A ratio therefore rises with advancing pregnancy from about 0.5 to close to 1 (Fig. 5.20(b)). In similar fashion to the left ventricle in early pregnancy, most of the right ventricular flow occurs in late diastole. This is in contrast to postnatal life, where the E/A ratio is normally around 1.5, indicating that most of the flow into the ventricle occurs in early diastole. The velocity of the E wave reflects the gradient between the right atrium and right ventricle, which is greater with advancing gestation, probably as a result of maturation in myocardial relaxation properties or an increase in the loading conditions. The velocity of the A wave reflects right ventricular end-diastolic pressure and is fairly constant between fetal and postnatal life. As in the mitral valve, a uniphasic pattern where the E and A waves are merged, sometimes occurs in the normal fetus.

Aortic valve

The Doppler sample volume should be positioned in the ascending aorta just distal to the valve leaflets (Fig. 5.21(a)). There is a short time-to-peak velocity (or sharp upstroke) with a single peak of forward flow in systole. There is no flow in diastole. The peak velocity of flow increases gradually from around 30 ± 5 cm/s at 12 weeks' gestation to around 80 ± 10 cm/s at term. The peak velocity is usually slightly greater in the aorta than in the pulmonary artery in the same

fetus but, as the velocities vary with fetal activity and cannot be obtained simultaneously, this is not invariable. The time to peak velocity or acceleration time (Fig. 5.21(b)) is slightly longer in the aorta than in the pulmonary trunk. This suggests that the resistance faced by the left ventricle – which "sees" the arch vessels, the isthmus and the descending aorta – is slightly lower than that faced by the right ventricle – which "sees" the branch pulmonary arteries, the duct and the descending aorta. Arterial Doppler velocities are independent of heart rate within the physiological range but can increase during fetal activity. Examining the details of flow characteristics as shown in Fig. 5.21(b) are mainly of use in research rather than of practical clinical use.

Pulmonary valve

The Doppler sample volume should be positioned in the pulmonary trunk just distal to the valve leaflets (Fig. 5.22(a)). There is a short time to peak velocity with a single peak of forward flow in systole. There is no pulmonary regurgitation seen in the normal fetus. The peak velocity of flow increases gradually from around 30 + 5 cm/s at 12 weeks' gestation to around 80 + 10 cm/s at term (Fig. 5.22(b)). In the same fetus, the aortic velocity is usually slightly higher than that in the pulmonary trunk but this is not always the case, as the velocities vary with fetal movement.

Arterial duct

The highest normal velocity in the heart is in the arterial duct. Fig. 5.23(a) illustrates aliasing of flow on the color flow map in the arterial duct in a sagittal view of the fetus. However, the Nyquist limit (the highest velocity which can be measured with color at the current settings) is only 56 cm/s. When the pulsed Doppler sample volume is positioned in the arterial duct (Fig. 5.23(b)), the velocity of flow is higher than this at nearly 1 m/s but this is within the normal range for the gestational age. The pulsed Doppler in the duct is always higher than in the pulmonary artery and there is always forward flow during diastole. However, some reverse flow into the duct in early diastole can occur in normal late pregnancy. The time to peak velocity is longer than in either the aorta or the pulmonary artery, reflecting the low resistance of the placental bed. The peak systolic velocity rises from about 50 cm/s at 16 weeks to around 1.8 m/s at term. The diastolic velocity increases during the same time period from 5 cm/s to around 12 cm/s.

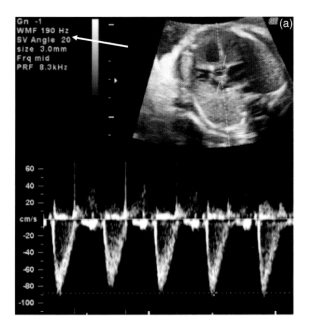

Fig. 5.21.(a). The Doppler sample volume is positioned in the ascending aorta just above the valve leaflets, with the ultrasound beam aligned with the flow, at an angle of less than 20 degrees (arrow). A typical aortic trace is seen. This has a single peak with a short time to peak velocity. There is no flow in diastole.

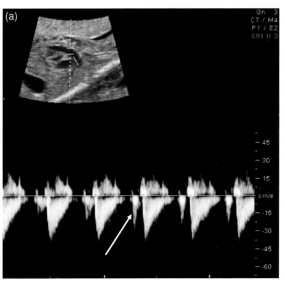

Fig. 5.22.(a). The Doppler sample volume is positioned in the main pulmonary artery just above the pulmonary valve leaflets with the beam aligned with the flow. A typical flow profile in the pulmonary artery is shown, which has a similar shape to the aortic valve, although the time to peak velocity is slightly longer on measurement. The spike (arrow), often seen preceding the pulmonary arterial flow, is derived from flow in the overlying right atrial appendage.

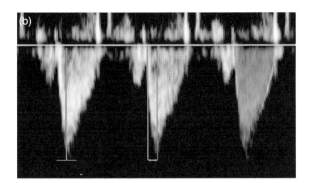

Fig. 5.21.(b). The flow in the arteries can be analyzed for functional characteristics in terms of peak velocity (left trace) time to peak velocity (middle trace) and flow velocity integral (right trace).

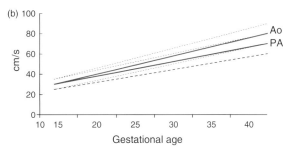

Fig. 5.22.(b). The aortic and pulmonary velocities are charted for gestation. The mean aortic velocity is shown in red and the mean pulmonary artery velocity is shown in blue. The dotted lies represent the 95th centiles.

Branch pulmonary artery flow

The pulsed Doppler sample volume can be positioned in either of the branch pulmonary arteries at their origin (Fig. 5.24). Color flow mapping helps to position the sample volume correctly. There is a characteristic flow profile showing a sharp rise to peak velocity, followed by a slow decline. There is a notch in the tracing and often a short wave of reverse flow, which coincides with pulmonary valve closure, followed by low-velocity forward flow in diastole. The systolic velocity of flow in the branch pulmonary artery increases with gestation and is lower peripherally than at its origin. In the proximal pulmonary artery, the peak velocity rises from a mean of about 55 cm/s at 18 weeks to a mean of around 90 cm/s at term. Diastolic flow is less in the proximal pulmonary artery than in peripheral vessels.

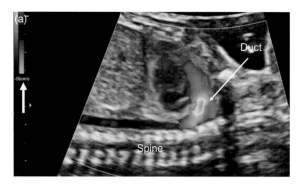

Fig. 5.23.(a). The color flow map in the long axis (sagittal) view of the fetus shows aliasing in the center of flow in the duct. However, the maximum velocity measurable by color flow at this depth with the current settings and transducer frequency is only 56 cm/s (broad arrow). To check that the velocity of flow is within normal limits, the pulsed Doppler sample must be positioned in the arterial duct (Fig. 5.23(b)).

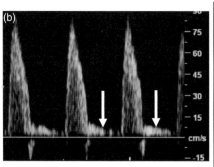
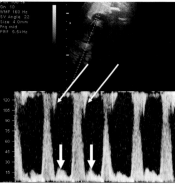

Fig. 5.23.(b). The Doppler sample volume is positioned in the arterial duct. The velocity in the arterial duct is always higher than that in the pulmonary artery, but here is within the normal range for the gestational age. There is always forward flow during diastole in the normal duct (broad arrows in both panels). However, towards the end of pregnancy, a small jet of reverse flow into the duct from the aorta can occur in early diastole (long arrows in the right-hand panel).

Isthmus

The isthmus is the distal portion of the transverse aortic arch between the left subclavian artery and the junction of the arterial duct. Normally, there is forward flow in this site both in systole and diastole but this changes with gestation. This is often easier to evaluate using color flow mapping, but pulsed Doppler may be useful to confirm a normal (Fig. 5.25) or abnormal flow pattern.

Estimation of volume flows and function

An estimate of volume flow can be made from the formula $Q = V\text{mean} \times \text{area}$, where Q = volume flow, V = velocity. The sample volume can be positioned in any of the four cardiac valves to obtain the mean velocity, and the area of the valve is calculated from the diameter of the valve ring, assuming a circular valve orifice and a "flat" flow profile. A flat flow profile indicates that, with the exception of a tiny portion of the blood flow being "dragged" at the vessel walls, all the blood moves forward at the same velocity. Thus, the sample volume positioned within, and parallel to, the stream of blood gives a profile which is representative of the whole. Alternatively, in the descending aorta, where the flow profile is pulsatile, the Doppler sample gate must be expanded to cover the whole vessel and record all the velocities within the flow stream.

The volume of left heart flow can be estimated at the mitral or aortic valves and of the right, at the tricuspid or pulmonary valves, with reasonable accuracy. The volume flow tends to be slightly greater if measured at the atrioventricular valves than at the arterial valves. This can be accounted for by measurement error. Accurate measurement is more difficult technically for the atrioventricular valves than for the arterial valves, and this is magnified by the fact that the diameter/2 is squared in the formula for area calculation. The mean velocity of flow through any of the cardiac valves changes little with advancing gestation from 16 to 40 weeks, with most of the increase in flow being accomplished by increase in the size of the valve orifice. The stroke volume of each ventricle increases about 10-fold between 20 and 40 weeks. As

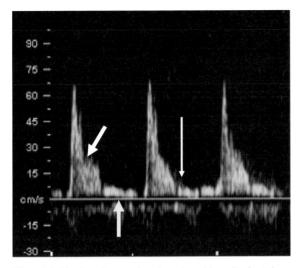

Fig. 5.24. The Doppler sample volume is positioned in the right pulmonary artery parallel with the flow. Branch pulmonary artery flow has this typical pattern of a sharp peak, followed by a notch (broad arrow) and a small reverse wave (thin arrow) at the end of systole before a small amount of forward flow during diastole (yellow arrow).

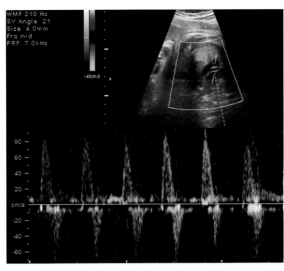

Fig. 5.25. The Doppler sample volume is positioned in the distal aortic arch in a normal fetus at 38 weeks of gestation. There is mainly forward flow in the arch (above the line), with a small jet of reverse flow (below the line) in early diastole.

the two ventricles function in parallel, output from both ventricles must be added together to give the combined cardiac output. Combined cardiac output is almost 500 ml/kg per min, which is close to what is expected from fetal lamb studies or from postnatal life. The right heart output is usually greater than the left, with a ratio of 55% : 45% respectively around 20 weeks of gestation. It changes to about 60% : 40% in the last 10 weeks of pregnancy. Volume flows are affected in late pregnancy by the fetal behavioral state, with an increase in left heart flow during active compared with passive sleep states. Contrary to established belief derived from the ovine model, a significant proportion of the combined cardiac output passes through the lung fields and returns to the left atrium as pulmonary venous return. The pulmonary blood flow rises from about 13% at 20 weeks, concomitantly with a fall in flow across the foramen ovale, until about 30 weeks when it stabilizes at about 25% of combined cardiac output. Because of the close position of the left ventricular outflow tract and mitral valve, a Doppler sample volume positioned in the left ventricle can display both flow profiles. This allows the isovolumic relaxation (IVRT) and contraction (IVCT) times and the ejection time (ET) to be measured simultaneously (Fig. 5.26). A fairly load independent index of function is the Tei index which is calculated from the formula,

IVRT + IVCT/ET. Doppler characteristics have also been used to calculate right and left ventricular force during gestation which increases 10-fold between 20 weeks' gestation and term but is similar for both ventricles.

Abnormal pulsed Doppler

Ductus venosus

An abnormal pattern of flow in the ductus venosus was first described in conditions of fetal hypoxia, where the "A" wave is reduced or even reversed (Fig. 5.27(a)). In the early fetus (<14 weeks), however, this appearance can be compatible with a normal outcome. In addition, the pattern can vary from normal, to absent flow in diastole to reversed flow in the same patient during the scanning time (Fig. 5.27(b)). Care should be taken, especially in the early fetus, not to confuse reverse flow with an overlying pattern of the hepatic vein (Fig. 5.27(c) and (e)). In **hypoxia**, the mechanism causing an abnormal flow pattern is probably dilatation of the duct, allowing the wave consequent on atrial contraction to be reflected further down the venous circulation. The depth of the notch is also influenced by **compliance and relaxation of the left ventricle, central venous pressure** as well as other factors. A reverse wave is commonly found in

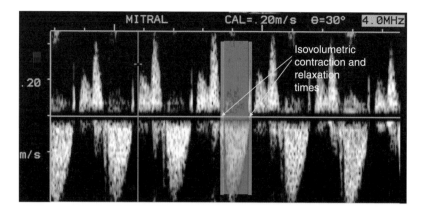

Fig. 5.26. The isovolumic contraction time (colored yellow) is the short interval between the end of atrial systole and the onset of ventricular contraction. The isovolumic relaxation time (colored pink) is the time interval between the end of ventricular systole and the onset of inflow into the ventricle (the E wave). The ejection time (colored blue) is the duration of ventricular systole. These time intervals are used in the Tei index, an index of ventricular function.

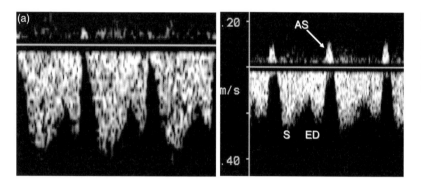

Fig. 5.27.(a). The ductus venosus tracing is abnormal in both panels with absent flow in atrial systole (AS) in the left-hand panel and reverse flow in the right-hand panel. Both these examples are in fetuses at 12 weeks' gestation. (S = systole, ED = early diastole)

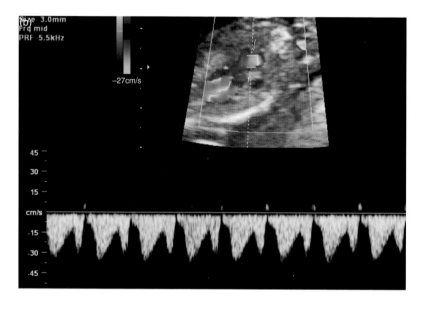

Fig. 5.27.(b). During the scanning time, the flow pattern in the ductus venosus in this fetus varied between forward, absent and reverse flow in diastole.

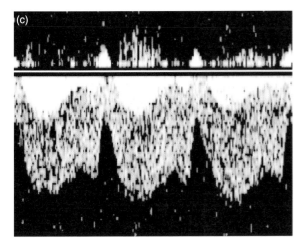

Fig 5.27.(c). Contd. The flow in the hepatic vein overlaps the tracing, which could be mistaken for reverse flow in the venous duct. Turning the gain down as shown allows the two separate flow profiles to be distinguished. Here the flow profile in the ductus venosus is normal.

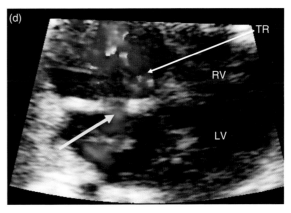

Fig. 5.27.(d). This fetus had pulmonary atresia with intact ventricular septum. There was high velocity tricuspid regurgitation (TR). In this malformation, all the venous return to the right atrium must cross the foramen ovale defect to the left atrium. The defect can be seen here to be quite small (yellow arrow).

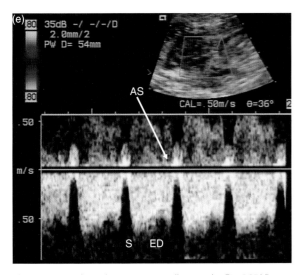

Fig. 5.27.(e). This is the same case as illustrated in Fig. 5.27.(d). There is reverse flow in the ductus venosus in diastole, in this case indicating a degree of restriction at the atrial septum to this excess volume of blood flow crossing it because of an obstructed right heart. (S = systole, ED = early diastole, AS = atrial systole)

right ventricular malformations such as tricuspid atresia and pulmonary atresia with intact septum and is due to relative restriction of the foramen ovale defect (Fig. 5.27(c)). In these conditions, all the blood returning to the right atrium has to cross the interatrial communication before proceeding through the heart. The foramen ovale defect therefore has to accommodate about twice its usual volume. If the defect is somewhat restrictive in this setting, this will be reflected in the flow pattern in the ductus venosus (Fig. 5.27(d) and (e)).

Pulmonary veins

An abnormal pulmonary vein flow pattern can occur in **left heart disease** associated with obstruction to the foramen ovale defect, and in **obstructed totally anomalous pulmonary venous drainage**. In left heart disease, such as critical aortic stenosis or the hypoplastic left heart syndrome, all, or nearly all, the pulmonary venous return must cross the foramen ovale to the right atrium. If the foramen ovale is widely patent, the pulmonary vein flow pattern will be normal. If, however, the foramen is restrictive or intact, the flow pattern will show varying degrees of abnormality (Fig. 5.28), which in turn will reflect varying degrees of venous congestion of, and subsequent damage to, the lungs. Occasionally, the pulmonary vein flow appears fairly normal and yet the atrial septum appears intact. This should alert the echocardiographer to look for a draining vein from the left atrium, the so-called levo-atrial-cardinal vein, which drains upwards to the innominate vein or superior vena cava. This vein is an embryonic structure which usually involutes, but can remain when the normal exits of the left atrium are obstructed. When the pulmonary veins drain anomalously, they usually come to a confluence behind the left atrium but very close to it, which can give the false impression that they drain normally (Fig. 5.29(a)–(c)). The Doppler

173

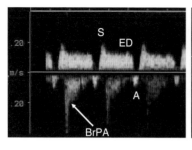
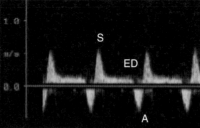

Fig. 5.28. In the left-hand panel, the flow profile in the pulmonary vein shows a lower wave than normal in early diastole (ED) and reverse flow during atrial systole (AS). This suggests mild restriction at the foramen ovale defect in a case of mitral atresia. As the pulmonary vein lies very close the artery, flow in the branch pulmonary artery (BrPA) is often seen on the same tracing as here. In the right-hand panel, the flow in early diastole is almost absent and there is a deep flow reversal wave. This indicates severe restriction at the foramen ovale in a case of the hypoplastic left heart syndrome.

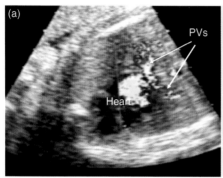
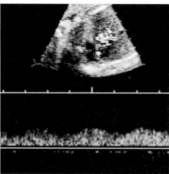

Fig. 5.29.(a). On the color flow map in the left-hand panel, the pulmonary veins come very close to the left atrium in the four-chamber view and join to a confluence. This then drained caudally, passing through the diaphragm in long-axis views (see Fig. 4.15) to join the portal system in the liver. The Doppler flow profile in the pulmonary vein shown in the right-hand panel does not demonstrate the typical notching characteristic of normal pulmonary vein flow (compare with Fig. 5.16), but shows continuous phasic flow. This flow pattern alone suggests a partially obstructed connection, which nearly always indicates that the veins connect to some other site than the atria.

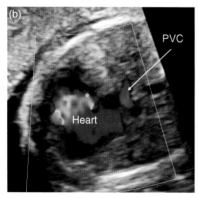
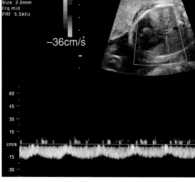

Fig. 5.29.(b). A pulmonary venous confluence is seen behind the heart in this fetus with right atrial isomerism. The flow profile on the right-hand panel indicated that the confluence did not connect to the atrial mass as it showed an obstructed pattern.

flow profile in this setting would usually be abnormal which should alert the echocardiographer to look for an ascending or descending venous channel. Usually the site of junction of a venous confluence, whether to the superior vena cava, innominate vein, portal system, or inferior vena cava, is partially obstructed, producing not only an abnormal pulsed Doppler tracing in the pulmonary vein itself, but also an area of flow acceleration in the upper thorax or abdomen.

Foramen ovale

The flow at the foramen ovale will be **reversed** in conditions of **obstruction to the left heart** such as mitral stenosis or atresia, critical aortic stenosis or the hypoplastic

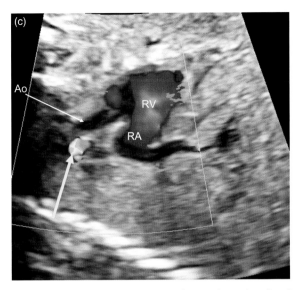

Fig. 5.29.(c). Contd. Imaging in sagittal views, showed an aliased area of flow in the upper thorax (yellow arrow). This was the narrow junction of the ascending vein, which drained the pulmonary venous confluence to the superior vena cava.

left heart syndrome. There may also be more reversal than normal in **coarctation of the aorta**. **Primary restriction** of the foramen ovale (in the absence of left heart disease) is a condition I have never knowingly seen in nearly 30 years of fetal heart scanning although it is reported in the literature. In order to make the diagnosis, there should be a high velocity jet between the right and left atria. This has been reported to lead to right heart dilatation and fetal hydrops.

Mitral valve

The E/A wave pattern of the mitral valve is very rarely abnormal in a clinically useful way. **Mitral regurgitation** is discussed in the chapter on the four-chamber view. **Stenosis** of the mitral valve is a rare abnormality in the fetus and would not be associated with an increase in the Doppler velocity of flow, as blood in the left atrium "off-loads" across the atrial septum instead of crossing the mitral valve.

Tricuspid valve

As with the mitral valve, the E/A wave pattern of the tricuspid valve is very rarely abnormal in a clinically useful way. **Tricuspid regurgitation** can be seen on color flow mapping and pulsed Doppler. The causes are discussed in Chapter 2 on the four-chamber view. The regurgitation jet will be at relatively low velocities (1–2 m/s) in the setting of a dilated right ventricle or in

a morphologically abnormal tricuspid valve (Fig. 5.30), but at higher velocity in pulmonary atresia with intact septum (Fig. 5.31).

In similar fashion to the mitral valve, **stenosis** of the tricuspid valve is a rare abnormality in the fetus and is not detected because of an increase in the Doppler velocity of flow, as blood in the right atrium would "off-load" across the atrial septum instead of crossing the tricuspid valve.

Ventricular septal defect

In utero, the pressure on both sides of the heart is more or less equal, unless there is obstruction in either the left or right ventricular outflow tract, when the obstructed side will obviously have a higher pressure. Usually therefore in an isolated ventricular septal defect, the flow across the defect will be from right to left at the beginning of the cardiac cycle, as the right ventricle contracts slightly before the left, and from left to right at the end of the cycle. This can be demonstrated on pulsed Doppler with the sample volume positioned in the defect (Fig. 5.32).

Aortic valve

There will be **no forward flow** across the valve in aortic atresia, but this must be confirmed by finding reversed flow in the arch. The **velocity** of flow in the aorta is **increased** in the setting of a stenotic aortic valve. This can be the only abnormal finding in mild to moderate degrees of **aortic stenosis**, with velocities up to 4 m/s. (Fig. 5.33(a)). In severe or critical aortic stenosis, there will be associated left ventricular hypertrophy initially, but, later in the disease process, diminished left ventricular function and lower velocities as a result (Fig. 5.33(b)). The velocity of flow in the aorta may be mildly increased in **tetralogy of Fallot** (Fig. 5.34). Continuous **reversed** flow in the **aortic arch** will indicate a **severely obstructed aortic valve**. Subaortic stenosis due to a membrane is very rare in the fetus (and neonate), although I have seen it once. An intriguing lesion causing subaortic stenosis is seen in Fig. 5.35(a) and (b). This was a brightly echogenic mass in the left ventricular outflow tract, with aliased high velocity flow in the ascending aorta. After birth, the mass was still seen but it was no longer causing significant obstruction. As the child has grown, the mass has not and there is now a normal aortic velocity on pulsed Doppler. The histology of the lesion is unknown. It really appeared too echogenic for a rhabdomyoma and there is no evidence of tuberose sclerosis in the child who has been thoroughly investigated for this. **Aortic incompetence** is an unusual finding in the fetus, and may indicate an **aorto-left ventricular tunnel** (see

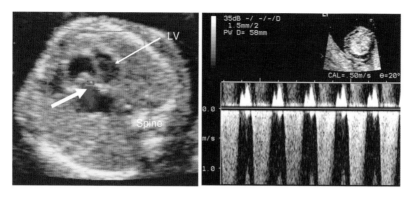

Fig. 5.30. There was a small jet of tricuspid regurgitation (thick arrow) seen on the color flow map. This was confirmed on pulsed Doppler to be holosystolic (throughout systole) and at a velocity of flow above 1 m/s. On the moving image, the right ventricle could be seen to be poorly contracting and the tricuspid valve somewhat dysplastic.

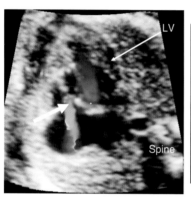
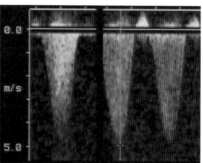

Fig. 5.31. There was tricuspid regurgitation in the four-chamber view. The Doppler sample volume positioned in the regurgitant jet, gave a velocity of over nearly 5 m/s (right-hand panel), indicating a right ventricular pressure of over 100 mmHg, which is very high for any gestational age. This was pulmonary atresia with intact ventricular septum.

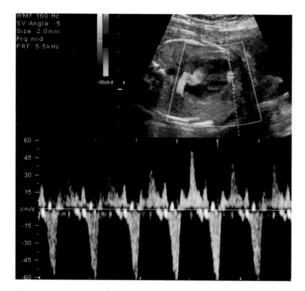

Fig. 5.32. The sample volume is positioned in a moderate-sized apical muscular ventricular septal defect. The flow from the right ventricle to the left is here represented by three small jets above the baseline, lasting through more of the cardiac cycle than the left to right flow. Left-to-right flow is shorter and at a higher velocity (below the baseline). The pattern of flow can be variable but is always bidirectional in the absence of outflow tract obstruction on one or other side of the heart.

Fig. 3.22(a) and (b)), **aortic valve disease**, or if mild, it may be **benign and transitory** (Fig. 5.36), although this is a very rare observation.

Common arterial trunk

The velocity of flow is usually mildly increased (up to 1.5 m/s) in a common arterial trunk but a velocity higher than this would indicate a degree of associated **truncal stenosis**, a poor prognostic feature (Fig. 5.37). A minor degree of **truncal valve regurgitation** is common but more significant regurgitation (see Fig. 3.28(a)) will affect the functional result, as this valve will become the aortic valve after surgical repair.

Pulmonary valve

There will be **no forward flow** across the valve in **pulmonary atresia**, and this will be confirmed by demonstrating reversed flow in the arterial duct. The velocity of flow in the pulmonary artery is **increased** in the setting of **pulmonary stenosis**. This can be the only abnormal finding in mild to moderate degrees of pulmonary stenosis (Fig. 5.38), with velocities which can reach as high as 4 m/s. In severe or critical pulmonary stenosis, there may be appreciable right ventricular hypertrophy

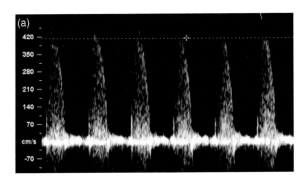

Fig. 5.33.(a). In this fetus, the left ventricular function was still good, generating a velocity of over 4 m/s across the valve. This is a severe case of aortic stenosis but a less critical example than that seen in Fig. 5.33(b), where left ventricular dysfunction has developed.

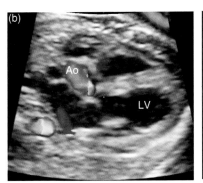 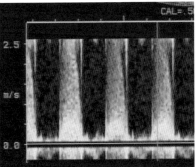

Fig. 5.33.(b). The aortic velocity is increased in the setting of aortic valve stenosis. On the left-hand panel, the left ventricle can be seen to be globular in shape. It was poorly contracting with little filling on the moving image. There was aliasing of the color flow map across the aortic valve. The obstruction at the aortic valve was severe, resulting in left ventricular dysfunction, such that only a peak velocity of 2.5 m/s was obtained on pulsed Doppler on the right-hand panel. At the end of pregnancy, the reserve of the ventricle in the fetus illustrated in Fig. 5.33(a) allowed a biventricular repair, whereas the fetus illustrated in 5.33(b) did not.

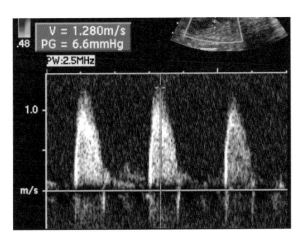

Fig. 5.34. There was a mildly increased Doppler flow velocity to 128 cm/s in the ascending aorta, in this case of tetralogy of Fallot at 22 weeks of gestation.

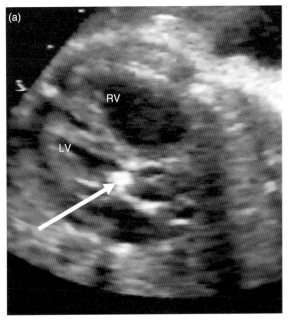

Fig. 5.35.(a). A mobile, echogenic mass was seen in the left ventricular outflow tract at 35 weeks of gestation.

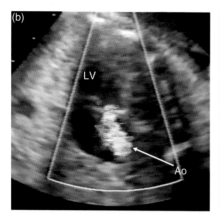

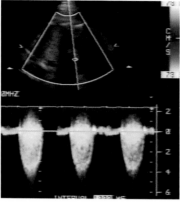

Fig. 5.35.(b). Contd. The lesion was partially obstructing aortic flow causing aliasing on color flow mapping of the aortic flow, and a velocity of almost 4 m/s on continuous wave Doppler (right-hand panel).

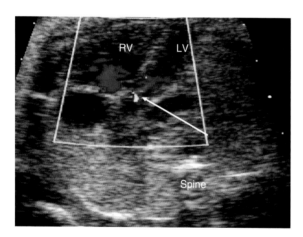

Fig. 5.36. There was trivial to mild but convincing aortic regurgitation (arrow) seen at 28 weeks' gestation. Careful examination of the left heart in particular did not appear to show any abnormality. At delivery, the heart was completely normal with no aortic regurgitation.

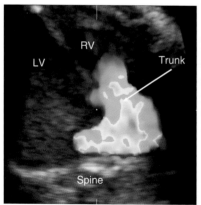

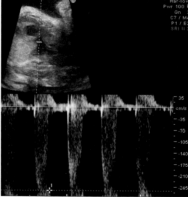

Fig. 5.37. On the left-hand panel, the common trunk arose predominantly from the right ventricle. There was aliasing of flow within the single great artery on the color flow map. On the right-hand panel, the Doppler sample volume is positioned just above the truncal valve. The velocity of almost 250 cm/s indicates mild to moderate truncal valve stenosis. The valve itself appeared thickened and doming during systole, with significant regurgitation on color flow mapping.

initially, or later, diminished right ventricular function and lower velocities as a result, but, except in twin-twin transfusion syndrome (see Fig. 3.22(e)), this picture of poor function is less commonly seen than in the left heart. **Reversed flow in the duct** will indicate a **severely obstructed or atretic pulmonic valve**. The velocity of flow in the pulmonary artery (and aorta) is often mildly increased in tetralogy of Fallot (see Fig. 5.34). Although there is usually moderately severe pulmonary stenosis in tetralogy, the blood flow can exit the aorta instead of going through the narrow pulmonary artery, so the degree of increase in the velocity does not reflect the degree of pulmonary narrowing. **Pulmonary incompetence** is uncommon and may indicate the **absent**

pulmonary valve syndrome, a **dysplastic pulmonary valve** (Fig. 5.39), **ductal constriction**, **high pressure** in **the peripheral vascular bed** or rarely it is seen in an otherwise normal heart when it may be **benign and reversible**. It may also occur in the so-called functional pulmonary atresia in the **twin–twin transfusion syndrome**. This is when the arterial pressure is very high in the recipient twin as a result of severe twin–twin transfusion syndrome. The right ventricle becomes thick and hypertrophied and eventually dysfunctional when it fails to produce forward flow across the pulmonary valve, therefore functional pulmonary atresia. The pulmonary valve however can be seen to be patent because of pulmonary incompetence (Fig. 5.40).

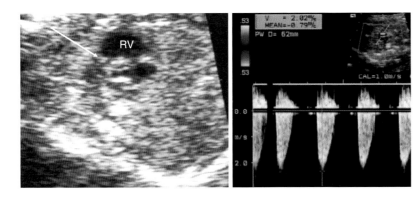

Fig. 5.38. The pulmonary valve appeared thickened on 2D images (arrow in left-hand panel) and the flow across the right ventricular outflow tract showed aliasing on color flow mapping. When the pulsed Doppler sample volume was positioned just above the valve leaflets, a velocity of just over 2 m/s was obtained (right-hand panel). This is indicative of moderate pulmonary stenosis.

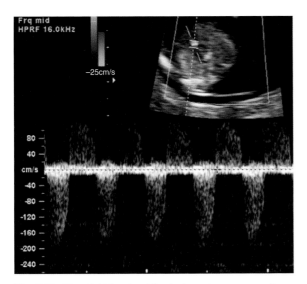

Fig. 5.39. There is bidirectional flow in the pulmonary artery in this fetus with a dysplastic pulmonary valve. Forward flow is below the zero line and reverse flow above it. The velocity of nearly 2 m/s across the pulmonary valve was found at 14 weeks' gestation, indicating severe pulmonary stenosis. A gradient of 80 mmHg was found in the neonate.

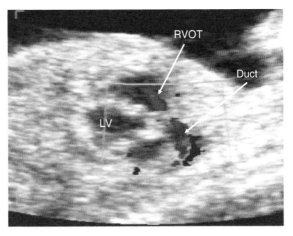

Fig. 5.40. The fetus is seen in a long-axis view of the arterial duct. There is reverse flow in the duct, which continues into the right ventricular outflow tract (RVOT), across the pulmonary valve. There was no forward flow into the pulmonary artery because of severe right ventricular dysfunction in this recipient twin in the twin–twin transfusion syndrome. This is functional pulmonary atresia.

179

Branch PAs

Although abnormal patterns of flow in the branch pulmonary arteries have been suggested as indicators of abnormal pulmonary parenchyma, such as can occur in diaphragmatic hernia or oligohydramnios, we have not found this to be reliable or clinically useful. Acceleration of flow in the branch pulmonary arteries has been reported occasionally in the fetus as a sign of branch stenosis. This would raise the possibility of Alagille's or Williams' syndrome.

Arterial duct

The velocity of flow in the arterial duct will be **increased** to over 2 m/s in the setting of **ductal constriction**. This is usually reversible if a stimulus, such as maternal ingestion of anti-inflammatory agents, is identified and stopped. The vessel will appear narrow in the 2D image and flow will be aliased on color flow mapping. Doppler velocities will be above the normal range. **Reversal of flow in the arterial duct** will be seen where there is inadequate forward flow across the pulmonary valve to supply the branch pulmonary arteries. It is best seen on color flow mapping but can be confirmed by pulsed Doppler (Fig. 5.41). This will occur in severe **pulmonary stenosis or pulmonary atresia, in severe tricuspid regurgitation, or in decreased right ventricular function.**

Isthmus

A coarctation shelf in fetal life does not cause an increase in flow velocity around the arch in the same way as it does postnatally, due to the large patent duct in utero. **Reversal of flow** in the isthmus will occur where there is inadequate forward flow across the aortic valve to supply the coronary arteries and the flow will be reversed throughout systole and diastole. This

will occur in **severe aortic stenosis**, in **aortic atresia** or with **diminished left ventricular function**. It will also occur in the setting of **placental insufficiency**, when there is redistribution of flow and dilatation of intracerebral vessels. A small amount of reverse flow in the arch is not uncommonly seen in normal late pregnancy (Fig. 5.25) but does not occur throughout the whole cardiac cycle as it does in aortic valve obstruction. Bidirectional flow can occur in the small fetus (see Chapter 6) in the arch or duct, usually in **trisomy 18. Bidirectional flow** in the arch (see Fig. 3.48(b)) can occur when there is an **intracranial arteriovenous malformation** (vein of Galen aneurysm).

The use of M-mode echocardiography

As the resolution of cross-sectional imaging has improved and pulsed Doppler has become available, M-mode has become less used in evaluating the heart, both in fetal and in pediatric cardiology. Its main current application is for:

(1) Measurement of cardiac structures.
(2) Estimation of left ventricular function.
(3) Evaluation of atrial and ventricular contraction sequence.

Normal M-mode

Measurements of chamber or vessel sizes using M-mode are more exact than those made from the cross-sectional image because of the very high sampling rate, but they must be made in a standard orientation (axial) to the structures being measured. This limits its usefulness in the fetus as, depending on the fetal position, the correct orientation cannot always be achieved. The correct position for measuring the left and right ventricular chamber sizes, the septal and left ventricular

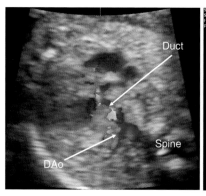
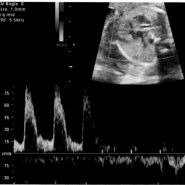

Fig. 5.41. On the left-hand panel on color flow mapping, a small tortuous arterial duct was found underneath the aortic arch in this case of pulmonary atresia. Reverse flow, originating from the descending aorta (DAo), was seen in the duct. On the right-hand panel, the pulsed Doppler sample volume positioned in the duct, confirmed reverse flow in the arterial duct.

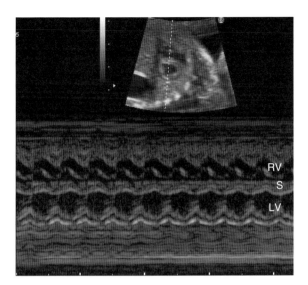

Fig. 5.42. In the 2D image shown above the tracing, the fetus is seen in the correct orientation for M-mode measurement of the shortening fraction of the left ventricle. The M-mode obtained from this view shows the right ventricle contracting anteriorly and the left ventricle posteriorly. The thickening of the septum (S) and walls of the ventricles during systole can be examined and measured.

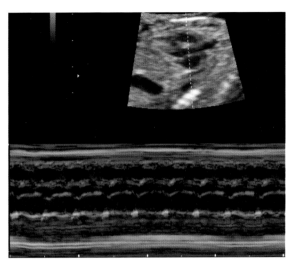

Fig. 5.43. The correct orientation for M-mode examination of the aorta and left atrium is either a long-axis view of the left ventricle as shown, or a short-axis view of the aortic origin.

free wall thickness, is a short-axis view of the left ventricle just below the mitral valve orifice (Fig. 5.42). This corresponds to the same site for measurement of the left heart in postnatal life. The contraction of the two ventricles is seen by examining the thickening of their walls and the septum during systole, as the walls move towards the septum. In order to obtain a correct aortic root and left atrial measurement, the M-line must be placed perpendicular to the aortic walls at the level of the valve orifice, in a long- or short-axis view of the aorta (Fig. 5.43).

M-mode is still useful in determining the shortening fraction of the left ventricle, as an estimate of systolic function. The M-line must be positioned in a standard fashion through the short-axis view of the left ventricle, as it is obtained in postnatal life. The left ventricular measurements are obtained from the left ventricular surface of the ventricular septum to the posterior free wall of the left ventricle (endocardial or inner surface), as close to end diastole (largest dimension) and end systole (smallest dimension) as possible. The right ventricular measurements are made from the right ventricular anterior free wall (endocardial surface) to the right ventricular surface of the ventricular septum. Shortening fraction (SF) is obtained from the formula SF = EDD – ESD/EDD, where EDD = end-

diastolic dimension and ESD = end-systolic dimension (Fig. 5.39). The left ventricular shortening fraction (or fractional shortening) ranges between 28% and 40%, as in postnatal life, and does not change between 18 and 40 weeks' gestation. It is appropriate to use this formula for the left heart because of the circular arrangement of muscle fibres, but not for the right ventricle. Values for the change in dimension during the cardiac cycle in the right ventricle can be estimated, but this is not the shortening fraction, strictly speaking. The usefulness of the right ventricular measurement is limited by the fact that the measurement is subject to error if exactly the same position across the right ventricle is not obtained every time. In practice, this is very difficult with variations in fetal position, so that measurements both between patients and in the same patient at different times are not reproducible or truly comparable. Abnormal left ventricular function can usually be appreciated by the experienced echocardiographer simply by observing the moving cross-sectional image of the left ventricle. However, a more exact estimation can be quantified by measuring the shortening fraction on M-mode (Fig. 5.44).

The main use for M-mode is in the evaluation of the cardiac rhythm, which is more fully discussed in Chapter 7. When the M-line is positioned through the atrial and ventricular wall or the atrial wall and aortic valve, the contraction sequence of the heart can be analysed. Every ventricular contraction is preceded

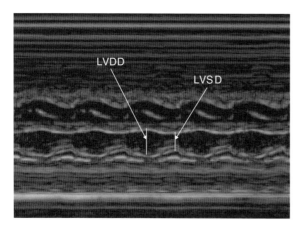

Fig. 5.44. The method of measuring the left ventricle on M-mode for calculating shortening fraction is shown. The left ventricular dimension in diastole (LVDD) is more or less the maximum dimension and the left ventricular systolic dimension (LVSD) is the smallest dimension. The change in right ventricular dimension between systole and diastole can also be measured in this view, but this is not strictly speaking the shortening fraction of the right ventricle.

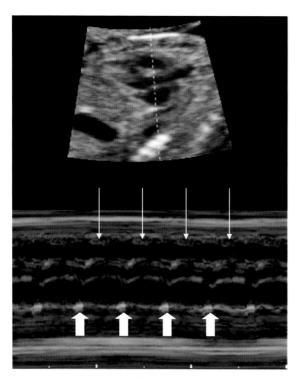

Fig. 5.45. The M-line passes through the right ventricle anteriorly, then the aortic valve and left atrial wall. The motion of the atrial wall and the ventricular wall, or the atrial wall and the opening of the aortic valve, can be used to determine the time interval between atrial and ventricular contraction. Although the timing of the exact onset of atrial and ventricular walls is difficult to determine, here there is clearly a one-to-one relationship between atrial (block arrows) and ventricular (thin arrows) contraction, with atrial contraction preceding ventricular contraction by a fixed time interval of less than approximately 140 ms.

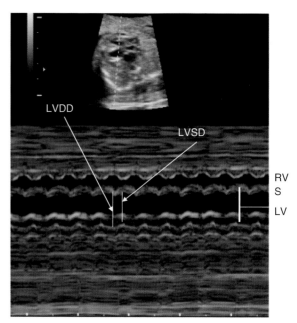

Fig. 5.46. The M-mode is recorded through the left ventricle in a case of critical aortic stenosis. The right ventricle is anterior and the wall moves well in contrast to the diminished excursion of the left ventricular wall. The bright echo within the left ventricle is the papillary muscle of the mitral valve, which is more echogenic than normal in this condition. The left ventricle is dilated and poorly contracting. The shortening fraction was measured at 12%, confirming the visual impression of diminished function. S = septum.

by an atrial contraction, approximately 80–120 ms before it, at the usual fetal heart rate of 140 beats/min (Fig. 5.45). The interval between atrial and ventricular contraction is the equivalent of the PR interval on the surface electrocardiogram. However, the same information on the sequence of atrial and ventricular contraction can also be obtained using Doppler techniques, often more easily, so even this use of M-mode is becoming obsolete.

Abnormal M-mode

Prior to the availability of Doppler flow mapping, the M-mode pattern of cardiac valve motion was recorded routinely, as abnormal patterns were used as an indication of valve obstruction. However, the correlation of valve thickening, and the shape of valve opening on M-mode, with the degree of stenosis was poor. By contrast, measurement of Doppler velocities through the cardiac valves can provide accurate information about valve stenosis. The patterns of M-mode valve tracings therefore are no longer used in current practice.

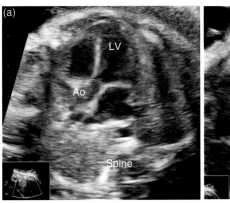
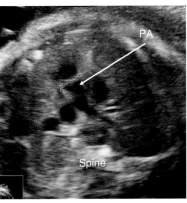

Fig. 5.47.(a). On the left panel, the aorta is measured at the valve ring in diastole (when the valve itself is seen). On the right panel, in the same patient, the pulmonary artery is measured at the valve ring in diastole. Ideally, the valves should be measured when the beam is perpendicular to the walls but the clarity of the walls in this image allow an accurate measurement. Note that the pulmonary artery appears slightly larger than the aorta in the same normal fetus.

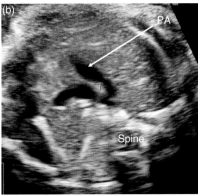
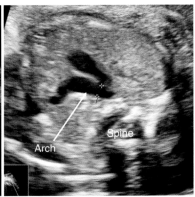

Fig. 5.47.(b). On the left-hand panel, the arterial duct is measured. On the right, the distal arch in the region of the isthmus is measured. We prefer this view of the isthmus for measurement, although a long-axis view can be used. The measurements obtained will be slightly different, however. Note that the transverse arch is usually slightly bigger than the duct in a normal mid-trimester fetus.

The importance of exact positioning of the M-line is a particular handicap in the fetus, when perpendicular alignment to each structure is not always possible, although some modern ultrasound machines have "steerable" M-mode. Thus, cross-sectional measurements of cardiac structures and chambers have superseded the original M-mode measurements. Diminished ventricular function can be appreciated visually on 2D images but it certainly is more accurately measured on M-mode and this remains useful. An example of diminished left ventricular function in aortic stenosis is seen in Fig. 5.46. Abnormal M-mode tracings in the context of arrhythmias are described in Chapter 7.

2D measurements

It is not essential to make measurements on 2D during a routine fetal echocardiogram. However, it can be useful to do so in order to confirm a normal size of the fetal heart structures and to remain familiar with the expected normal size at the usual gestational age for fetal heart evaluation. The possible measurements to be made in a four-chamber view have been shown in Chapter 2, although we do not make these measurements as a routine. We do, however, routinely measure the aorta and pulmonary artery, the arterial duct and isthmus. All measurements should be made in a standard fashion (Fig. 5.47(a) and (b)). The measurements should be compared to normal ranges, which are nowadays imbedded into the common databases in use in fetal medicine (Fig. 5.48(a)–(d)). However, these should not be interpreted too literally as some of the data currently used are not always accurate, especially at later gestations. Some more recent publications of Z scores may be more useful and a useful website for this is www.parameterZ.com. Measuring the size of the pulmonary artery branches can be useful in some abnormalities and the method of measurement and the growth over gestation are shown in Fig. 5.49.

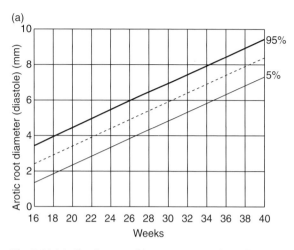

(a)

Fig. 5.48.(a). The diameter of the aorta, measured as in Fig. 5.47(a), is plotted against gestational age.

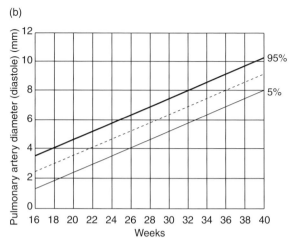

(b)

Fig. 5.48.(b). The diameter of the pulmonary artery, measured as in Fig. 5.47(a), is plotted against gestational age.

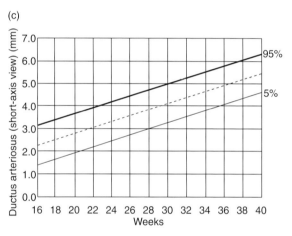

(c)

Fig. 5.48.(c). The diameter of the arterial duct, measured in a transverse view as in Fig. 5.47(b), is plotted against gestational age.

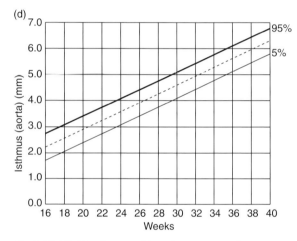

(d)

Fig. 5.48.(d). The diameter of the isthmus, measured in a transverse view as in Fig. 5.47(b), is plotted against gestational age.

Rendering

We only recently acquired a machine capable of volume rendering. It involves quite a lot of off-line work for limited gain in terms of understanding the defect. The rendering is handicapped if image quality has been poor at acquisition, although this is exactly the situation when you would like rendering to add information. However, it can produce some beautiful images. Figure 5.50 shows "broad-slice" rendering of the left and right ventricular apex, which clearly demonstrates the difference in trabeculation between the two. Rendering of the crux in broad-slice can allow an "en face" view of the atrioventricular valves in the

normal fetus (Fig. 5.51), in an atrioventricular septal defect (Fig. 5.52), or in cases where the integrity of the crux is in doubt (Fig. 5.53(a)). Rendering can provide a better appreciation of the depth and volume of some defects (Fig. 5.53(b) and (c), Fig. 5.54(a) and (b)). It can allow the relative positions of the arterial valves in transposition to be determined (Fig. 5.55(a)–(d)), which have some correlation with the frequency of coronary artery abnormalities and therefore ease of surgical repair. It can allow arch reconstruction (Fig. 5.56) but, in our fairly limited experience so far, we have not found it helpful in diagnosing or refuting coarctation, which is always a difficult diagnosis prenatally. It can

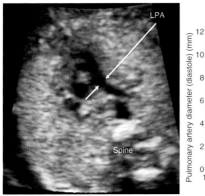
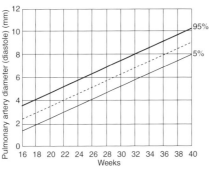

Fig. 5.49. On the left-hand panel, the heart is seen in a three-vessel view, slightly angled in order to image the left pulmonary artery. It can be measured at its origin (between the arrowheads) as shown. The growth during gestation is shown on the right-hand panel. Both branches of the pulmonary artery should be similar in size, so the chart can be used for either.

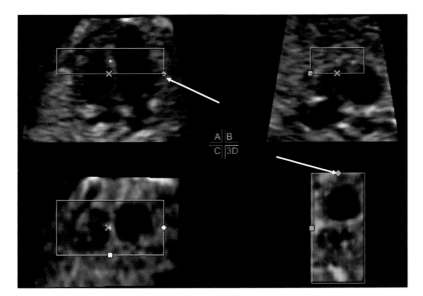

Fig. 5.50. Both apices are viewed from the vantage point of the green line. The left ventricular apex looks "empty," whereas the right is filled with coarse muscle bundles. The diamond (arrow) indicates the left side.

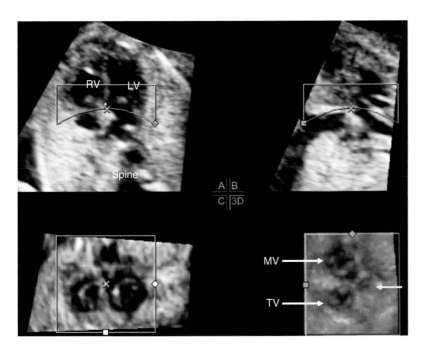

Fig. 5.51. The atrioventricular valves are viewed from the green line, as if from the atria. In the rendered image, the leaflets of the closed atrioventricular valves can almost be discerned with the aortic valve in the normal "wedged" position between them (yellow arrow) in this normal heart.

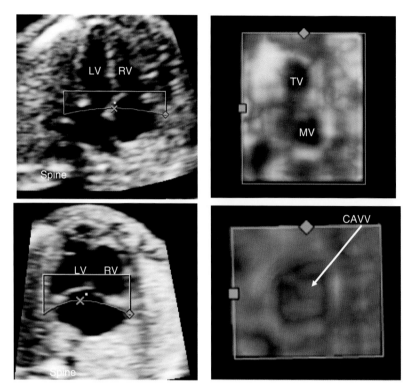

Fig. 5.52. In the upper panels, the atrioventricular junction is normal, with two discrete valve orifices in the right-hand rendered image. In the lower panels, there is a common atrioventricular valve (CAVV), which is seen as one orifice in the right-hand rendered image.

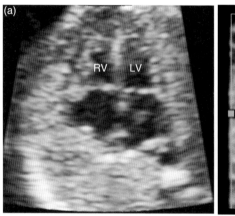
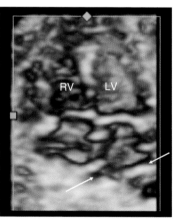

Fig. 5.53.(a). In this fetus, the crux in the 2D image, seen on the left-hand panel, was suspicious for loss of off-setting, which could indicate a small atrioventricular septal defect. The atrioventricular junction appears rather "straight." However, the rendered image in the right-hand panel, clearly demonstrated normal off-setting. Note that the structure of the foramen ovale defect and the pulmonary veins (arrows) are seen well in this type of image.

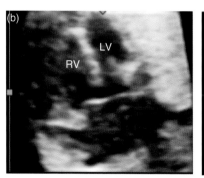
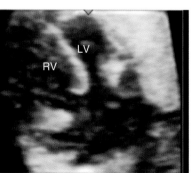

Fig. 5.53.(b). In this fetus with an atrioventricular septal defect, the defect was clear in the four-chamber view from normal 2D imaging. However, the rendered image gives a different appreciation of the defect in the systolic (left-hand panel) and diastolic frames (right-hand panel).

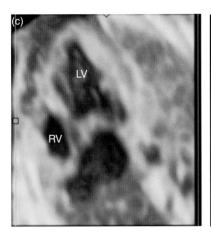 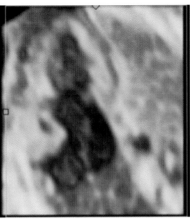

Fig. 5.53.(c). Contd. In the rendered four-chamber view, the atrioventricular valve lies straight across the crux and there is a hypoplastic right ventricle. When the atrioventricular valve is open in diastole (right-hand panel), it can be seen that most of the common valve opens into the left ventricle.

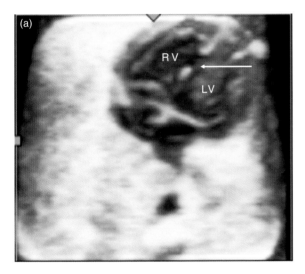

Fig. 5.54.(a). There was an apical muscular ventricular septal defect well seen in 2D views. The rendered image, however, gives a better impression of the depth of the defect (arrow).

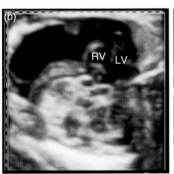 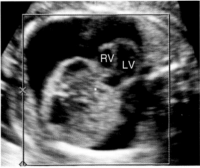

Fig. 5.54.(b). The rendered image (right-hand panel) of the teratoma seen on the left, adds some depth and volume information to the understanding of the lesion. The cystic nature of the tumor mass is emphasized.

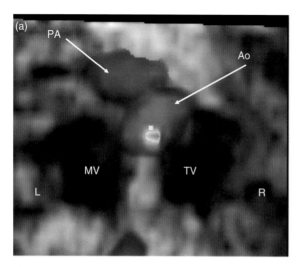

Fig. 5.55.(a). The 4 cardiac valves are rendered in an "en face" view in order to display the relative positions of the great arteries. Which valve is which in terms of right–left orientation has to be determined in the "A" plane on Voluson rendering. The normal relationship of the great arteries to the atrioventricular valves is shown. Note that the aorta is normally "wedged" close between the two atrioventricular valves whereas the pulmonary artery lies above and to the left of the aorta.

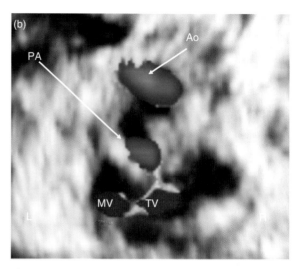

Fig. 5.55.(b). The relative positions of the arterial valves in a case of transposition is shown. This is the most common arrangement seen in transposition, with the aorta anterior and to the right of the pulmonary artery. As the relative positions of the great arteries has some correlation with the incidence of coronary artery anomalies, this may be of some usefulness, although the relative great artery positions can also be determined by standard 2D views (see Fig. 3.31(c)).

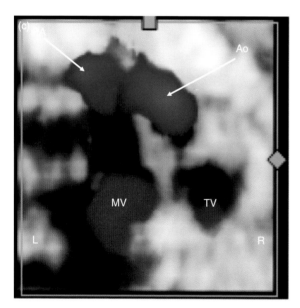

Fig. 5.55.(c). In a less common form of transposition, the aorta and pulmonary artery lie side-by-side with each other.

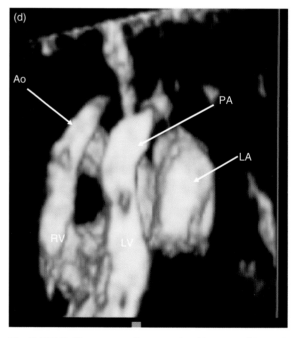

Fig. 5.55.(d). The great arteries are rendered in transposition and viewed from the front left side. The aorta arises anterior and to the right of the pulmonary artery. Compare this image with the normal spiral arrangement of the great arteries as seen in Fig. 3.2(f).

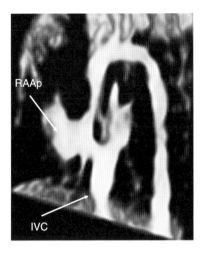 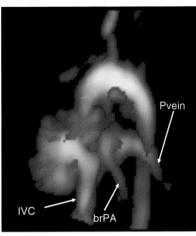

Fig. 5.56. The aortic arch has been rendered in inversion mode on the left and in color on the right. In both cases the aortic arch is viewed as if looking from the left side. The outlines of the vessels are not smooth in the left panel because of fetal movement during acquisition. It is almost impossible to obtain images where fetal movement does not occur. RAAp = right atrial appendage, Pvein = pulmonary vein, brPA = branch pulmonary artery.

be used to generate volume data of ventricular sizes, but this has limited usefulness in terms of the prediction of outcome.

Summary

Evaluation of the heart with color flow mapping is an essential part of cardiac analysis. It is important to develop and maintain skill in obtaining pulsed Doppler tracings and to be able to recognize the patterns of flow in different sites in the vascular system. Understanding the basic principles of Doppler analysis will allow the correct positioning of the ultrasound beam as close as possible to parallel to the direction of flow for both color and pulsed Doppler. They both provide confirmation of abnormal flow in specific malformations. Although M-mode is now of limited usefulness, the ultrasonographer should be familiar with its appearance and with the (few) situations in which it is appropriate and provides useful information. Measurement data, measured on the 2D image, can be useful as a routine and is often essential in the documentation of a particular cardiac malformation. Rendering is likely to become easier with advancing technology and increasingly used to aid the understanding of both the normal or abnormal heart structure.

First trimester fetal heart scanning

Fetal echocardiography is typically carried out between 18 and 23 weeks of gestation. In the past, it was our practice to follow up the first echocardiogram with a repeat examination at around 28 weeks of gestation when technically superior images could be expected. With improvements in ultrasound technology and evidence that few cardiac abnormalities are overlooked in the mid-trimester, late gestation scans are no longer scheduled as a routine. Our current practice is for late scans to be limited to specific situations, such as late presentation of a high-risk patient, follow-up of known abnormalities, or where the initial indication was for a family history of a condition such as aortic or pulmonary stenosis, which may evolve as the pregnancy progresses. Instead, attention has turned towards performing fetal echocardiography additionally at earlier gestations for some specific indications.

Fetal heart examination using transvaginal probes has been performed as early as 7–9 weeks of gestation in normal fetuses (Fig. 6.1). There are now several series reporting experience of fetal echocardiography and the reliable detection of major cardiac defects in the range of 11 to 15 weeks of gestation. Both transabdominal and transvaginal scanning have been reported to be successful. Those favoring the transvaginal route stress the advantage of higher resolution images obtained with high frequency transducers close to the fetus. Most of those regularly performing transvaginal fetal echocardiography have experience and skills in gynecological scanning. A vaginal position of the transducer limits its movement and therefore the range of views that can be obtained. This limitation can be overcome by external manipulation of the uterus about the probe with a hand on the maternal abdomen. However, these maneuvers are restricted at gestational ages less than 13 weeks, when the uterus remains within the pelvis. Transabdominal scanning allows more scope for manipulation of the probe around the uterus to achieve the multiple views required to establish normal connections or to assess an abnormality. Our experience is that restricted views, rather than lack of resolution, are the most frequent limiting factor in early fetal echocardiography. However, there are particular circumstances, such as in obese women, or in those with a retroverted uterus, where transvaginal scanning might be expected to have a clear advantage. As with any technique, practice and experience have a

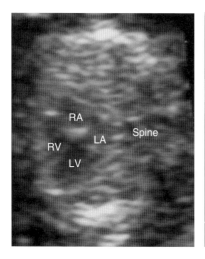 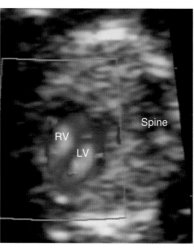

Fig. 6.1. The heart is imaged by the transvaginal route between the ninth and tenth weeks of gestation. The four chambers of the heart can be readily seen on 2D imaging and the color flow map shows filling of both ventricles across patent atrioventricular valves.

major impact on success. The favored methods of individual operators are probably determined by their own familiarity with the different techniques rather than by the intrinsic strengths and weaknesses of the modes of scanning. Figure 6.2(a) and (b) illustrate the type of images which can be obtained in an early fetus by the transabdominal route.

Indications for early fetal echocardiography

The rationale for performing fetal echocardiography early is that women at particularly high risk may be spared the anxiety of having to wait until 20 weeks for the first information about their baby's heart. In addition, where a severe defect is diagnosed, the mother may have the option of a surgical rather than medical

termination, which most women find less distressing. Detailed cardiac scanning before 14 weeks of gestation is technically demanding and will normally be carried out in addition to, rather than instead of, a 20–23-week scan. At the present time, it is appropriate to restrict a detailed study to those cases where there is a clear indication for it. A family history of severe congenital heart disease in a first-degree relative (a parent or sibling of the fetus) is one such indication. The recurrence rate in this situation is around 2%, and there is significant value in providing some early guarded reassurance that all seems well in the pregnancy, for a family previously traumatized by their experience with congenital heart disease. For a less clear-cut family history of congenital heart disease, maternal diabetes, or exposure to potentially teratogenic drugs, it has been our own usual practice to offer the first cardiac scan at

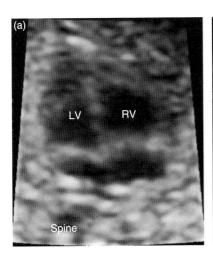
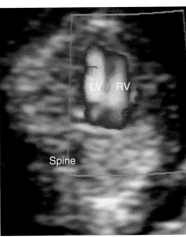

Fig. 6.2.(a). The fetus lies in an ideal position for cardiac scanning at the 12-week transabdominal nuchal scan. The four chambers of the heart are seen, with equal ventricular filling on the color flow map.

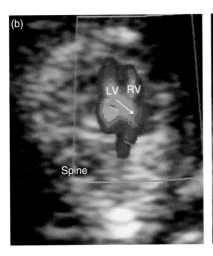
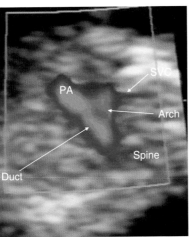

Fig. 6.2.(b). Just cranial to the image obtained in Fig. 6.2(a), the left ventricular outflow tract is seen on the left-hand panel arising from the left ventricle and directed rightwards. Immediately above the view obtained in the left-hand panel, the image on the right-hand panel is seen, which shows the pulmonary artery crossing over the aortic origin. It joins the transverse arch just in front of the spine via the arterial duct. Although the great arteries measure just over 1 mm at this gestation they are readily seen with color flow.

191

20 weeks. Early cardiac scanning, on the other hand, is routinely offered to those with increased nuchal translucency above the 99th centile (or over 3.5 mm), as these patients are at particularly high risk, depending on the degree of increase (Fig. 6.3). In our setting within a Fetal Medicine Unit, fetal echocardiography is normally performed at the same clinic visit as the nuchal scan and prior to chorion villous sampling (CVS) if this is to be performed. However, in centers where the fetal echocardiographer is not so readily available, it may be more appropriate to delay the cardiac scan until the result of rapid karyotype testing is available, as the incidence of chromosomal abnormality in this group is high. In addition, scanning at

14 weeks is substantially easier than at 12 weeks because of the rapid fetal growth during this period of time. This is illustrated by the pathological specimens seen in Fig. 6.4.

Whilst detailed heart examination is not indicated universally, a basic assessment of the fetal heart should be included as part of routine 11–14-week scans, in addition to assessment of the general anatomy and measurement of the nuchal translucency. As this practice has become more widespread, suspicion of cardiac abnormality at the routine 11–14-week scan on the part of the obstetric sonographer has become an increasingly common indication for referral for early fetal echocardiography (Fig. 6.5).

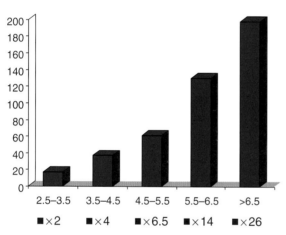

Fig. 6.3. The relationship between the nuchal translucency (NT) measurement and the incidence of cardiac malformation is seen. The incidence increases with increasing NT measurements, from twice the background rate when the measurement is between the 95th and 99th centiles to 26 times the normal rate when the NT is over 6.5 mm.

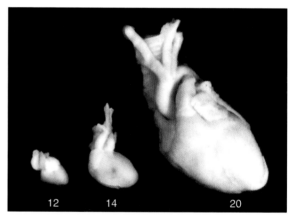

Fig. 6.4. Whole cardiac specimens are displayed at 12 weeks, 14 weeks and 20 weeks' gestation, respectively. The heart at 12 weeks is about the size of a grain of rice, at 20 weeks the size of a one euro or one pound coin. Note that the heart almost doubles in size between 12 and 14 weeks. Thus, defining the intracardiac anatomy is substantially easier at 14 than at 12 weeks.

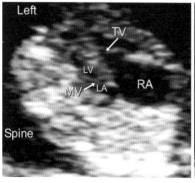
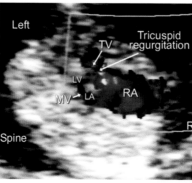

Fig. 6.5. In this fetus, the nuchal translucency measurement was normal but the sonographer noticed the abnormal appearance of the heart in the four-chamber view during the NT study. At detailed fetal echocardiography, the heart was enlarged due mainly to right atrial enlargement. This was due to displacement of the tricuspid valve into the right atrium. Color flow mapping showed tricuspid regurgitation. This was a case of Ebstein's anomaly of severe degree.

Technique

The basic principles of early fetal echocardiography are similar to those used at later gestation, but there are some differences in emphasis. Image resolution and clarity in relation to the size of the structures being demonstrated is more limited at the early scan. A single plane image may not provide enough detail to allow the operator to identify positively the structures within it. Slow continuous transverse sweeps through the upper abdomen and chest allow a better appreciation of the way in which structures in adjacent slices relate to each other (Fig. 6.2(a) and (b)). The acquisition of 3D volumes using STIC technology may prove to be particularly useful in this setting, although the degree of movement of the early fetus compromises the quality of the volumes obtained. Color flow mapping has a more dominant role in first trimester echocardiography, improving the delineation of chambers and vessels as well as demonstrating flow direction. Rapid switching between 2D and color flow images allows confirmation of structures as vascular, and aids in the identification of chambers and vessels. Velocities encountered in the normal heart at 11–14 weeks are significantly lower than those at 20 weeks and the Doppler velocity range should be adjusted accordingly, anticipating velocities up to about 35 cm/s. An important limiting factor in obtaining diagnostic images is the fetal position, which may be fixed in a sick fetus with an increased nuchal measurement, for example. On the other hand, sometimes the main difficulty in obtaining good images or good Doppler tracings is the degree of mobility of the fetus at this early stage.

The early cardiac scan starts with an assessment of fetal position and orientation. The position of the abdominal aorta and inferior caval vein at the level of the diaphragm may be clear enough to indicate the atrial situs, but this is not always the case. The stomach and cardiac apex can nearly always be identified, however, and abnormalities of their position may indicate underlying abnormalities of atrial situs. An abnormal position of the heart may also be seen in association with diaphragmatic hernia, which may present at this early stage (Fig. 6.6). As at later gestational ages, a perfect, orthogonal four-chamber plane is necessary in order to assess heart size, position, chamber sizes and the crux. Ideally, the four-chamber plane should be viewed from at least two different aspects, an apical and a lateral orientation. It will normally be possible to identify two ventricles of similar size on the cross-sectional image. Color flow mapping demonstrates flow into both ventricles and also the amount of filling gives some indication of their relative sizes. The implications of a difference in ventricular size are the same as those at the 20-week scan (Figs. 6.7(a)–(c), 6.8). The atria can also be compared in size, but the color flow map is less helpful in this as the velocities are usually too low to outline the cavities with color. The sensitivity for detection of isolated ventricular septal defects at the first trimester is low because of the technical limitations. However, it is generally possible to identify a normal crux and therefore to exclude an atrioventricular septal defect (Fig. 6.9(a) and (b)), although some subtle cases may be overlooked. It is our usual practice to obtain pulsed wave Doppler of

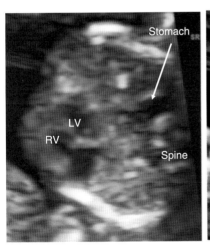
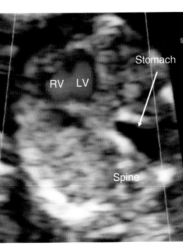

Fig. 6.6. The transverse section of the thorax shows the heart displaced into the right chest. The stomach bubble could be seen in the left chest due to a diaphragmatic hernia.

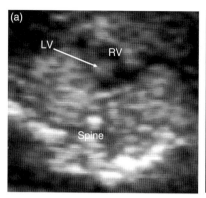 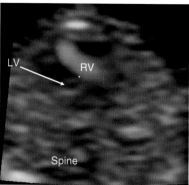

Fig. 6.7.(a). In the four-chamber view, the right ventricle could be seen but only a small echogenic "lump" was seen in the position of the left ventricle. On color flow mapping, only flow through the tricuspid valve was seen.

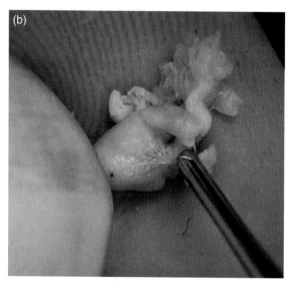

Fig. 6.7.(b). The tiny nature of the correlating heart specimen is seen.

both atrioventricular valves, although in general, the inflow Doppler waveform is not markedly altered by either cardiac defects or chromosomal abnormalities. Exceptionally, a monophasic or otherwise abnormal inflow pattern is seen and when this does occur it may indicate trisomy 18 in the fetus (Fig. 6.10). Atrioventricular valve regurgitation occurs in some normal fetuses, in most fetuses with a chromosomal abnormality, and in association with some specific cardiac defects. Regurgitation from the left atrioventricular (mitral) valve occurs less commonly than that of the right-sided valve. It is occasionally seen in the normal heart, but is most commonly seen with atrioventricular septal defects or aortic atresia. Tricuspid regurgitation occurs in a small proportion of normal fetuses, but is significantly associated

with chromosomal abnormality as discussed below. However, it is also associated with an increased incidence of structural heart defects, including atrioventricular septal defect, Ebstein's anomaly, hypoplastic left heart syndrome, and pulmonary atresia with intact ventricular septum. Bidirectional flow in one or other or both of the great arteries may occur, a finding which is highly associated with chromosomal anomalies, particularly trisomy 18, at this gestation (Fig. 6.11(a) and (b)).

As with later scans, a slow sweep upward towards the head from the four-chamber plane is helpful in identifying the great arteries. On such an upward sweep, the left outflow appears first and continues as the aorta, initially directed to the fetal right shoulder. At a slightly higher level, the pulmonary artery arises anteriorly from the right ventricle and passes almost directly posteriorly, in continuity with the arterial duct. Slightly higher still, the aortic arch is seen close to the right of the arterial duct as the two converge to meet the descending aorta (Fig. 6.2(a) and (b)). Conventional color flow mapping, with velocity range set at around 30 cm/s may be helpful in delineating the great arteries. Power Doppler, in which the intensity (energy) of flow, rather than its velocity, determines the signal on the map may also be sensitive and helpful, especially on those systems that are able to give directional information on the power Doppler flow map. Deviation from the normal appearance of the outflow tracts should raise the suspicion of an underlying abnormality. If only one great artery is identified, this usually indicates that the other great artery is smaller than normal or may point to common arterial trunk as the diagnosis. Thus, a large and well-seen pulmonary trunk with no obvious aorta is typical of aortic atresia or severe coarctation. This appearance should prompt a more detailed search for a small

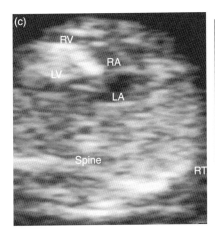

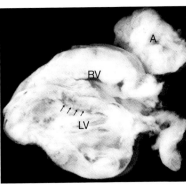

Fig. 6.7.(c). Contd. The left ventricle in this example was also abnormal, poorly contracting on the moving image and hyperechogenic. The matching pathological specimen seen on the right-hand panel showed that the increased echogenicity corresponded to calcium deposition in the septum (arrows).

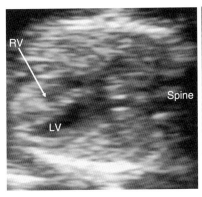

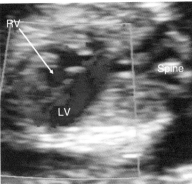

Fig. 6.8. The right ventricle was thick-walled resulting in a small ventricular cavity on the right side. It was poorly contracting in the moving image. On the color flow map seen in the right-hand image, there is flow to the apex of the left ventricle but very little filling of the right ventricle. This appearance is characteristic of pulmonary atresia with intact ventricular septum.

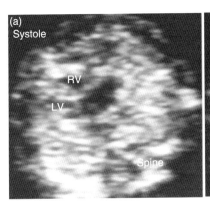

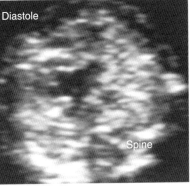

Fig. 6.9.(a). In the systolic view on the left-hand panel, the crux does not appear intact. There appears to be a defect in the primum portion of the atrial septum. When the valve opens in diastole (right-hand panel), it is clear that this is a common atrioventricular valve with a complete defect at the atrioventricular junction.

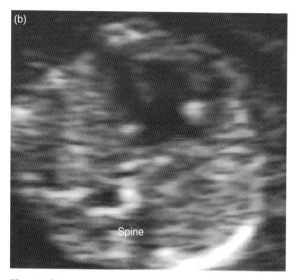

Fig. 6.9.(b). Contd. In an apical four-chamber view, differential insertion and an intact crux are usually readily identifiable. However, in this fetus, there is a large atrioventricular septal defect.

aortic arch. As in later pregnancy, retrograde flow in a small arch is typical of aortic atresia (Fig. 6.12). A large aorta with no pulmonary artery evident is characteristic of pulmonary atresia. Further views of the left outflow tract may demonstrate the large outlet ventricular septal defect typical of tetralogy of Fallot. A marked discrepancy in size of the great arteries has similar implications as a later fetus. A small aorta, with forward flow preserved, may indicate coarctation of the aorta. A small pulmonary artery may indicate pulmonary atresia with intact ventricular septum or more commonly tetralogy of Fallot (Fig. 6.13(a) and (b)). If both great arteries are identified and are similar in size, but have lost their normal "crossover" relationship, transposition should be suspected (Fig. 6.14). Whenever a great artery abnormality is suspected, it is important to consider not only the common conditions described above but also the possibility of more complex defects (Fig. 6.15).

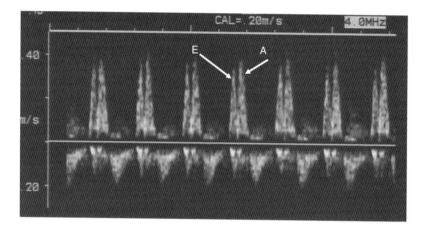

Fig. 6.10. The tricuspid valve flow profile is shown in a case of trisomy 18 at 12 weeks' gestation. The E and A wave are almost equal in velocity, a pattern not usually seen before the end of pregnancy. Although not a consistent finding in all cases of trisomy 18, on the other hand, I have not seen it in other settings, so it is highly suggestive of this diagnosis.

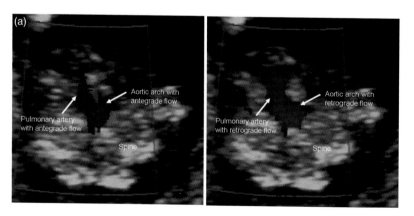

Fig. 6.11.(a). The aortic arch, pulmonary artery and duct are seen in the upper thorax in this 12-week fetus with a nuchal translucency of 5.2 mm. In different phases of the cardiac cycle, both antegrade and retrograde flow are seen on color flow mapping. This could be confirmed on pulsed Doppler. This is highly associated with chromosomal defects, particularly trisomy 18.

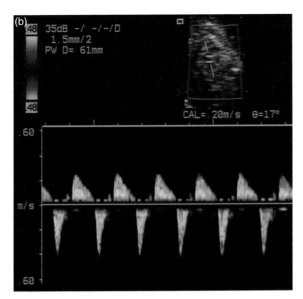

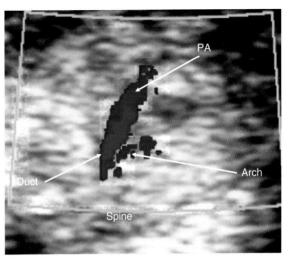

Fig. 6.12. In this fetus only one great artery was seen arising from the heart. This was the pulmonary artery. Reverse flow was seen in the transverse aortic arch, confirming the diagnosis of aortic atresia.

Fig. 6.11.(b). Contd. The pulsed Doppler waveform confirms bidirectional flow in the pulmonary artery in a 12-week fetus who proved to have trisomy 18. Forward flow is above the baseline, retrograde flow below.

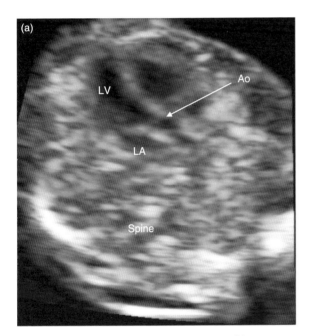

Fig. 6.13.(a). Despite the limitations in resolution of these tiny structures, the aorta can normally be seen to be wholly arising from the left ventricle.

Tricuspid regurgitation

At the 11–14-week gestation period, tricuspid valve regurgitation has been found to be associated with chromosomal anomalies. Because of this, examination for tricuspid valve regurgitation using pulsed wave Doppler has been introduced in some centers, as part of the first trimester risk assessment. This requires an accurate four-chamber plane cut, viewed from an aspect that optimizes the angle for the Doppler as well as allowing correct placement of the sample volume. The Doppler sample volume must be positioned correctly across the tricuspid valve, so that it lies partially in the right atrium and partially in the right ventricle. The ultrasound beam should be almost parallel to the flow into the right ventricle. Incorporating assessment of the tricuspid valve into the nuchal evaluation also leads to the recognition of some major four-chamber view abnormalities. Tricuspid regurgitation occurs in about 4% of normal fetuses at 12 weeks of gestation but is more common in fetuses with a chromosomal abnormality. This is due to a number of factors. Atrioventricular septal defect is common in fetuses with a chromosomal abnormality, especially trisomy 21, and there is a very high incidence of atrioventricular valve regurgitation in fetuses with an atrioventricular septal defect at 12 weeks (although, perhaps surprisingly, this is not true in later gestation). Polyvalve dysplasia may occur in chromosomally abnormal fetuses, mainly fetuses with trisomy 18 and 13, and may lead to regurgitation. Tricuspid regurgitation occurring in fetuses with normal hearts (whether with a normal or abnormal karyotype) may be a consequence of delayed delamination of the septal leaflet of the tricuspid valve,

197

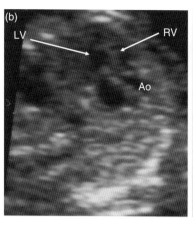

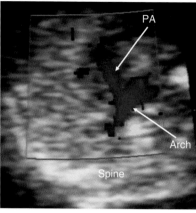

Fig. 6.13.(b). Contd. In contrast to Fig. 6.13(a), the aorta is seen arising astride the crest of the ventricular septum in the left-hand panel. Examination of the pulmonary artery demonstrated that it was smaller than the aorta in size, which was particularly appreciable on color flow mapping (right-hand panel). This combination of findings indicates tetralogy of Fallot.

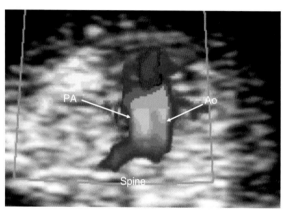

Fig. 6.14. Despite difficult images in this patient, who was less than 12 weeks' gestation, the two great arteries clearly arose from the heart in parallel arrangement. This is transposition.

which is only completed between 10–12 weeks in the normal, and is known to be delayed in the anatomical specimen in Down's syndrome. Tricuspid regurgitation must be distinguished from the normal valve closure "artifact" (Fig. 6.16) and from normal forward flow in the left ventricular outflow. For the purposes of first-trimester risk assessment, tricuspid regurgitation must have a duration of almost half of systole to be counted as positive. An additional requirement that the maximum velocity of regurgitation should be at least 60 cm/s, helps avoid the inadvertent identification of normal forward flow in the left ventricular outflow as tricuspid regurgitation, as the arterial flow will nearly always be less than 60 cm/s whereas true tricuspid regurgitation will nearly always have a velocity of greater than 60 (Fig. 6.17). Abnormal findings in the heart, either a structural or functional

abnormality, are found in the majority of all the chromosomal anomalies (Fig. 6.18).

An additional marker for Down syndrome is the presence of an aberrant right subclavian artery and the identification of this anomaly increases the risk determined by the nuchal scan by a factor of at least ten. The right subclavian artery, whether normal or aberrant, is more easily seen at the 20-week scan (Fig. 4.42 and 4.45) but with practice can be identified between 11–14 weeks' gestation and therefore incorporated into the nuchal risk assessment.

Pulsed Doppler recording of the ductus venosus at the early scan is an additional method of assessment of the well-being of the fetus. However, it can be difficult to obtain, difficult to interpret (see Chapter 5) and inconsistent during the same scan. It can be abnormal in some forms of CHD without the implication that this indicates a compromised fetus. On the other hand, when it is consistently convincingly abnormal, as in Fig. 6.19, it increases the risk of a karyotype anomaly or fetal loss.

Pitfalls in early scanning

We have learnt from experience with 20-week scanning that some types of cardiac abnormalities do not become evident until later pregnancy, such as complete heart block, cardiomyopathies, and cardiac tumors. It has also been shown that some forms of CHD can progress into more severe malformations with advancing gestation. This has been found in aortic or pulmonary stenosis, progressing to more severe stenosis or even atresia, in valve regurgitation, and in coarctation, where poor growth of the left ventricle or arch leads to a more difficult surgical repair than would be expected from the initial scan. However,

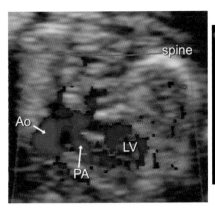

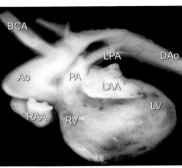

Fig. 6.15. On the color flow map, despite a rather unusual shape to the aorta, the pulmonary artery crossed over it in a normal fashion. However, it was seen to be smaller than the aorta. The pathological specimen confirmed the echocardiographic findings of complex heart disease; there was tricuspid atresia with a small pulmonary artery arising from the rudimentary right ventricle.

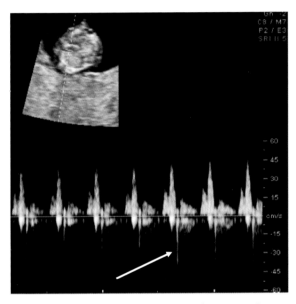

Fig. 6.16. The Doppler sample volume must be positioned across the tricuspid valve so that regurgitant flow is included in the flow profile. However, it is common to detect a sound reverberation artifact from the valve cusps themselves, termed valve click (arrow). This occurs immediately after tricuspid valve closure, therefore during the isovolumic contraction period (see Fig. 5.26) is very sharp, short in time and usually no higher than 40 cm/s in velocity as shown here. It is a normal finding and can be distinguished from tricuspid regurgitation. Compare this tracing with that of true tricuspid regurgitation seen in Fig. 6.17.

to be uncommon from our experience with over 2000 early scans, but there certainly have been examples of progressive disease both in our series and in that of others. This has involved the development of aortic or pulmonary atresia from apparently normal or from minor abnormality (Fig. 6.20(a)–(f)), the identification of a small atrioventricular septal defect which was not evident earlier and the diagnosis of coarctation, which was not suspected on the initial 12-week scan, the last even on retrospective review of the videotaped recording. In the fetus shown in Fig. 6.20, the abnormal cardiac findings were such that a karyotype anomaly was anticipated. I failed to realize when the karyotype had come back as normal, that the patient had been rebooked for 20 weeks, as is our usual practice. Now that I know that this degree of tricuspid regurgitation is not compatible with a normal fetus, I would re-examine the patient at 14 weeks. As it was, the patient opted for termination of pregnancy for pulmonary atresia with intact ventricular septum when the diagnosis was made at 20 weeks. An earlier examination could have saved the patient this wait of 6 weeks and the termination procedure performed at less risk, although, of course, it is possible that the complete picture of pulmonary atresia may not have been fully developed at 14 weeks either.

In summary, early detailed fetal heart scanning, though technically more challenging than later scanning, can yield a wealth of information, not only about the fetal heart itself, but also about extracardiac anomalies. However, image quality is limited at this early stage and progression of minor to more severe disease can occur in later pregnancy. A follow-up echocardiogram at 20 weeks is therefore always recommended.

the conditions which develop from a normal study at 20 weeks to a serious malformation later are relatively uncommon and the cases of mild disease which progress dramatically are relatively few. In contrast, we still do not have enough data to know how frequently the fetal heart appears normal at around 12 weeks and something significant is seen at 20 weeks. It appears

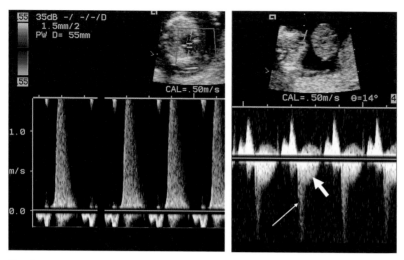

Fig. 6.17. In contrast to valve click, tricuspid regurgitation occurs during ventricular systole. In the left-hand panel, the fetus lies with the back up so that forward flow in the tricuspid valve is below the baseline. There is clearly holosystolic tricuspid regurgitation (above the baseline) at a velocity of over 1.5 m/s. This pattern is suggestive of trisomy 18. In the right-hand panel, the tricuspid regurgitation jet (thin arrow) is much shorter in duration. The peak velocity of about 80 cm/s distinguishes it from the aortic flow, which overlaps into the tracing (thicker arrow). The tricuspid regurgitation jet is broader (longer in time) and higher velocity than the valve click seen in Fig. 6.16. Note that the velocity of regurgitant flow is over 1.5 m/s on the left, higher than the normal velocity of arterial flow at any gestation and about 70 cm/s on the right, higher than the normal velocity of arterial flow at this gestation. The flow pattern on the right-hand panel is typical of trisomy 18, on the left-hand panel typical of trisomy 21, although neither is diagnostic. The pattern on the right-hand panel could be compatible with a normal fetus but the pattern seen on the left, in my experience, is not compatible with a normal fetus.

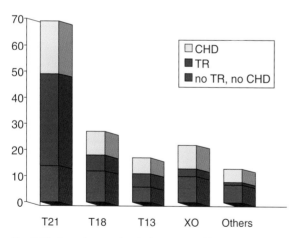

Fig. 6.18. It can be seen that, in the majority of fetuses with chromosomal anomalies, either structural heart disease or tricuspid regurgitation will be found on detailed heart scanning at 11–14 weeks of gestation. There will be abnormal cardiac findings in over 80% of fetuses with Down's syndrome.

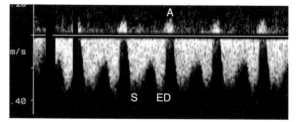

Fig. 6.19. The flow in the ductus venosus is unequivocally abnormal with reversed flow during atrial systole (A). S = systole, ED = early diastole. This type of tracing is highly associated with fetal anomalies although it can occur in a normal fetus.

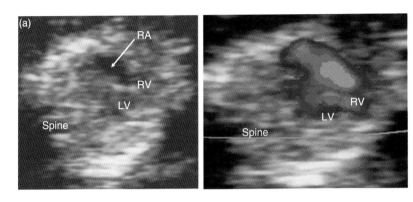

Fig. 6.20.(a). At the study performed at 13 weeks' gestation, the four-chamber view appeared abnormal (left-hand panel) due to right atrial dilatation, which was particularly noticeable on color flow mapping. However, there appeared to be equally good filling of both ventricles on color (right-hand panel).

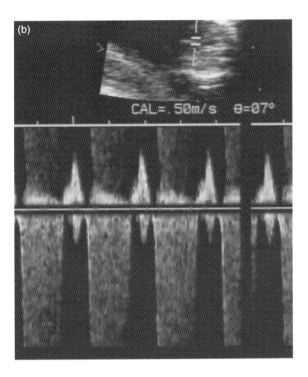

Fig. 6.20.(b). On pulsed Doppler there was holosystolic tricuspid regurgitation. The velocity of regurgitant flow could not be measured accurately but was in excess of 2 m/s.

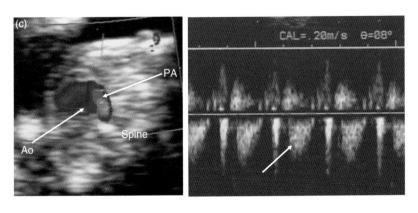

Fig. 6.20.(c). Still at 13 weeks, the pulmonary artery appeared to be a good size with convincing forward flow on both color and pulsed Doppler (arrow on right-hand panel).

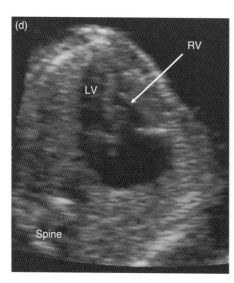

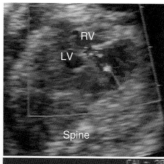

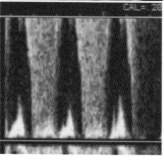

Fig. 6.20.(d). Contd. At 20 weeks, the right ventricular walls appeared thick and poorly contracting and the cavity appeared smaller than the left. There was mild to moderate tricuspid regurgitation on color flow mapping (upper right panel) and it was holosystolic and at high velocity on pulsed Doppler (lower right panel).

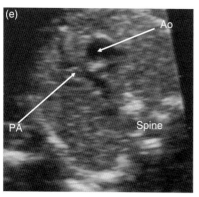

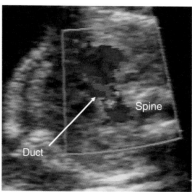

Fig. 6.20.(e). The pulmonary artery was clearly smaller than the aorta (left panel). The pulmonary valve was thickened and there was no forward flow detected across it on color flow mapping. On the transverse view (right panel) and the long-axis view.

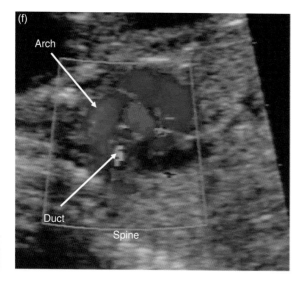

Fig. 6.20.(f). Reverse flow was seen in the arterial duct. These findings are typical of pulmonary atresia with intact ventricular septum. Although the echocardiogram at 12 weeks was not completely normal, this very serious diagnosis had not yet evolved.

Arrhythmias

Background

Rhythm disturbances are a fairly frequent finding on the routine anomaly scan but most of these will be benign and self-limiting. Important, life-threatening arrhythmias are much less common, but everyone performing routine scans should be able to recognize them as such, in order to know when to seek specialist advice for assessment and treatment. Arrhythmias are virtually the only group of conditions encountered in fetal cardiology where prenatal treatment, rather than only counseling and planning for postnatal treatment, is well established, rather than experimental. Most arrhythmias will be immediately obvious on examination of the four-chamber view of the heart but M-mode echocardiography and pulsed-wave Doppler provide additional information about the exact nature of the arrhythmia. The majority of both benign and serious arrhythmias occur in the setting of a structurally normal heart, but some arrhythmias are associated with particular structural heart defects.

Although the science underlying arrhythmias is complex, their basic assessment need not be complicated. A simple understanding of the conduction system is helpful in understanding rhythm disturbances (Fig. 7.1). An arrhythmia may be indicated by a heart rate which is either too fast or too slow, or a rhythm which is irregular. It is important to distinguish between variations in heart rate which are out of the normal range, but occurring as a physiological response to factors external to the heart, and those which arise primarily because of a disturbance of the rhythm-generating mechanisms within the heart itself. The former (sinus tachycardia and sinus bradycardia) may be important indicators of extra-cardiac disease and the fetal condition, but it is the latter that are of primary concern to the cardiologist. Increases or decreases in heart rate due to primary arrhythmias are typically more extreme than those occurring as a physiological response to external factors.

Techniques for the assessment of the fetal heart rhythm

Cross-sectional ultrasound

A qualitative assessment of the heart rate and rhythm can be made on the real-time four-chamber cross-sectional image. The fetal heart rate may be noted to

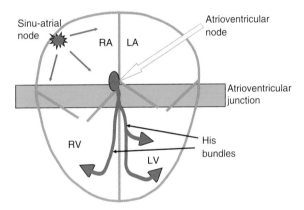

Fig. 7.1. The cardiac conduction tissue is illustrated in a basic diagram. The sinu-atrial node lies in the right atrial wall and the atrioventricular node lies on the right atrial side of the atrioventricular junction. The sinu-atrial node fires an impulse which spreads throughout the atria and which triggers the atrioventricular node. The electrical impulse is then conducted through the His bundles to the right and left ventricles to cause ventricular systole. The atrioventricular junction normally acts as a barrier to direct conduction between the atria and ventricles or vice versa. Looking at the diagram, one can visualize all the forms of arrhythmia in simple terms. Ectopic "or extra" beats can arise from anywhere in the myocardium, most often the atria but also the ventricles, to produce an irregular rhythm. This "irritable focus" can cause one, many, or coupled extra beats. A coupled ectopic occurs regularly a short time interval after the sinus beat so that they form a pair of beats or a couple. Heart block can either be found in left isomerism (when there is no right atrium and usually a hypoplastic sinus node), in some other forms of CHD when the conducting tissue takes an abnormal course, or when there is inflammatory damage to the specialized conducting tissue itself. Tachycardias usually arise when there is an unusual focus in the atrial mass (flutter) or where some of the tissue at the AV junction, instead of blocking the electrical impulse as it usually does, allows the ventricular impulse to re-enter the atria and form a conduction circuit.

be normal, too slow, or too fast. The rhythm may be assessed as regular or irregular and the presence of synchrony or asynchrony between atrial and ventricular contraction may be discernible. Thus, in the context of a routine scan, examination of the four-chamber view over a period of time may be sufficient to exclude arrhythmia or to indicate that more detailed assessment is required. Cross-sectional imaging in the four-chamber and other planes is obviously essential to rule out an associated structural heart defect. In addition, cross-sectional imaging is useful in assessing the consequences of an arrhythmia in terms of cardiac function, such as cardiac dilation, reduced contractility, and accumulation of excess fluid within the pericardium, pleural spaces or abdominal cavity or within the subcutaneous tissues.

M-mode echocardiography

Detailed analysis of the cardiac rhythm requires accurate measurement of the heart rate, the time intervals between specific events in the cardiac cycle and, in particular, an appreciation of the relationship between atrial and ventricular contractions. M-mode echocardiography is one method of obtaining this important information. In M-mode, echoes returning from a single static scan line are plotted against time. This contrasts with cross-sectional imaging in which echoes from multiple scan lines are built up to form a sector image, which is continually updated to form a real time image. A sector image is usually used to aid the optimum placement of the M-mode cursor so that the scan line passes through the appropriate structures to be examined. The cursor will usually be placed in such a position that atrial and ventricular activity can be recorded simultaneously and their timing compared. Recording atrial activity requires that the cursor passes through the free wall of one or other atrium at an angle sufficiently near to the perpendicular to give a clear and distinct signal on the M-mode trace. Ventricular activity can be recorded either by tracing movement of the ventricular wall itself or by placing the cursor line through one of the arterial valves. In the latter case, the onset of valve opening corresponds to the beginning of ventricular ejection (Fig. 7.2).

Doppler echocardiography

The fetal heart rate is readily determined from a Doppler trace obtained with the sample volume placed just distal to one of the arterial valves. A trace obtained with the sample volume including the left ventricular

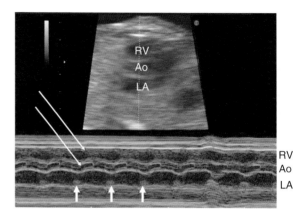

Fig. 7.2. The M-mode tracing is seen with the cursor positioned through the right ventricular free wall anteriorly, the aortic valve and the left atrial free wall posteriorly. There is a one-to-one relationship between atrial (broad arrows) and ventricular (long arrows) contraction with a normal time interval between them. In this tracing therefore, ventricular contraction can be seen from the right ventricular wall movement or from the opening of the aortic valve. Note, however, that the precise time of onset of ventricular contraction is easier to see from the aortic valve opening than from the ventricular wall movement.

inflow and adjacent outflow will demonstrate the E wave of early passive filling of the ventricle followed by the A wave of filling augmented by atrial contraction and then, in the opposite direction, ejection into the aorta (Fig. 7.3, left-hand panel). In the presence of normal sinus rhythm, this type of trace can be used to estimate the interval between the onsets of atrial and ventricular contraction (A–V interval), which is the mechanical equivalent of the electrical P–R interval on the ECG. When the heart is not in sinus rhythm, the trace is often difficult to interpret, as atrial contractions during ventricular systole will not be detectable in the atrioventricular inflow profile (Fig. 7.4).

Of more practical value in the presence of an abnormal rhythm are Doppler traces which include signals from both a central artery and a central vein. Suitable sites are the ascending aorta and superior vena cava (or adjacent transverse aortic arch and innominate vein) and a proximal branch pulmonary artery and adjacent pulmonary vein as shown in Fig. 7.3. In a fetus in sinus rhythm, there is biphasic forward flow in the superior vena cava, which is preceded by a brief spike of reversed flow brought about by atrial contraction. The beginning of this flow reversal corresponds in time to the onset of atrial contraction and the onset of forward flow in the adjacent aorta, in the same direction on the trace, corresponds to the onset of ventricular ejection (Fig. 7.3, middle tracing). The pattern of flow obtained

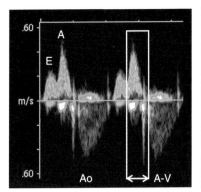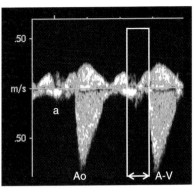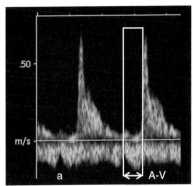

Fig. 7.3. A pulsed wave Doppler trace of the atrioventricular valve inflow at the mitral valve and adjacent left ventricular outflow tract is shown on the left-hand panel. The first peak of forward flow through the mitral valve is due to passive filling of the ventricle (E-wave) and the second peak is due to ventricular filling augmented by atrial contraction (A-wave). Flow in the opposite direction is ejection in the overlapping left ventricular outflow tract (Ao). The regular biphasic form of the inflow is consistent with normal sinus rhythm and the interval between the onset of the A-wave and the onset of ventricular ejection (A–V interval) will approximate to the P–R interval of the ECG. In the middle panel, a pulsed wave Doppler recording from the superior vena cava (SVC) and ascending aorta (Ao) is shown. Forward flow in the SVC is above and forward flow in the aorta is below the baseline. During systole and early diastole there is biphasic venous filling of the atria followed by a brief period of reversed flow (a) brought about by atrial contraction.
On the right-hand panel, a pulsed wave Doppler tracing obtained from an adjacent central pulmonary artery and vein is shown. Forward flow in the branch pulmonary artery is above the baseline and has the characteristic form of a narrow spike which marks the onset of ventricular ejection. Flow below the baseline is in the pulmonary vein. During atrial contraction, flow in the pulmonary vein ceases or is transiently reversed (A-wave). From these two combined recordings, the relative timing of atrial contraction and ventricular ejection can be compared, and are consistent with normal sinus rhythm.

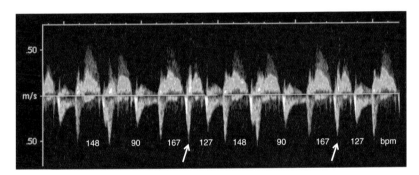

Fig. 7.4. A pulsed wave Doppler recording from the mitral valve (below baseline) and aortic outflow (above baseline) in a fetus with frequent atrial ectopic beats. The time interval between two normal heart beats (A-waves) corresponds to an underlying heart rate of approximately 148 bpm. Two conducted atrial ectopic beats result in a fusion of the preceding E and A waves (arrows), an aortic outflow profile occurring sooner than expected (167 bpm) and a following compensatory pause (127 bpm). The two time intervals corresponding to a heart rate of 90 bpm are due to non-conducted atrial ectopic beats, that depolarize and reset the sinu-atrial node but do not conduct to the ventricles as they arrive at the atrioventricular node whilst it still in its refractory state. These beats do not result in any A-waves as atrial contraction occurs during ventricular systole when the mitral valve is closed.

from the pulmonary artery and adjacent vein is fairly similar, with a less obvious reversal of venous flow during atrial contraction (Fig. 7.3, right-hand tracing), but frequently easier to obtain in practical terms. In the absence of sinus rhythm the pattern of flow, as well as the timing of events, is altered and this is discussed under the individual rhythm abnormalities.

Non-echocardiographic methods

Non-invasive fetal electrocardiography is hindered by interference from the much stronger electrical activity of the maternal heart and muscles. Although various methods have been devised to subtract these stronger signals, the quality of the fetal ECG obtained is not of sufficient quality to be of much value in the management of arrhythmias. Magnetocardiography is potentially a much more useful means of assessing fetal heart activity and can define the electrical events in the fetal heart with arrhythmia to an extent which is not possible by any other means. Its use remains restricted to a very few centers where the technique is available, but it may become more accessible as issues of cost and portability are addressed.

Benign arrhythmias

Ectopic beats

The most common arrhythmia is that caused by ectopic beats. This typically presents to the fetal echocardiographer because irregularity of the heart rhythm has been noted during routine auscultation or a scan. The exact incidence is hard to establish because the observed incidence increases according to the duration and intensity of heart rate monitoring, but it is undoubtedly very common. It is most often noted during the last trimester of pregnancy, is sometimes seen during the routine 20–23-week scan but rarely at the 11–14-week scan. At least one study suggested a small excess above the expected rate of structural cardiac defects in fetuses

referred for ectopic beats, but ectopic beats much more usually occur in the context of a normal heart.

An ectopic beat is an extra beat arising prematurely from a site other than the heart's natural pacemaker. The site of origin is most commonly in one of the atria, but may also be in one or other ventricle. An individual atrial ectopic beat may be conducted to the ventricles or non-conducted (Fig. 7.4). A conducted atrial ectopic beat, or an ectopic beat of ventricular origin, will be manifest as ventricular contraction, or ejection, occurring sooner than expected, based on the underlying heart rate. The contraction will be less vigorous than the preceding contraction because the ventricles will have had less time to complete their filling before the premature onset of the contraction (Fig. 7.5). A non-conducted atrial ectopic beat is one that arrives at the atrioventricular node whilst it is still in its refractory state and therefore is not conducted to the ventricles. Such an ectopic beat will, however, "reset" the pacemaker back to the beginning of its cycle so that the next ventricular beat occurs approximately one normal cycle length after the atrial ectopic beat (rather than the preceding ventricular beat). A non-conducted or "blocked" ectopic beat thus appears to be a "missed" beat (Fig. 7.6). The contraction following the missed

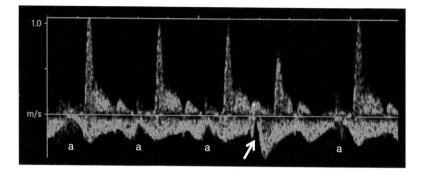

Fig. 7.5. Conducted atrial ectopics. A pulsed wave Doppler tracing from a central pulmonary artery (above baseline) and adjacent pulmonary vein (below baseline). During normal atrial rhythm there is a decrease in venous flow during atrial contraction (a) followed by a typical flow profile in the artery. The atrial ectopic beat (arrow) occurs sooner than expected and is followed by a smaller arterial profile, as the ventricle has less time for diastolic filling before the premature onset of ventricular contraction. The following beat has more time for filling and also a somewhat larger profile than during normal rhythm.

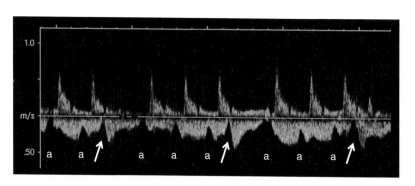

Fig. 7.6. Blocked atrial ectopics. Flow velocities in the branch pulmonary artery (above baseline) and adjacent pulmonary vein (below baseline) were recorded simultaneously. The normal regular pattern with a decrease in venous flow (a) followed by arterial pulmonary flow in the other direction is interrupted by non-conducted atrial ectopic beats (arrows).

beat will usually be increased in intensity and ejection volume. In most cases the diagnosis of ectopic beats will be fairly obvious from simple observation in the four-chamber view of the 2D image and can be confirmed by M-mode or Doppler studies. The distinction between ventricular ectopic beats and conducted atrial ectopic beats requires careful examination of a Doppler trace showing venous and arterial flow. With an atrial ectopic beat, the extra ventricular beat will be preceded (with a delay of around 100 ms) by atrial contraction, whereas with a ventricular ectopic beat, it will not (Fig. 7.7). This distinction, however, is not usually of any clinical importance, so in practice we do not spend a lot of time making this distinction echocardiographically.

The correct recognition of ectopic beats becomes more challenging when the beats occur with some degree of regularity, giving rise to a regularly irregular rhythm. For example, a bigeminal rhythm may arise when ectopic beats arise alternately with sinus beats (Fig. 7.8(a) and (b)). If the ectopic beats are not conducted to the ventricles, the appearance will be that of a regular bradycardia almost as slow as half of the expected sinus rate for the gestational age. This situation may be very difficult, but very important, to distinguish from genuine 2:1 heart block, as transplacental steroid treatment of antibody-mediated incomplete heart block might prevent progression or even reverse the block. This treatment is, however, not without risks and should not be given to fetuses with blocked atrial bigeminy, which will resolve spontaneously without any hemodynamic problems. Regular or irregular ventricular bradycardia resulting from blocked atrial ectopic beats has frequently been misinterpreted on the cardiotocogram trace as evidence of fetal distress,

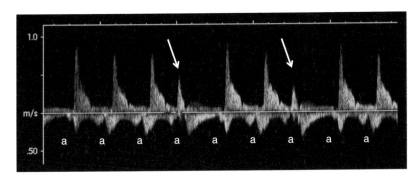

Fig. 7.7. Ventricular ectopic beats. The flow velocity tracing from a branch pulmonary artery (above baseline) and adjacent pulmonary vein (below baseline) is shown. Despite premature ventricular contractions (arrows) the atrial rate (a) remains regular and there is no decrease in venous flow preceding the ventricular ectopic beats.

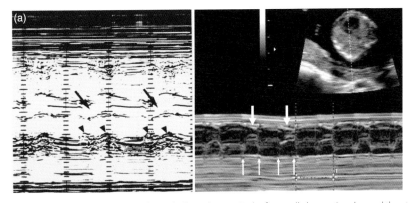

Fig. 7.8.(a). The M-line passes through the right ventricular free wall, the aortic valve and the atrial wall in a fetus with alternate blocked atrial ectopic beats. On the left-hand panel, the diagnosis of coupled ectopic beats is relatively easy, as two atrial beats occur followed by a pause. The ventricles (as seen from the aortic valve opening indicated by the larger arrows) respond only to the sinus (first) atrial beat but are refractory when the ectopic atrial beat (the second) occurs. This is in contrast to complete heart block where the atrial rate is usually completely regular and bears no relationship to the ventricular response (see Fig. 7.15). On the right hand panel, a much more difficult example to diagnose is shown. The appearance closely resembles sinus rhythm with 2:1 heart block as the ventricular rate (thicker arrows) appears regular at half of the atrial rate (thinner arrows). However, close inspection and measurement of the time intervals reveal that the atrial rate is not truly regular, every second beat actually being a slightly premature ectopic beat, which fails to conduct to the ventricles.

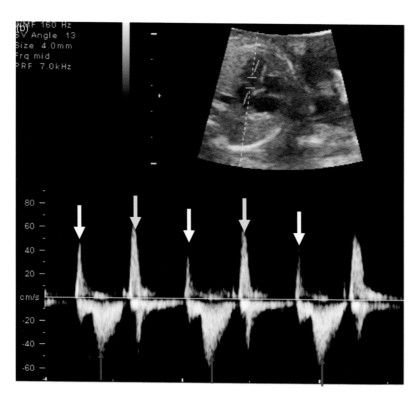

Fig. 7.8.(b). Contd. The Doppler sample volume is positioned in the mitral valve overlapping the left ventricular outflow tract. Although the atrial rate (above the line) appears regular, the ventricles (red arrows) are only responding to alternate atrial contractions (white arrows). The premature atrial contractions are hidden within the ventricular contractions and therefore are not visible. Only the passive filling wave of the premature beat is seen (yellow arrows).

sometimes leading to inappropriate emergency delivery. Sometimes the only way to be sure of distinguishing between blocked ectopics and second-degree heart block is to take blood for anti-Ro antibodies and bring the mother back a week later. Blocked ectopics are likely to have disappeared spontaneously and the antibody test will be negative, whereas heart block will have persisted and the antibody test will be positive.

Fetuses presenting with ectopic beats do appear to be at increased risk (of the order of 2%–5%) of subsequent supraventricular tachycardias. In fetuses with blocked atrial bigeminy, the risk is probably somewhat higher. Similarly, fetuses on anti-arrhythmic treatment for supraventricular tachycardia sometimes exhibit frequent apparent ectopic beats on initial conversion to sinus rhythm. One possible explanation for this association is that the apparent ectopic beats involved arise from retrograde activation of the atria via an accessory pathway and are thus abortive "attempts" at initiating a re-entry supraventricular tachycardia.

Ectopic beats do not normally cause significant hemodynamic compromise, even when they are very frequent. They eventually resolve spontaneously and permanently during pregnancy or within a few weeks after birth although they may come and go many times

before doing so. Thus, drug treatment or intervention in the pregnancy is not indicated. However, their presence should prompt increased caution in interpreting the cardiotocogram and increased vigilance in observing for supraventricular tachycardias before and immediately after birth, including a postnatal ECG to check for pre-excitation.

Tachycardias

The heart rate in the early embryo increases to a maximum of around 175 bpm between 8 and 9 weeks of gestation, then progressively decreases. At 12 weeks of gestation, the mean heart rate is 164 bpm (95th centile 175 bpm). By 14 weeks, the mean heart rate falls to 156 bpm (95th centile 167 bpm) and by 20 weeks to 140 bpm. Subsequently, the mean heart rate decreases more slowly to about 130 bpm by term. It is important to distinguish between a sinus tachycardia occurring as a response to external influences on the heart and a tachycardia resulting from electrical derangement in the heart itself. Sinus tachycardia is rare in the fetus but causes include infection and fever in the mother, hypovolemia and shock, drugs and hyperthyroidism. A mild increase in heart rate is seen in the 12-week gestation fetus with trisomy 21 or Turner's syndrome.

A persistently elevated heart rate of 170 bpm in mid-gestation can be seen with no apparent cause. It is unusual for a sinus tachycardia to exceed 180 bpm. Likewise most tachycardias that have a primary arrhythmia as their basis will have a rate in excess of 180 bpm (and usually over 200 bpm), but there will be occasional exceptions to both. It is conventional to divide the primary arrhythmias into the two categories of ventricular and supraventricular tachycardias.

Supraventricular tachycardia

Supraventricular tachycardia describes any tachycardia with an origin which is not confined to the ventricles. Supraventricular tachycardias are much more common than those of ventricular origin. The origin of a supraventricular tachycardia may be from an ectopic focus within the atrial junctional tissue, from a re-entry circuit within the atria themselves, or most commonly a re-entry circuit which crosses between atria and ventricles. A clinically important and easily made distinction is between supraventricular tachycardias with 1:1 atrioventricular conduction (i.e. atrial rate equal to ventricular rate) and those with some degree of second-degree block, commonly 2:1 conduction, as found in atrial flutter. The former type is the most common and the unqualified term supraventricular tachycardia is sometimes used to indicate solely this type, although strictly speaking the definition includes atrial flutter and fibrillation as well as sinus tachycardia.

In any supraventricular tachycardia, mild cardiomegaly and tricuspid regurgitation is not uncommon, mitral regurgitation less so. Although atrioventricular valve regurgitation is more commonly seen with fetal hydrops, it does not necessarily indicate that the fetus will progress to hydrops (Fig. 7.9).

Supraventricular tachycardia with 1:1 conduction

In a fetus with supraventricular tachycardia with 1:1 conduction, the atrial rate is typically in about 240–260 bpm, although rates of between 200 and 280 are possible. By definition, atrial and ventricular rates will be equal, and atrial and ventricular contractions will have a fixed relationship with each other, a fact best demonstrated on M-mode, with the cursor passing through an atrial and ventricular free wall or through an atrium and the aortic valve (Fig. 7.10). The basis of most tachycardias of this type is an atrioventricular re-entry

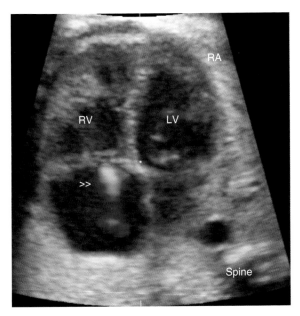

Fig. 7.9. This fetus was in atrial flutter. There was mild cardiomegaly and mild to moderate tricuspid regurgitation (arrowheads) but despite maximum drug therapy, the rhythm disturbance persisted, without hydrops developing, for five weeks until delivery.

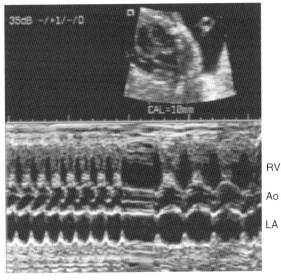

Fig. 7.10. The M-mode cursor passes through the right ventricle anteriorly, then through the aortic valve and left atrial wall. There is one-to-one conduction between the atria and ventricles at a rate of 240 bpm, which breaks to a normal rate during the tracing. Sudden onset and termination of a tachycardia is typical of a re-entry tachycardia.

circuit. The classical example is that described as part of the Wolf–Parkinson–White syndrome. This is characterized by an accessory pathway crossing the normally electrically insulating atrioventricular junction and providing an electrical connection between atria and ventricles in addition to the AV node. In the tachycardic state, conduction usually occurs in a normal antegrade direction at the atrioventricular node, but as the ventricular muscle becomes excited, the accessory pathway becomes activated and conducts back to the atria. The delay in the excitation getting back to the atrial side of the atrioventricular node allows the AV node time to recover from its refractory state and to conduct the impulse back to the ventricles to continue the cycle. Re-entry tachycardia may occur in association with several alternative types of accessory pathway and also in the absence of a separate accessory pathway, where tracts within the AV node itself have sufficiently dissimilar properties to allow a re-entry circuit to be maintained. Characteristic features of re-entry tachycardias in general are that the heart rate is regular and constant and that the onset and cessation of the tachycardia is abrupt, with a typical rate of around 240 bpm. Rarely supraventricular tachycardia with 1:1 conduction occurs from a mechanism other than AV re-entry, such as an atrial ectopic tachycardia. This may be difficult to distinguish from sinus tachycardia except for a tendency towards a rate of around 200 bpm.

Clues as to the mechanism underlying a particular case of supraventricular tachycardia may be obtained from estimation of the VA and AV intervals using M-mode or Doppler methods as described above. In a typical AV re-entry tachycardia, such as in the Wolf–Parkinson–White syndrome, retrograde atrial activation follows soon after ventricular activation and the VA interval is short (VA/AV <1) (Fig. 7.11(a) and (b)). In postnatal life, this leads to a retrograde P wave typically buried in the QRS complex of the ECG. In the unusual condition of a permanent junctional reciprocating tachycardia (PJRT) the accessory pathway conducts exceptionally slowly so that atrial activation occurs very late, the retrograde P wave of the ECG arises close to the following QRS and the VA interval is long (VA/AV >1). Atrial ectopic tachycardia (Fig. 7.12) and sinus tachycardia are also associated with a long VA interval. Consideration of the VA interval will not usually determine the optimum initial drug therapy, but does help to predict which tachycardias are likely to prove difficult to control.

Supraventricular tachycardia with 2:1 block

Atrial flutter arises from a re-entry circuit, which is confined to the atria themselves. The rhythm is regular, with an atrial rate of almost 500 bpm or even higher.

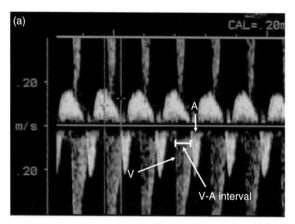

Fig. 7.11.(a). This tracing is obtained when the aortic and superior vena caval flow is recorded simultaneously. There is 1:1 conduction at a rate of 260 bpm. The aortic flow is below the zero line. Flow in the superior vena cava is above the line in systole and early diastole but reverses during atrial systole. The time relationship between ventricular (V) and atrial (A) contraction can thus be measured. The time between the onset of these two peaks is the VA interval (here, 110 ms) and the VA/AV ratio is 110/120 =0.92. This is a short VA tachycardia.

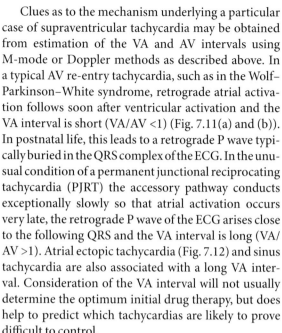
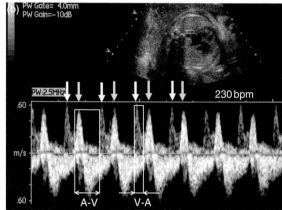

Fig. 7.11.(b). This tracing is obtained from the pulmonary artery and vein, with the venous flow below the zero line. Ventricular contraction (white arrows) is occurring at a short interval before atrial contraction (yellow arrows). This is a short VA tachycardia.

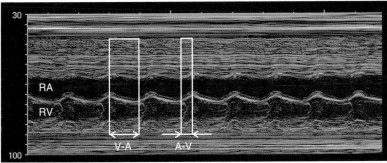

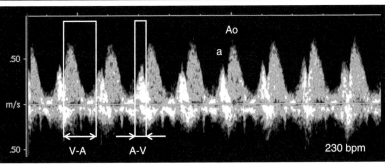

Fig. 7.12. Recordings from a fetus with atrial ectopic tachycardia of 230 bpm. Both M-mode (on top) and Doppler recordings from the superior vena cava and aorta (at bottom) demonstrate that the V–A interval is longer than the A–V interval corresponding to a long retrograde P wave tachycardia. In addition, it could be demonstrated during the examination that the tachycardia had a gradual onset (not seen on the picture), distinguishing it from persistent junctional reciprocating tachycardia.

The AV node is unable to conduct at such a high rate and typically alternate flutter beats will be blocked to give a ventricular rate of exactly half of the atrial rate (about 240–250 bpm). The relationship between atrial and ventricular activity may be demonstrated by M-mode or combined arterial and venous Doppler (Fig. 7.13). Atrial fibrillation is rarely seen in the fetus (I have never seen it in nearly 30 years of practice), but it would be characterized by a fast and disorganized atrial activity with irregular conduction to the ventricles at a slower rate.

Ventricular tachycardia

Ventricular tachycardia is rare in the fetus but a positive diagnosis may be made by careful examination of M-mode and Doppler tracings. Ventricular tachycardia is diagnosed when the ventricular rate exceeds the atrial rate (Fig. 7.14). Characteristically, a ventricular tachycardia tends to be slower than a supraventricular tachycardia, around 200 bpm as opposed to around 240 bpm, but this is not always the case.

Management of tachycardia

The nature and mechanism of any rhythm abnormality must be assessed, using the methods previously described, before embarking on any treatment. Expectant management may be an option where the

tachycardia is very intermittent or transient, or where the rate is relatively low. However, close vigilance is required in the management of such cases as the situation may rapidly deteriorate and it is usually more difficult to control an arrhythmia with drugs once fetal compromise is evident, than to prevent compromise by timely treatment in the first place. For a fetus presenting with an important tachycardia at a viable gestation age, the option of early delivery and ex-utero treatment may be considered. For a fetus in good condition and already close to term (>36 weeks) this may be a good option. However, for a fetus that is hydropic and/or significantly pre-term, the risks of early delivery are considerable and in-utero management with drugs in the first instance is often the better option. A decision about the best management in an individual case will depend on the current state of the mother and fetus, the gestational age, the type of arrhythmia, local experience and results in the management of the sick pre-term infant, and experience in prenatal drug therapy. Most anti-arrhythmic therapy is given orally to the mother (transplacental therapy), but direct therapy, into the fetal umbilical vein or into muscle has also been used. Most fetal cardiologists reserve direct therapy for exceptional cases as there is no clear evidence that it is generally more effective than transplacental treatment, and the risks to the fetus of repeated direct

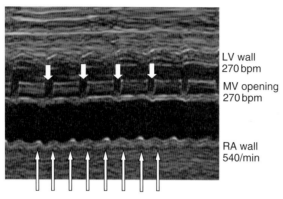

Fig. 7.13. The M-line passes through the left ventricular wall, the mitral valve (thick arrows) and the right atrial wall (thin arrows). The atrial wall appeared to be "shivering" in the moving image, as the rate was 540 bpm. The ventricular wall and aortic valve are responding to every second atrial beat so that the ventricular contraction is exactly half the atrial rate (2:1) conduction. This is atrial flutter.

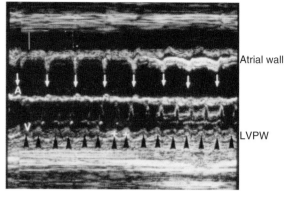

Fig. 7.14. Due to the rarity of this condition, this figure is courtesy of a friend (Dr. Lillian Lopes) and dates from 1991. The ventricular wall (LVPW) indicated by the black arrowheads, can be seen contracting at 210 bpm. The atrial rate on the other hand is normal at 140 bpm (white arrows).

access are significant. In addition, the use of intramuscular digoxin in particular in the neonate and child gives notoriously unreliable serum drug levels and for this reason is not usually advocated by the pediatric arrhythmia specialist.

Transplacental anti-arrhythmic therapy

Transplacental anti-arrhythmic treatment of fetus inevitably involves exposure of the mother herself to the drug and therefore to possible adverse effects. Potential harm that may arise includes the induction of arrhythmias in the mother's heart (pro-arrhythmia), although this is more likely if she herself has a pre-existing cardiac pathology. The nature of the proposed treatment including possible side effects and adverse consequences for the mother as well as the fetus, and any alternatives should be discussed. Before embarking on any such treatment, the mother must be assessed for factors which might increase her risk of complications. This will include enquiry about possible cardiac symptoms and any history of structural or functional cardiac abnormality. Any suspicious findings may warrant further investigation by an appropriate expert but in the absence of any suggestive history, investigation of the mother can be limited to a 12-lead electrocardiogram (ECG). The purpose of the ECG is to detect both latent cardiac disease in the mother and to act as a baseline for future ECGs that may be required to monitor the action of the anti-arrhythmic treatment on the maternal heart, or to evaluate potential adverse symptoms.

A wide range of different anti-arrhythmic drugs has been used to treat fetal arrhythmias with varying degrees of success. Case series show that the more commonly used drugs do appear to be effective in controlling arrhythmias, but there is a paucity of good data on the relative efficacy of the different agents. Adequate transfer across the placenta between the maternal and fetal circulations is essential for a drug to be effective as a transplacental agent. Information about placental transmission of many drugs is available from animal studies, in-vitro human studies and from simultaneous cord blood and maternal blood sampling in vivo. Many variable factors such as relative pH, albumin levels and umbilical venous pressure may influence the efficacy of transfer and this may explain why some data is apparently conflicting. Fetal hydrops has a major influence on the placental transfer of some drugs. Both clinical responses recorded in case series and fetal–maternal blood level comparisons indicate that with digoxin in particular, transfer is usually adequate in the non-hydropic fetus, but is poor when fetal hydrops is established.

Digoxin

Digoxin is the usual first-line treatment for supraventricular tachycardias. Drug absorption is decreased and drug elimination and blood volume is increased in pregnancy, therefore larger doses are required than in the non-pregnant patient. A typical starting dose is 250 µg three times daily. Some authors prefer to start with a loading dose of 1.5–2.0 mg over the first 24 hours, although this is not our usual practice. Many women will experience some nausea initially, but this will usually improve over time and is not an indication for an immediate reduction in dose. However, visual symptoms including blurred vision and seeing abnormal colors are usually associated with toxic serum levels. The timing of blood sampling for digoxin levels should take into account the fact that several days are required before tissue levels approach a steady state following a change in dose and that serum levels only reflect the tissue level 6–8 hours after ingestion of each dose of the drug. The serum level aimed at in the mother should be in the range of 1.6–2.5 µg/l. The main value of serum levels is in determining whether there is leeway for an increase in dose (usually to three and four times on alternate days, but occasionally to 250 µg four times a day) if a clinical response is lacking. The clinical response to digoxin may take a week or more and this, as well as its poor placental transfer in the setting of hydrops, is a reason for not relying on digoxin alone in a fetus that is already showing evidence of compromise or for giving it as a direct intravenous bolus in this setting.

Flecainide

Flecainide is a Class I (membrane stabilizing) antiarrythmic agent. Placental transfer of flecainide is good and, unlike digoxin, usually remains adequate even in the presence of fetal hydrops. Clinical response to flecainide in the fetus is generally more rapid than with digoxin, but may still take several days. A significant disadvantage of flecainide is that, in certain circumstances, it has been shown to have an important and dangerous pro-arrhythmic effect. Although there are no reports of serious pro-arrhythmic effects in the mother in the context of transplacental fetal therapy, this remains a theoretical possibility. It is therefore mandatory to minimize the risk by excluding pre-existing maternal cardiac disease and by strictly monitoring blood levels and adjusting the dosage accordingly. For fetal therapy of supraventricular tachycardias, a typical starting dose is 100 mg three times daily. A flecainide level should be obtained urgently after 3 days and the dose adjusted according to the maternal blood level and the clinical response. Although a higher therapeutic range has been used in the past, we would not normally let maternal levels much exceed 700 mcg/l. In the presence of a good clinical response we would not normally increase the dosage on the basis of blood levels alone. Blood levels should continue to be monitored

and maternal ECGs repeated whilst treatment is continued and especially when any change in dose is made. Flecainide can reduce the flutter rate of atrial flutter with potential dangerous consequences. The flutter rate may decrease to the extent that 1:1 conduction of the flutter waves to the ventricles (rather than the typical 2:1 block) becomes possible. If this were to happen, the ventricles would be driven at such a high rate that cardiac output would be compromised and possibly ventricular arrhythmias induced. It is therefore recommended that digoxin always be given with flecainide when treating atrial flutter to help raise the threshold rate against 1:1 conduction.

Sotalol

Sotalol belongs to Class II (beta blocking) as well as Class III (action potential prolonging) groups of antiarrhythmic drugs. It has been used to control SVT successfully in the fetus, including cases where fetal hydrops was present, although it is only efficacious in about the same proportion of cases as flecainide (about 70%). As with flecainide, sotalol can have a pro-arrhythmic effect. In particular, sotolol prolongs the corrected QT interval on the ECG and this may pre-dispose to the dangerous ventricular arrhythmia "torsade de pointes." The increase in QT interval is to a large extent dose dependent and may be easily monitored on serial maternal ECGs. QT interval prolongation may be exaggerated by interaction with other drugs including erythromycin, clarythromycin, and domperidone. It is therefore vital that the mother on sotalol communicates this fact to anyone who prescribes for her. A typical starting dose of sotalol for transplacental treatment is 80 mg twice daily. This may be adjusted according to clinical response, maternal ECG changes, and serum levels if they are available. Placental transfer is good even in the presence of hydrops, with fetal levels very similar to maternal levels. Sotalol is reported to be successful in the treatment of fetal atrial flutter, but its effectiveness in 1:1 supraventricular tachycardias has been questioned in at least one study, although a later study by the same authors is more positive about its use. There are no randomized trials comparing it with flecainide, which is the main alternative.

Amiodarone

There are some reports of successful second-line treatment of fetal tachycardia with amiodarone, but it has been less widely used than flecainide. It has been given as a loading dose of 1800 to 2400 mg per day in divided doses for 2–7 days. The dose was reduced to 800 mg per day thereafter for up to a further week. However, once the fetus was in sinus rhythm, the dose was decreased to a true maintenance dose of 200–400 mg/day. The maternal ECG should be repeated on a daily basis, with particular attention paid to the QT interval. Amiodarone may induce hypothyroidism in the fetus. Although this is reversible on cessation of therapy, it occurs at a time critical to normal neurological development and the neurological effects may not be reversible. Amiodarone therefore should be reserved for treatment of refractory fetal arrhythmias which have failed to respond to the other drug options and where the fetus is too premature for delivery as an alternative.

Drugs in combination

In principle, the use of combinations of anti-arrhythmic drugs together without good reason is best avoided as drug interactions may complicate the maintenance of satisfactory levels and it may be difficult to attribute any adverse effect to a specific one of the drugs used. One rational use of multiple drugs is the management of atrial flutter using digoxin as well as flecainide, where digoxin alone has failed or is deemed unlikely to be effective because of hydrops. Used alone, flecainide may reduce the atrial flutter rate low enough to allow 1:1 conduction to the ventricles, rather than the usual 2:1 block, and thus cause a very high and unsustainable ventricular rate. Digoxin acts to reduce the maximum rate of conduction through the AV node and thus prevent this potentially dangerous complication. In other circumstances, digoxin started as first-line therapy is sometimes continued when a second-line therapy such as flecainide or sotalol is added, but there is no clear evidence of benefit or otherwise in doing this. The use of anti-arrhythmic drugs in combination is also an option in unusual cases where the more tried and tested regimes have failed, but the possibility of adverse reactions should be carefully considered and treatment should be supervised by an expert familiar with the drugs to be used.

Bradycardia

Bradycardia in the fetus is generally defined as a fetal heart rate of less than 100 bpm but the gestational age

should also be taken into account as the normal heart rate is higher in the early fetus than at term.

Benign bradycardia

It is quite a common occurrence during the mid-trimester scan to observe a dramatic slowing of the fetal heart rate, sometimes almost to the point of asystole, followed by a progressive recovery in heart rate. In some cases, this may be the result of vagal stimulation brought about by pressure on the fetus itself, or more likely on the umbilical cord, from the transducer. At this gestation, the vagal response is unopposed by a less well-developed sympathetic nervous system, resulting in a short-lived but fairly profound bradycardia. The phenomenon is quite specific for gestation age, in that it is, in our experience, never seen at the nuchal scan and much less common after 28 or so weeks.

Once this benign transient bradycardia has been ruled out, the following causes of bradycardia should be considered.

(1) Severe hypoxia
(2) Sinus node dysfunction
(3) Blocked atrial ectopic beats
(4) Second degree heart block
(5) Complete heart block
(6) Long QT syndrome

Bradycardia, whether transient or sustained, may be an indication of severe fetal distress and therefore an indication for urgent delivery. The other causes of bradycardia should be considered, however, in order to avoid an unnecessary and potentially dangerous urgent delivery. Interpretation of a suspicious cardiotocogram (CTG) tracing should be supplemented with direct auscultation, and by ultrasound scan in selected cases, as the CTG trace does not give full information as to the nature of the rhythm.

Sinus node dysfunction

Sinus node dysfunction in the fetus is recognized most commonly in the fetus with left atrial isomerism. In this condition, the sinus node may be abnormally positioned and function at a slower rate than normal. The anatomical features, including interruption of the inferior caval vein are the clue to the underlying diagnosis. The heart rate is typically 80 to 120 beats per minute. Sinus node dysfunction is distinct from complete heart block, although both may occur together in left isomerism.

Blocked atrial ectopic beats

Blocked atrial ectopic beats have been discussed in a previous section above. The heart block which occurs in the setting of ectopic beats is physiological and entirely appropriate. It is not an indication of disease or abnormality of the conducting tissues.

First-degree heart block

Although this conduction abnormality does not cause a bradycardia, it is appropriate to mention it at this point, as it is the precursor for second and third degree block. The heart rate is normal but the time between atrial and ventricular contraction is prolonged (Fig. 7.15). The normal range is approximately 80–140 ms. When observed in the context of maternal anti-Ro antibodies, treatment with beta- or dexamethasone has been reported as preventing the progression to higher degrees of block, although the evidence for this is still weak. The patient illustrated in Fig. 7.15 had a prolonged P–R interval from 26 weeks of gestation. She had clinical systemic lupus and anti-Ro antibodies but was reluctant to take steroids prenatally. The neonate had a completely uncomplicated course, required no treatment and remains in first-degree heart block at a year of age.

Second-degree heart block

Second-degree heart block describes the situation where some but not all atrial beats are transmitted to the ventricles. For example, in 2:1 heart block, only alternate atrial beats will conduct and the ventricular rate will be half that of the atria (Fig. 7.16). There will, however, be a fixed relationship between atrial and ventricular beats. It may be difficult to distinguish second-degree heart block from blocked atrial ectopic ectopic beats (Fig. 7.8) and from complete heart block where the rate of the ventricular escape rhythm is coincidentally half that of the atrial rate, although careful mesurement of the time intervals will usually give the correct diagnosis. True second-degree heart block generally does indicate conduction system disease.

Complete heart block

In complete heart block, there is no conduction between atria and ventricles (Fig. 7.17(a)–(c)). Ventricular contraction is dependent on an escape rhythm intrinsic to the ventricles. The ventricular rhythm is usually regular but much slower than normal, with rates typically between 40 and 90 bpm. There may occasionally be super-added ventricular ectopic beats causing irregularity of the rhythm. The hallmark of complete heart block is that there is complete dissociation of atrial and ventricular rhythms. Sometimes in complete heart block, the initial impression may be of 2:1 heart block as a ventricular contraction appears to follow every other atrial contraction. However, a longer period of observation will reveal that the relationship between atrial and ventricular contractions is not truly fixed, but that the AV interval changes progressively as

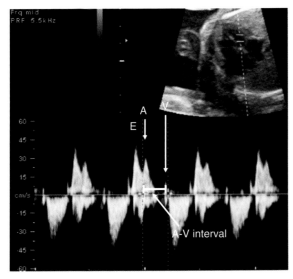

Fig. 7.15. The time between the onset of the A wave and the onset of ventricular contraction was prolonged at 210 ms. Note the reversal of the E–A ratio in the mitral valve probably implying a degree of left ventricular dysfunction.

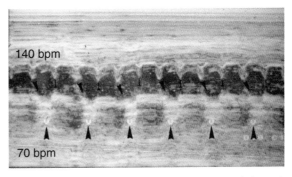

Fig. 7.16. The M-line passes through the atrium anteriorly (on top) and the ventricles posteriorly (below). The atrial rate is regular, but at 140 bpm exactly twice that of the ventricles. This is second-degree heart block where only alternate atrial beats are conducted.

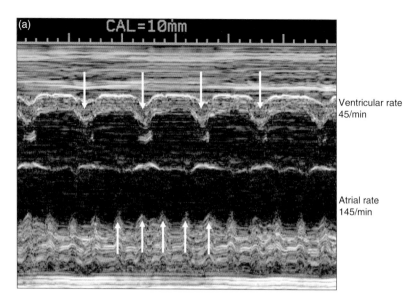

Fig. 7.17.(a). The atrial and ventricular contractions are completely dissociated from each other, with here the ventricular rate at 45 bpm and the atrial rate at 145 bpm.

Ventricular rate 45/min

Atrial rate 145/min

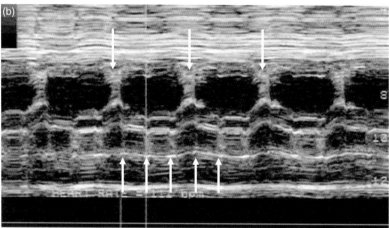

Fig. 7.17.(b). The atrial and ventricular rhythms are completely independent of each other but the atrial rate (below) has fallen to 111 bpm and the ventricular rate (above) to 38 bpm. This was recorded just a few days prior to intrauterine death in a case of left atrial isomerism with hydrops and a complex heart malformation.

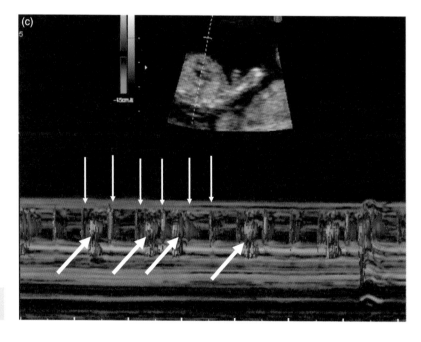

Fig. 7.17.(c). Sometimes color M-mode, if it is available on your ultrasound machine, can be helpful in defining arrhythmias. The red blocks represent atrial contraction, which is regular and occurring at about 140 bpm. The blue blocks represent ventricular contraction which is completely dissociated from atrial contraction and much slower. It is difficult to measure the ventricular rate accurately because there are frequent ventricular ectopic beats, producing an irregular slow rhythm between 50 and 60 bpm.

the ventricular rate only approximately, rather than exactly, matches half of the atrial rate.

Complete heart block may occur in association with structural heart disease or in isolation. The heart defects that are particularly associated with complete heart block are most commonly left atrial isomerism, but also atrioventricular discordance and double inlet left ventricle. Complete heart block may be a presenting feature with a cardiac defect or it may develop during follow-up in fetal or in postnatal life. Complete heart block associated with complex structural heart disease such as left isomerism with an atrioventricular septal defect carries a very poor prognosis. The atrial and ventricular rates tend to fall progressively (Fig. 7.17(b)) resulting in fetal hydrops. When this happens, spontaneous intrauterine death is very frequent.

When complete heart block occurs in the absence of structural heart disease, anti-Ro (SSA) and anti-La (SSB) antibodies are found to be present in the blood of more than 90% of mothers. Only a minority of these women will have a previously diagnosed connective tissue disease. Anti-Ro and anti-La antibodies start to cross the placenta from about 16 weeks of gestation and it is unusual to see complete heart block attributable to these antibodies presenting before about 18 weeks of gestation. Having crossed the placenta, antibodies may bind to cardiomyocytes in the fetus and initiate an inflammatory process in the conducting tissue resulting in progressive apoptosis, replacement by fibrous tissue and loss of function. However, it is of interest to be aware that even monochorionic twins can respond differently to circulating maternal antibodies with one developing heart block and the other not, so there is some element of substrate susceptibility.

The inflammatory nature of the process invites the possibility of suppression with steroids or other drugs to prevent progression to complete heart block. There are anecdotal reports which support the idea that fluorinated steroids may halt or even reverse the progression of the disease if given early enough. Attempts have been made to predict the onset of complete heart block with a view to starting treatment at the earliest signs. The recurrence risk for complete heart block in a future pregnancy in a woman who has had both a previously affected fetus and is known to have anti-Ro and anti-La antibodies is about 1 in 5. This risk is generally not considered high enough to justify the use of prophylactic steroid therapy of unproven value and with potential adverse effects, including neurodevelopmental delay. Pregnancies at such a risk can be intensively monitored from about 18 weeks' gestation onwards.

Increase in the AV interval using M-mode or Doppler indicating first-degree heart block, or the onset of second-degree heart block might be considered indications to start therapy with steroids. Any benefit of such treatment in the possible prevention of complete heart block would need to be balanced against the adverse consequences of long term steroids in the developing fetus. The majority of cases with heart block in association with maternal antibodies present as established complete heart block, which seems irreversible and steroid treatment has not been demonstrated to restore sinus rhythm in these cases. In established complete heart block, there is at least mild cardiomegaly (Fig. 7.18), which will increase if hydrops develops. There can also be patchy increased echogenicity of the myocardium of the atria or ventricles, which appears alarming but is not necessarily associated with a poor prognosis. In addition, a small pericardial effusion is commonly seen but this does not always indicate that hydrops will develop. In a few cases of complete heart block with a structurally normal heart, no maternal antibodies are found. In some of these cases antibodies have been found in the mother even some years later but, in the remainder, the cause is unknown and some appear to be familial.

Management of complete heart block

The prognosis for complete heart block varies according to the clinical state, gestation, and associated

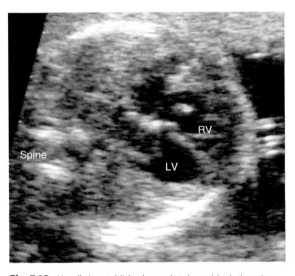

Fig. 7.18. Usually in established complete heart block, there is a degree of mild cardiomegaly as seen here. There is also sometimes patchy increased echogenicity of the myocardium which was seen here in the moving image and which tends to, but does not always, equate with a poor outcome.

structural heart defects. Where hydrops is already evident and/or there are major structural heart defects, the prognosis is generally very poor, with a high risk of spontaneous intrauterine or early neonatal death, and termination of the pregnancy is an option that may be considered. The prognosis for isolated complete heart block, without structural abnormality and where the fetus does not become hydropic in utero is rather better, but a lifelong requirement for an artificial pacemaker is to be expected. For a fetus that has reached viability and is deteriorating, preterm delivery and ex-utero pacing may be considered. However, in many fetuses deteriorating in this way there is impaired ventricular function, the response to pacing is limited and the prognosis for survival is poor. There is no firm evidence that drug or other interventions in-utero can influence the course of the disease. One fairly large study showed that the overall prognosis for antibody-associated complete heart block was improved in a later cohort where prenatal steroids (and sympathomimetics) were used frequently compared with an earlier cohort where they were used only rarely. However, this type of study is subject to bias from confounding factors and the results reported were not significantly better than those in at least one other large center where steroids are not generally given. Deterioration in cardiac performance in fetuses with heart block may be due to associated immune myocarditis and this would be a rationale for steroid therapy, but proof of benefit remains lacking.

Beta-sympathomimetic drugs such as salbutamol or terbutaline have been administered as transplacental therapy in order to boost fetal heart rate in complete heart block. Although a significant increase in heart rate may be achieved in the short term, tolerance develops rapidly in the fetus. Escalating doses, which may not be tolerated by the mother, are often required to maintain a sustained response making treatment for longer than 2–3 weeks impractical. In all cases of complete heart block consideration must be given to the most appropriate method and site for delivery. The mode of delivery will depend to a large extent on the experience of the obstetrician involved. A normal delivery is achievable in complete heart block as the rhythm maintains its variability to some extent to allow monitoring. However, many obstetricians would prefer to go straight to cesarean section. If active management for complete heart block is to be pursued postnatally,

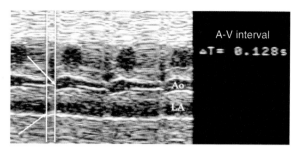

Fig. 7.19. There was normal one-to-one conduction between the atria and ventricles, with a normal P–R interval of 128 ms measured here. However, a heart rate of 80 bpm was consistent from 12 weeks of gestation throughout pregnancy. Postnatally, a long QT syndrome was found on ECG.

facilities for pacemaker insertion should be available even though early pacemaker insertion will not be necessary in all cases.

Long QT syndrome

This is a rare condition of which I have only seen one example to my knowledge. There was a persistent bradycardia, first noticed at 12 weeks' gestation at the nuchal scan. The heart was structurally normal and the inferior vena cava intact, so that left isomerism was more or less excluded. The P–R interval was normal and there were no abnormal antibodies detected in the mother. (The early detection of bradycardia virtually excluded it being antibody mediated anyway.) The atrial and ventricular rates were the same and consistently around 80 bpm (Fig. 7.19). The fetus progressed normally during gestation and there were no other findings. At birth, the neonate had a long QT syndrome, which required placement of a pacemaker. A recent publication found a persistent fetal heart rate below 120 bpm when they looked retrospectively at a small group of neonates with long QT syndrome. When there is a sustained rhythm below 120 bpm, therefore, this diagnosis should be considered and excluded by a postnatal ECG.

Summary

An abnormal heart rhythm is either too fast, too slow, or irregular. The irregular rhythms are the most common, are self-limiting and usually require no intervention. A sustained slow rhythm or a tachycardia requires referral for detailed fetal echocardiography and managed as outlined above.

Chapter 8

Counseling and outcome of individual cardiac malformations

Counseling

Despite counseling being a difficult and important aspect of fetal cardiology, it receives little attention and training. Some general principles common to all ultrasound scanning should be followed. The parents should be advised at the start of the scan that it takes some time and concentration to check all the different parts of the fetal heart, so that they are not intimidated by long silences. Giving partial information before the examination is complete must be avoided as it may be misleading, therefore the parents should be advised that all their questions will be answered at the end. If trainees or other observers are in the room during the scan, only essential features of the images should be pointed out, in order to minimize distress to the parents. I prefer to turn off the Doppler volume in the presence of a fetal anomaly, as hearing the fetal heart beat is a particularly emotional bonding experience for the parents. I also prefer that they cannot see the ultrasound screen if there is an abnormality, although in some cases using the images to point out the abnormal findings at the end may be helpful, although personally I prefer to draw diagrams for the patient instead.

It is more difficult to counsel parents when they are unprepared for bad news, for example, at an expectedly "routine" scan, or if they have not understood that they were being seen as a high-risk patient. The initial anger, numbness, and failure to take in information, which is the usual reaction to finding a problem, will then have to be played through and overcome. Often, by the time the parents are referred to the fetal cardiologist, they are expecting some sort of problem and this helps counseling. However, the counselor should be aware that anxiety and fear may be manifest as hostility and anger and be understanding of this reaction. Ideally, counseling should not take place in the scan room, but in a quiet uninterrupted setting, with the parents seated face-to-face with the doctor. The aims of counseling are

- to provide an accurate diagnosis of the malformation

- to outline the management and treatment options available
- to provide a clear and truthful picture of the prognosis
- to outline alternatives of management if they are available
- to help the parents reach the form of management which is best for them in their individual situation

The specifics of counseling then will depend on the precise cardiac diagnosis, the security of diagnosis, the gestational age, the association with extracardiac malformations, the natural history of the malformation in fetal life, and the surgical options, including the local and "best" surgical results. There is no ethical dilemma if the counselor, first, has a clear grasp of the facts of a particular lesion, and second, offers a thorough and complete picture of what the future holds concerning it. The natural history of the cardiac defect from the time of fetal diagnosis is often quite different from pediatric experience and anyone involved in fetal counseling should be aware of where differences apply. The usual and most likely outcome should be explained, but the worst and best outcomes should not be ignored. One of the weakest areas of our knowledge is long-term results. Surgery for many complex forms of heart disease has only been successful in recent years and the long term is as yet unknown. In addition, the long-term outcome of today's surgery is likely to be much better than that of 20 years ago so, even if 20-year follow-up data are available, they are only useful as a guide rather than a really comparable prediction. Expectant parents are hoping for a normal 70-plus year lifespan for their child; therefore it is important that they understand the limitations of our knowledge in this respect.

Cardiac diagnosis

There is a wide range of severity in congenital heart malformations, from lesions which require no treatment, such as small ventricular septal defects, to lesions which can only be treated with palliative surgery, such

Table 8.1 Suggested scale of CHD on a 1–10 basis, 1 with best prognosis, 10 with worst

(1) Small VSDs

Mild PS

(2) ASD, PDA (neither are detectable prenatally),

VSD moderate

Bicuspid aortic valve

(3) Severe PS

Large VSD

Moderate AS

TOF

Simple TGA

Simple corrected TGA

(4) Atrioventricular septal defect

Coarctation

Double outlet RV (some forms)

TAPVR

Mild Ebstein's anomaly

(5) Common arterial trunk

TOF with pulmonary atresia

Pulmonary atresia with IVS (some forms)

(6) Common arterial trunk

TOF with pulmonary atresia

Severe aortic stenosis

Double outlet RV

Complex TGA

Corrected TGA, complex

(7) Tricuspid atresia

Double inlet ventricle

(8) Pulmonary atresia with IVS (some forms)

Mitral atresia

Severe Ebstein's with cardiomegaly

Critical aortic stenosis

(9) HLHS

Right isomerism

(10) AVSD with CHB and left isomerism

Any CHD with intrauterine congestive heart failure

Myocardial dysfunction with congestive heart failure in utero

as the hypoplastic left heart syndrome. Unfortunately, the majority of malformations detected during fetal life fall into the more severe end of the diagnostic spectrum. The concept of "fatal" or "non-fatal" is not relevant in cardiac anomalies, as almost all lesions can now be approached surgically, although some have a very high risk of mortality. It should be explained to the parents that quality of life and longevity are more important concepts to understand. It can be useful to consider cardiac lesions on a scale of one to ten, with one being the least severe (Table 8.1). Between 3–6

would fall lesions where the heart structure can be restored, although with varied degrees of difficulty, to a "normal" or near normal anatomy. Most "one ventricle repairs" would fit in the 7–10 range, depending on the precise anatomy. Alternatively, malformations can be divided into "good" – those which are easily treated and will not affect the child in the long term, "intermediate" – those which can be successfully repaired surgically but which are likely to affect long-term survival, and "bad" – those lesions likely to have a profound effect during childhood and on the chance

Table 8.2 Suggested grading of CHD detectable prenatally

"Low risk" CHD – may not need surgery or low risk surgery

VSD

"Moderate risk" CHD - low mortality for surgery but likely to affect long-term survival

TOF

Simple TGA

Simple corrected TGA

AVSD

Coarctation

Double outlet RV (some forms)

Isolated TAPVR

Ebstein's anomaly without severe cardiomegaly

"High risk" CHD - a high mortality for surgery or repeated surgeries likely during childhood or likely to be compromised cardiologically as young adults

Common arterial trunk

TOF with pulmonary atresia

Pulmonary atresia with IVS (some forms)

TOF with pulmonary atresia

Severe aortic stenosis

Double outlet RV (some forms)

Complex TGA

Complex corrected TGA

Tricuspid atresia

Double inlet ventricle

Pulmonary atresia with IVS, Mitral atresia

HLHS

AVSD with DORV and right isomerism

AVSD with CHB and left isomerism

Ebstein's anomaly with severe cardiomegaly

TAPVR with obstruction or with isomerism syndrome

of reaching healthy adult life (Table 8.2). The reason all one-ventricle (or Fontan) repairs are in the range of poorest prognosis is that it is generally accepted that, although this type of circulation can function well for 20–30 years, there is an increasing attrition in these patients over time. A failing Fontan circulation cannot usually be salvaged by surgical revision, leaving cardiac transplantation as the only option, However, these patients are often poor candidates for transplant and in the competition for scarce organs, other patients with a better chance of survival are often preferred. Parents should be warned of this possible loss of their child in young adult life. Tables 8.1 and 8.2 are only intended to be rough guidelines to aid the concept of counseling. Every pediatric cardiologist would compile a slightly different list of severity, depending on his or her experience and personal level of optimism.

The term "counseling" indicates a dialog, not a monolog, and it is often useful to start by asking the parents what they understand about the problem so far.

This gives the counselor a chance to assess their level of understanding and their reaction to the information they have gained before reaching the tertiary center. Research has demonstrated that parents in the neonatal intensive care setting are offered "euphemisms, vague statements, and half-truths" by physicians, and that they are assumed to be "too overwhelmed to assimilate information or make rational decisions." This is a source of resentment and anger to parents. There is no excuse for avoiding informing the parents directly when a malformation is detected in fetal life. Although patients vary in their desire for information and involvement, there is evidence that physicians frequently underestimate it. Parents should be offered clear information, even if they reject or deny it. Using diagrams to explain the defect, giving written information of the diagnosis and an outline of surgical management is helpful, and aids the parents in remembering what has been said after they have left the doctor. Language should be used that is within the understanding of the individual parent.

221

Part of the skill of talking to parents is in making them understand, without condescension, whatever their level of education. Common questions such as why a cardiac defect has happened and whether it will happen again in a future pregnancy, should be anticipated and answered with current knowledge. Many fetal cardiologists favour a multi-disciplinary approach involving the obstetrician, geneticist, and surgeon as a group, to supply supportive or additional information. However, to some families this is intimidating and an additional session with any of these colleagues individually may be preferable. A common problem, which complicates counseling nowadays, is the parents accessing the Internet for information, before or after counseling. Sometimes this extra source of information can be beneficial and helpful, but more often it is misleading, biased, and inappropriate for the precise circumstances of the individual patient. None of the information online is subject to any form of review, so has the potential to be totally inaccurate. Conflicting information can be a major source of confusion for the parents and the counselor must be prepared to explain any possible differences in information. It is useful for the counselor to compile a list of useful and valuable websites appropriate to the lesion and direct the patient to them for back-up information.

Security of diagnosis

The ability to discuss a specific diagnosis accurately will depend on the completeness of the fetal echocardiogram and how much detail was obtained. If image quality is poor, for example, in very early or in late pregnancy, or in an obese patient, the details of a malformation may be more difficult to define and this may influence the precision of prognostication. This may not make a lot of difference in some cases – for example, with poor images it may be difficult to differentiate between a common arterial trunk and tetralogy of Fallot with pulmonary atresia but visible confluent central pulmonary arteries. However, counseling is not very different for these two lesions as both are complex forms of malformation, that have a significant mortality at surgical repair and which require repeated surgical intervention to replace conduit material. In contrast, simple transposition of the great arteries has a good prognosis for one-stage surgical repair (at least in the short term) but if complicated by pulmonary stenosis and a ventricular septal defect, or a straddling atrioventricular valve, for example, a quite different surgical route with less good results may be

the outlook. Such complicating lesions may not always be detected initially, especially in early pregnancy or if image quality was poor. In each case, the fetal cardiologist should try to think of what could have been missed or misinterpreted, which would make a significant difference to the diagnosis and counseling. If a decision concerning the continuation of the pregnancy rests on an incomplete or unsatisfactory study, it should be repeated within a short time interval, or the patient should be referred to a more experienced fetal cardiologist. Unnecessary delay before definitive counseling is inexcusable, as it will only increase parental anguish.

Gestational age

The gestational age of the patient can influence the counseling in two ways. First, it will have an impact on the management options. These will be discussed below. Second, it is important in terms of the potential for evolution of the malformation. It is well recognized that cardiac malformations can change or progress with advancing gestation (Table 8.3). For example, any vessel or chamber which is obstructed can fail to keep pace with growth of the rest of the fetus, resulting in hypoplasia of the affected part. This has been seen in pulmonary stenosis resulting in right ventricular hypoplasia, or in aortic stenosis or coarctation of the aorta, resulting left ventricular hypoplasia. Pulmonary or aortic stenosis can progress to pulmonary or aortic atresia, respectively. Atrioventricular valve regurgitation and cardiomegaly can increase, and even result in fetal hydrops with advancing gestation. In a case of tetralogy of Fallot or coarctation of the aorta, to give two examples, presenting at 18 weeks' gestation, the

Table 8.3 Malformations which have been seen to change, develop, or progress during the second half of pregnancy

Pulmonary stenosis
Aortic stenosis
Coarctation
Pulmonary artery hypoplasia in pulmonary atresia or TOF
Right ventricular hypoplasia in PS
Pulmonary atresia from PS
Left ventricular hypoplasia in AS
Aortic atresia from AS
AV valve regurgitation with or without Ebstein's anomaly
Arch hypoplasia in coarctation
Cardiac tumors
Complete heart block
Myocardial dysfunction

possibility of evolution must be included and explained in the counseling. This would not be necessary in the case of either lesion seen for the first time at, for example, 36 weeks.

Association with extracardiac malformations

It is important that the pediatric cardiologist performing fetal scanning is aware of the associations of cardiac anomalies with extracardiac malformations, particularly those which are not well recognized in pediatric practice or those which may not be entirely identifiable antenatally. The association of Down's syndrome with an atrioventricular septal defect is well known, but the association of a large inlet ventricular septal defect or mitral atresia, double oulet right ventricle with trisomy 18, is less recognized. Tetralogy of Fallot is particularly commonly associated with chromosome anomalies and with structural extracardiac lesions such as tracheo-esophageal fistula or exomphalos. In one study, almost 50% of cases of fetal tetralogy of Fallot were not isolated. Overall, chromosomal anomalies were found in nearly 20% of fetal cardiac malformations (Table 8.4), in contrast to a rate of 12.8% in live births with congenital heart disease. A further 10% have additional extracardiac malformations. The presence of extracardiac malformations may indicate a chromosomal defect or syndrome diagnosis (e.g. VATER syndrome). Combinations of defects may impact the parents' decision concerning the management of the pregnancy or the prognosis for surgical repair or in some cases the cardiologist's plans for management – for example, surgical treatment for

any cardiac malformation is not usually offered in the setting of trisomy 18. A particularly difficult situation is that presented by the finding of a microdeletion of chromosome 22 indicating the Di George or velocardiofacial syndrome. This chromosome anomaly occurs particularly with interrupted aortic arch, common arterial trunk, or tetralogy of Fallot but the phenotype is very variable, especially in relation to neurodevelopmental delay, which can vary from mild to severe. In addition, there is a variable degree of immune deficiency and a strong association between 22q11 deletion and the development of schizophrenia in young adult life. When this chromosomal defect is found, it is essential that the parents have detailed counseling, ideally from a geneticist, on the extracardiac implications for the child.

Natural history of the cardiac malformation in fetal life

The course of an individual cardiac malformation in fetal life is often different from what would be expected from postnatal experience. There is an increased incidence of fetal loss in any fetus with a chromosome defect, but it is particularly high in Turner's syndrome. Unexpected spontaneous fetal loss has also been seen in Ebstein's malformation, tetralogy of Fallot, and common arterial trunk. Fetal loss is common in fetuses with isomerism of the left atrial appendages, particularly when there is the combination of an atrioventricular septal defect with complete heart block. It is also important to have a clear idea of the incidence of perinatal loss, which occurs under a particular diagnostic heading, as many reports in the literature exclude

Table 8.4 Association of fetal CHD with chromosomal anomalies

Diagnosis	% with chromosomal anomalies
VSD	48
AVSD	35
Coarctation	29
TOF	27
Mitral atresia	18
Trunk	14
DORV	12
Tricuspid dysplasia	5
Pul atresia/PS	5
HLHS	4
Tricuspid atresia	2

Chromosomal anomalies were not found in simple transposition, corrected transposition or double inlet ventricle in this series.

cases which do not reach surgery. For example, the Baltimore–Washington Infant study reports a medical (non-surgically treated) mortality of 10% for infants with tetralogy of Fallot or transposition of the great arteries. This loss may be improved by prenatal recognition of the disease or, alternatively, these cases may represent neonates with multiple malformations or the worst anatomical types of these diagnoses. In one series of 26 fetal cases of the hypoplastic left heart syndrome where the pregnancy continued with the intention to treat all cases surgically, only 18 cases reached surgery and 9 cases survived, representing an overall survival rate of 35% from an intention-to-treat position, which is much lower than concurrently reported surgical mortality. Much of the mortality could be explained by extracardiac features, only some of which were predictable prenatally, such as chromosome malformations, tracheo-esophageal fistula, neurological damage, or prematurity.

Surgical options, local and "best" surgical results

Over the last 20 years, surgical options and results have changed dramatically under all diagnostic headings and this can only continue in a positive direction. However, results do vary between centers and in different parts of the world. When counseling a patient with congenital heart disease, it is important to know what surgical options are available, both locally and elsewhere. For example, transplantation is one accepted method of treatment for the hypoplastic left heart syndrome, but it may not be available locally. This may need to be explained and discussed. It is also important to know the results of surgery performed locally and how they compare with results in other centers. These data can only be obtained by continuous monitoring of one's own center's results, and familiarity with the presented and published results of others. It is important for the fetal cardiologist to keep in touch with this continually changing picture. Published results must be viewed critically, however, as case selection can alter the "true" picture and only the best results tend to be published, which does not represent a real reflection of the outcome of all cases under a diagnostic heading.

It is important not only to inform the parents of the cardiac aspects of long-term results but also of possible neurodevelopmental implications. It is a common question from parents whether the "lack of oxygen" in some cardiac conditions can affect brain development in their child. There is increasing evidence that some techniques associated with cardiac surgery, repeated, or prolonged surgeries, and some specific conditions such as the hypoplastic left heart syndrome, are associated with a significant impact on motor skills and IQ scores. In addition, some forms of surgical repair are associated with a significant incidence of neurological complications such as stroke, which is reported in up to 10% of cases after the Fontan operation.

Management options

Management options include the possibility of termination of pregnancy or re-organization of perinatal care. Termination of pregnancy is a legal option for fetal malformations in most of the developed world, but the gestational age limit is variable. In general, it is allowed up to 24 weeks' gestation, but late termination, even up to term, can be obtained in some countries or in certain States in the USA, for major malformations. The counselor must be able to discuss the options of termination of pregnancy, whatever his or her own beliefs, and present them in a factual manner without introducing their own bias. In practice, termination of pregnancy is an increasingly difficult decision for the mother to make as gestation advances. The earlier the diagnosis of fetal malformation can be achieved, which is now possible from as early as 12 weeks' gestation, the more safely termination of pregnancy can be accomplished physically, and with least emotional trauma. The maternal sensation of fetal movement does not begin before 16 weeks and the pregnancy is not usually obviously visible, therefore, still a private matter for the parents. By 20 weeks' gestation however, most parents have already invested thoughts, hopes, and dreams in the future of the fetus, particularly the mother, who can feel fetal movement by this time. No matter what the parental beliefs concerning termination, this is never a decision that is taken lightly by the parents and is one which causes a great deal of anguish. Parents who choose to interrupt a pregnancy for a fetal anomaly, do so as the advocate of the child, because of an expected quality of life they find unacceptable on his or her behalf. They deserve the counselor's unreserved support, whatever his or her own opinion of the decision. Termination is a procedure that is associated with some risk for the mother, something which she must also be encouraged to consider and understand. It is the duty of the counselor to help the parents reach the decision that is correct for them. This involves listening to both partners and observing their interaction, in order to help them find the "best" solution to what may be the most important decision of their life. Many physicians suggest that it is impossible to be unbiased in counseling parents. This may be true to an extent, but bias should be consciously minimized. The options are usually clear, and presenting them is straightforward. Under an individual diagnostic heading, there are facts available concerning the prenatal and postnatal course and, although they may be interpreted differently by different advisors, such as a 5% mortality means 95% survival, they are still the same for everyone to present. In addition, most parents have thought about the termination issue long before they reach this point in their lives. Most have clear views of where they stand on it, and for many, the stance is immutable. Termination of pregnancy is never "recommended" or definitely indicated in any circumstances. The parents should be encouraged to think carefully of the option of termination in the light of the prognosis that has been described. Even those parents who ask what the physician would do in the circumstances, should be told that he or she cannot and should not make this decision for them, although occasionally after repeated counseling sessions, it may be clear that this is what the patient needs in order to come to a decision. However, the counselor will not personally be taking the risk to the mother that termination of pregnancy entails, nor will watch his or her own child go through repeated surgeries, or care for the young adult with an uncertain future. It is not unfair or biased, however, to describe one's experience of counseling or how often other parents have elected termination with similar disease. Of over 3000 sets of parents counseled in my experience, about half have chosen termination and the other half have continued, offering two large equal groups for comparison. Those who were able to accept termination did recover from it in time and ended up, in the vast majority of cases, with a normal healthy family. In contrast, many of those continuing lost the affected child, always after much anguish, sometimes after many years, and not infrequently after the breakdown of the whole family unit. That is not to say there are not some successes, at least in the short term. Also, there are some forms of congenital heart malformation that have become much better surgical risks during the nearly 30 years of my experience of fetal echocardiographic diagnosis and thus the counseling has changed over time. But the parents should feel confident that they will be supported fully whatever their decision.

If termination of pregnancy is not an option legally, or if the parents elect to continue, the further management of the pregnancy must be considered. All on-going cases of fetal congenital heart disease must have a thorough scan of the rest of the fetal anatomy to search for associated extracardiac malformations and this may need to be repeated at later gestations. An amniocentesis should be considered in all cases, although there are some categories of heart disease, such as the isomerism syndromes, or simple transposition, where chromosome anomalies are very rare and a karyotype may not be essential. The finding of additional malformations or chromosomal anomalies may signficantly change the prognosis, such that the option of termination of pregnancy may have to be re-addressed with the parents after these investigations are completed. In a continuing pregnancy, it may be useful to have the parents talk to a previous patient who has been diagnosed prenatally with a similar lesion, and whose child has undergone surgery. This can provide real support and friendship for the parents during this difficult time, when feelings of isolation are often very prominent. If the cardiac malformation is "duct dependent" (Table 8.5), that is, either the systemic or pulmonary circulation is supported by ductal flow, it is optimum to deliver the mother at, or near, the cardiac center where surgical intervention will take place. Duct-dependent lesions include aortic or pulmonary stenosis or atresia, coarctation or interruption of the aorta. The importance of "duct dependence" is that the patency of the duct can be maintained by prostaglandins in the immediate post-delivery period until surgical intervention can take place. This protects the newborn from the potentially damaging effects of either severe hypoxia in the setting of inadequate pulmonary blood flow, or organ damage in the setting of inadequate systemic output. Other lesions where early decompensation can occur, and delivery in the surgical center is essential, include transposition of the great arteries and total anomalous pulmonary venous drainage. Balloon atrial septostomy can be performed as an emergency procedure for transposition where necessary and total anomalous pulmonary venous drainage is the only remaining condition in pediatric cardiology where surgery may be urgently required and life-saving. In contrast, many forms of cardiac malformation are not associated with early decompensation and these fetuses can be safely delivered locally and seen by the cardiologist at leisure in the first weeks of life, for example, where

Table 8.5 Suggested lesions which may be "duct-dependent" – delivery in a cardiac center may be recommended

Pulmonary circulation dependent on duct
- Severe pulmonary stenosis (isolated or with any underlying anatomy)
- Pulmonary atresia (isolated or with any underlying anatomy)

Systemic circulation dependent on duct
- Severe aortic stenosis
- Aortic atresia (HLHS)
- Coarctation of the aorta

Other lesions subject to possible early decompensation
- TGA
- TAPVR

the fetus has an atrioventricular septal defect. When the decision has been made to deliver in the tertiary center, transfer is usually arranged between 30 and 34 weeks' gestation, to minimally inconvenience the mother, but at the same time to allow her to become familiar with a new obstetrician and hospital in time for her delivery. At this time, it can be useful to have the parents meet the surgeon, or someone from his or her team, who can familiarize them with the details of plans and arrangements for surgery. It is rare for premature delivery to be indicated for a fetal cardiac lesion. Perhaps a fetus who is deteriorating in terms of myocardial function, such as in aortic stenosis, or becoming increasingly hydropic but has reached at least 35 weeks' gestation, may be considered as a candidate for early delivery. This, however, must be weighed against the complications of prematurity or low birthweight in a neonate destined for surgery. Ideally, delivery of the fetus with a cardiac malformation should be induced close to term, in order to take place during the week and during the day, at a time when resuscitation is readily available if needed urgently. Cesarean section is almost never indicated for cardiac reasons and should be avoided if possible, especially if the cardiac malformation is expected to be associated with a high mortality.

Some parents, who are either diagnosed too late for termination or who are unable to choose this option for personal reasons, ask about the possibility of not intervening surgically and "allowing nature to take its course." This option is still available in some centers for the hypoplastic left heart syndrome but, in general, not for other lesions, even for malformations such as pulmonary atresia with intact septum or complex heterotaxy sydromes, which probably have about the same 5-year mortality as the hypoplastic left heart syndrome. This is not perhaps very logical, but it is often the current state of affairs. Even where parents have decided before birth that they do not want surgery, it can be extremely difficult for them to maintain a "non-intervention" stance after the baby is born, if there is a known surgical option available. This is particularly so if the newborn does not die soon after birth, which can happen if the arterial duct remains patent naturally. Health-care workers surrounding the newborn are particularly liable to offer their opinion, however well meant and irrespective of their level of information about the case, thereby intensifying the guilt and doubt felt by the parents in this situation. In addition, some doctors could not support parents who would prefer not to have their child surgically treated, and would even take steps to take the care of the child out of the hands of the parents, which results in a horrible situation for all concerned. Parents should be advised of the difficulty of a non-intervention route if they are considering this as an option in the prenatal period.

In summary, there are many different aspects of counseling for the fetal cardiologist to consider when approaching the parents of a fetus with congenital heart disease. The counselor can only give correct information if the diagnosis is accurate and secure and he or she is truly familiar with the whole picture of the defect in fetal life, not just in postnatal life. In general, the types of congenital heart disease detected prenatally will significantly change the life experience for the child, and the parents deserve to have a clear picture of this. Making a decision concerning interruption of pregnancy will change the parents' lives however they choose. The task of the fetal cardiologist is to help them make the "best" choice for their particular circumstances and family.

Prognosis and outcome in specific diagnostic categories

The outcome data represents pooled fetal data from Guy's Hospital, London between 1980 and 1997, from Columbia Presbyterian Hospital, New York between 1993 and 1997 and from King's College Hospital, London between 1998 and 2006. The outcome data therefore covers a 27-year period and involves around 3790 cases, approximately 2100 in the first 18 years and 1651 in the last 9 years. The accuracy of the data is better and the details more complete for the last 6 years or so. The last 9 years' data are more heavily weighted towards fetuses with multiple malformations and karyotypic anomalies, partly because of performing fetal echocardiography at the time of finding increased nuchal translucency, and partly because in this period we have been working in a fetal medicine setting. This is exemplified by the fact that the mean gestational age at diagnosis in the first 18-year block is 23 weeks and 19 weeks in the last 9-year block. Note also the comparison between the timing of diagnosis in the two series, illustrated in Figs. 8.1 and 8.2. The diagnostic categories which were most commonly seen are illustrated in Fig. 8.3. Note that the main diagnostic categories remain similar, although there are some slight changes seen over the 27-year period, reflecting an increase in the detection of great artery abnormalites. The types of chromosomal anomalies which were found in the later series is shown in Fig. 8.4 (data are too incomplete

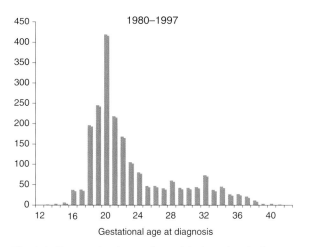

Fig. 8.1. The gestational age at diagnosis in the early series is shown. Note that 20 weeks is the most frequent time of diagnosis. Diagnosis prior to 24 weeks was made in 68% of cases.

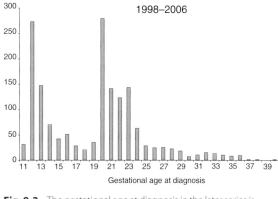

Fig. 8.2. The gestational age at diagnosis in the later series is shown. Note that there are now two peak times for diagnosis, 12 weeks, around the time of the nuchal scan, and 20 weeks. Diagnosis prior to 24 weeks was made in 84% of cases.

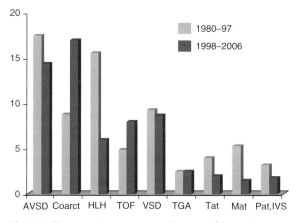

Fig. 8.3. The two series are compared in terms of the most common diagnostic categories, expressed as proportions of each series. Note the slight trend towards a higher proportion of great artery abnormalities in the later series.

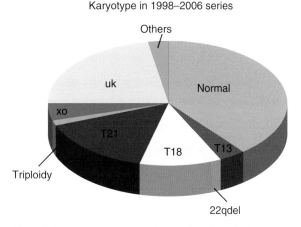

Fig. 8.4. The types of karyotype abnormalities found in the later series are shown. Known karyotype anomalies occurred in 38.6% of the series.

227

Outcome in 1980–1997 series

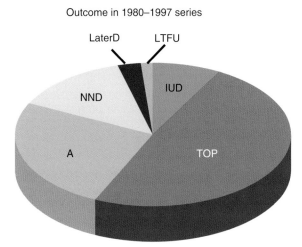

Fig. 8.5. The outcome in the early series is illustrated. Of the continuing pregnancies, about half were alive at short-term follow-up.

Outcome in 1998–2006 series

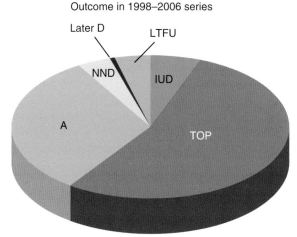

Fig. 8.6. The outcome in the later series is shown. Now about two-thirds of the continuing pregnancies survive in the short-term.

in the early series). Note the high rate of chromosome anomalies in this series, emphasizing the biased group preferentially seen in fetal life. For comparison, the background rate for chromosomal anomalies in live births, in a population-based geographical area reported in the 1980s in the Baltimore–Washington Infant study, was around 12%.

The outcome data for each series are illustrated in Figs. 8.5 and 8.6. It is important to understand that the outcome data are short term. As we work in a referral center, it is extremely difficult to obtain outcome, although despite that, there are fewer than 60 of the 1651 recent cases lost to follow-up. What we do obtain, however, is usually purely short-term survival in the first month or so of life, and therefore this is not an accurate reflection of the survival of the affected fetus into childhood or young adulthood. Despite the unsatisfactory nature of our follow-up, the force of numbers does provide some sort of picture of the whole.

Each diagnostic category will be described and our experience of the condition and outcome detailed.

Total anomalous pulmonary venous drainage

This is a rare lesion *per se* and also one which is difficult to diagnose prenatally. It can be recognized in fetal life as an isolated lesion or as part of more complex heart disease, especially in right atrial isomerism. The pulmonary veins will not drain to either side of the left

atrium in the usual pattern but anomalously to the coronary sinus, or to an ascending or a descending channel. Chromosomal anomalies are very rarely found in association. In its isolated form, it can be successfully repaired surgically with a low mortality and fairly good results. However, the site of drainage and the degree of obstruction will influence the success rate and, in addition, a few cases have a poor result due to more peripheral venous hypoplasia in the lung fields or restenosis at the surgical site. The outlook for fetuses with total anomalous pulmonary venous drainage in the setting of right atrial isomerism is very poor.

Outcome data

Only five cases of isolated total anomalous pulmonary venous drainage have been seen over the study period, diagnosed at gestational ages between 18 and 29 weeks. A further two cases were missed. One of these two was seen prior to the availability of color flow mapping, but one was recent and the pulmonary vein flow identified mistakenly as draining to the left atrium (see Chapter 2, Fig. 2.48(a)). Strictly speaking, this case was not isolated as there was associated left atrial isomerism, an unusual combination. Of the total group of seven cases, there was one termination of pregnancy, four neonatal or infant deaths and there are only two survivors. However, two of the four deaths were due to extracardiac problems, rather than to the heart lesion itself. This is too small a group for any conclusions to be drawn about the outcome.

Nowadays, particularly if the veins drain above the diaphragm, one would be cautiously optimistic that this condition can be successfully repaired surgically at one operation and with a good functional result and outlook, at least into early adult life, which is as far as our data extends.

Mitral stenosis

This is a rare lesion in isolation and difficult to diagnose in the fetus. The mitral valve will appear restricted in motion and is often coupled with abnormal papillary muscles. Less than normal flow across the mitral valve leads to a small left ventricle. The pulsed Doppler flow profile is not helpful but a significant left to right shunt at the foramen would be considered unfavourable. Mitral stenosis occurs much more commonly in association with aortic stenosis or atresia. It can occur with coarctation and in left ventricular outflow obstruction as Schone's syndrome, but may be difficult to diagnose in this setting. Congenital mitral stenosis if symptomatic may be suitable for balloon valve dilation or repair or may require valve replacement. If this last becomes necessary in childhood, this entails successive replacement of an artificial valve with growth, and long-term anticoagulants, both of which have a significant risk in children. If the mitral valve is significantly abnormal in aortic stenosis or coarctation, the left ventricle may be considered "unusable" and a one-ventricle (or Fontan) repair undertaken because of the high morbidity associated with a biventricular approach. The severity of mitral valve malformation associated with other left heart disease may not become evident until after birth, resulting in a much more complex postnatal course than anticipated.

Outcome data

Mitral stenosis has been diagnosed in its isolated form in only five cases, seen between 18 and 29 weeks' gestation, one having an associated ventricular septal defect. There were three terminations of pregnancy and one infant death. There is one survivor with mild mitral valve dysplasia. Again, the numbers are too small to draw conclusions, but if a significantly abnormal mitral valve with a small left ventricle and convincing papillary muscle abnormality was seen, the outlook for a good result would be poor. Repeated intervention may be necessary with a poor functional result, until a large enough valve replacement can be offered. As indicated above, valve replacement is a last resort in children because of the complications of anti-coagulant therapy.

Mitral atresia

This is where there is no flow across the mitral valve. This can occur with aortic atresia in the hypoplastic left heart syndrome, which is quite common and will be discussed in more detail below, or with double outlet right ventricle, which is less common, or with a concordant aorta and a ventricular septal defect, which is still less common. The outcome data here only apply to the last two situations. In all cases, a one-ventricle repair is the only possible surgical approach.

Outcome data

In the combined data, there are a total of 139 cases of mitral atresia (3.6% of the total CHD), diagnosed at gestational ages between 11 and 31 weeks. The majority (103) had a double outlet connection, in 11 the great arteries are not specified and in 19, there was a concordant aorta with a ventricular septal defect. The rate of karyotype anomalies ranged from 11%–35% in the different series. Most of the abnormal karyotypes were trisomy 18 with a few trisomy 13. Termination of pregnancy took place in 100/139 cases, there was an intrauterine death in 8, neonatal death in 17, infant death in 3 and there were 8 who survived the immediate neonatal period. The remaining 3 were lost to follow-up.

Mitral valve dysplasia

This is rarely seen except in association with dysplasia in other cardiac valves in trisomy 18.

Mitral regurgitation

This is rare in the fetus as an isolated finding. It appears to be of different significance in the 12-week fetus from when it is detected later in pregnancy (see Chapter 6). Mitral regurgitation may be seen on pulsed or color flow Doppler, in the four-chamber view. It rarely causes left atrial enlargement except when the foramen ovale is restrictive, as may occur when mitral regurgitation is associated with aortic stenosis. It is usually benign and transient in the later fetus, but it is sufficiently unusual to warrant follow-up. Other left heart disease such as aortic valve disease should be carefully excluded as it is a common associated lesion with aortic stenosis. Mitral and tricuspid regurgitation can occur as a functional response to tachycardia, cardiomyopathy, anemia, or twin–twin transfusion syndrome.

Outcome data

If the cases of secondary mitral regurgitation, in, for example, cardiomyopathy, twin–twin transfusion syndrome, anemia, etc. are removed, there have only been 13 cases of mitral regurgitation seen in our series. One fetus had a dwarfism syndrome, which the mother also had, there were four cases of trisomy 21, two of trisomy 18 and one of trisomy 13. The remaining six fetuses had a normal outcome, all apparently well. However, there were two additional cases of apparently isolated mitral regurgitation initially, where aortic stenosis developed in later pregnancy.

Tricuspid stenosis

This is a rare lesion and one which is difficult to diagnose in the fetus in isolation. The valve may appear abnormal and restricted and the right ventricle small. It occurs more commonly as part of pulmonary atresia with intact ventricular septum. If it is not severe, it is better tolerated postnatally than prenatally. If severe, it may require a one-ventricle repair.

Outcome data

This diagnosis has only been made prospectively in one case and retrospectively in a couple of others. The outlook will depend on the severity of stenosis and the size of the right ventricle. The prospectively diagnosed case survived. One of the cases diagnosed in retrospect died.

Tricuspid atresia

This is a relatively uncommon but well-recognized condition, where there is no flow across the tricuspid valve. There is always a small right ventricle and a ventricular septal defect in association. Chromosomal anomalies are rarely associated with this condition. The only possibility for surgical intervention is a one-ventricle repair but this should be one of the "best" forms of one-ventricle repair, in that the single pump is a left ventricle. Despite this, results in early adult life are still not ideal. In about 20% of cases of tricuspid atresia, the great arteries are also transposed, which makes surgical treatment more complex.

Outcome data

There have been a total of 115 cases of tricuspid atresia (3% of the total CHD), diagnosed between 12 and 37 weeks of gestation. Of these, 36 had transposed great arteries (31%), 4 had pulmonary stenosis or atresia in addition and 3 associated coarctation of the aorta. Two fetuses had a karyotype anomaly, one XXY and one trisomy 18. There were 79 terminations of pregnancy, 3 intrauterine deaths, 3 neonatal deaths, 4 infant deaths and 26 were alive at the last follow-up. This represents a 27% short-term mortality in the ongoing pregnancies, but the data do extend back to the 1980s.

Tricuspid dysplasia

This can occur as an isolated lesion. The valve is thickened and nodular, there is tricuspid regurgitation of varying severity and this can lead to right atrial enlargement of variable degree. It can lead to functional or anatomical pulmonary stenosis or atresia as a secondary phenomenon. If very severe, it can lead to fetal hydrops and intrauterine death. Alternatively, long-standing cardiomegaly can lead to secondary lung hypoplasia and early neonatal death. In less severe forms of tricuspid dysplasia, the valve can become less regurgitant after birth when the pulmonary artery pressure falls. Isolated tricuspid dysplasia is uncommonly associated with chromosomal anomalies, but tricuspid dysplasia in association with dysplasia of other cardiac valves can be a sign of trisomy 18.

Outcome data

There have been 70 cases of tricuspid dysplasia, diagnosed between 12 and 41 weeks of gestation. There were 36 with additional forms of cardiac malformation, 25 with pulmonary atresia in addition, 6 with pulmonary stenosis, 3 with a ventricular septal defect, one with coarctation and one with mitral stenosis. Only a minority of cases had karyotyping, usually because of associated extracardiac malformations. Of these, there were 2 cases of trisomy 21, and one each of triploidy, trisomy 13, trisomy 18 and unbalanced translocation. Termination of pregnancy occurred in 32 cases, intrauterine death in 11, neonatal death in 14, and 11 were alive at early follow-up. Two cases were lost to follow-up.

Ebstein's anomaly

This is a fairly uncommon, but well-recognized, condition, one which varies considerably in severity. It is a failure of delamination (or separation) of the septal leaflet of the tricuspid valve from the septal surface of the right ventricle. Delamination is an embryological process which finishes quite late in fetal life, around 10–11 weeks of gestation. As a result of the septal leaflet being adherent to the septal surface, the site of coaptation of the tricuspid valve cusps is displaced into the right ventricle to a varying degree. The valve is usually, but not always, dysplastic to some degree and regurgitant. The right atrium is dilated. There may be associated pulmonary stenosis or, less commonly, atresia, which may be functional or anatomical. Chromosomal anomalies are not commonly found in association with this condition. The prognosis will depend on the anatomical severity of the malformation. If there has been severe cardiomegaly since early pregnancy, inadequate lung development is usually the cause of early death. This is analogous to an early and severe diaphragmatic hernia. If the neonate is severely cyanosed due to associated right ventricular outflow tract obstruction or severe tricuspid regurgitation in the first days and weeks of life, the prognosis is poor. However, if ventilation and stabilization can be achieved in the neonatal period, things tend to improve as the pulmonary resistance falls after birth. In childhood, symptoms vary from mild, exercise-induced cyanosis to severe exercise restriction, with arrhythmias and other complications. Fetal diagnosis tends to be in the most severe range of the disease with a resulting high rate of termination or early mortality, although the outcome seems to be improving, perhaps because of fetal recognition of milder disease. Surgical treatment can improve the quality of life, although it is usually better if any surgical procedure can be delayed until after growth is completed, in the event that valve repair is not possible and valve replacement necessary.

Outcome data

There have been 71 cases of Ebstein's malformation seen in the series (1.8% of the total cases of CHD), diagnosed at gestational age range between 12 and 38 weeks. Of the 71 cases, 12 had pulmonary atresia, 14 had pulmonary stenosis, 5 had ventricular septal defects, one aortic atresia, and one a right aortic arch as associated lesions. Trisomy 21 was found in three cases. Karyotyping was normal in the remaining cases tested, but was not frequently performed in the absence of extracardiac malformations, as it is known to be an uncommon association. Termination of pregnancy took place in 33 cases, there was an intrauterine death in 6, neonatal death in 9, infant death in 2 and there are 20 early survivors. One patient was lost to follow-up.

Common atrioventricular junction

This is where the valves on both sides of the atrioventricular junction share leaflets. A common valve usually occurs with an associated interatrial defect and a ventricular septal defect, at this specific point in the centre of the heart. Common leaflets with an atrial defect alone is a well-recognized less frequent, variation, sometimes called a partial atrioventricular defect or an ostium primum defect. Common leaflets with an inlet ventricular septal defect alone (without the atrial defect) is a rare variant. A common atrioventricular junction can occur in one of two settings: with normal atrial situs or with situs ambiguous. Normal atrial situs is the most common, making up at least 60% of the total cases seen in utero. Within this group with normal situs, the majority of cases (>80%) will have trisomy 21, although a common atrioventricular junction can occur in other chromosomal anomalies. The remaining cases, who have normal situs and normal chromosomes, have a high incidence of associated left heart disease, such as coarctation of the aorta.

Surgical repair of a complete defect is nowadays undertaken between 3–9 months of age. The prognosis for successful surgical repair of an atrioventricular septal defect at a low mortality (<5%) in the child with Down syndrome is good, although the mortality from associated lesions is often surprisingly high in this group. Those children with normal chromosomes and left heart disease tend to fare less well at surgical repair, and may be more liable to residual left sided atrioventricular valve stenosis or incompetence. Associated cardiac malformations are fairly common with an atrioventricular septal defect and will complicate the prognosis. On the other hand, an uncomplicated partial atrioventricular septal defect in a normal child can be readily repaired between 2 and 4 years of age with good results.

When a common atrioventricular junction occurs with abnormal situs, this can be either left or right atrial isomerism. Chromosomal anomalies are very rarely seen in association with abnormal situs. In fetal life, left isomerism tends to be seen more commonly than right, perhaps because of the detection of the frequently associated rhythm disorder. An atrioventricular septal defect is common in left atrial isomerism but if it is associated with complete heart block, the prognosis is poor, with intrauterine or early postnatal death, despite treatment. One case of left isomerism had what was thought to be a normal heart, but was found postnatally to have total anomalous pulmonary venous drainage directly to the right atrium. Anomalous veins are rare in left isomerism (in contrast to right isomerism) and direct connection of the veins to the right atrium is uncommon in any setting. Despite successful cardiac surgery, this neonate died as a result of biliary atresia, a known association with left atrial isomerism. An atrioventricular septal defect is almost invariable in right atrial isomerism and almost always occurs in association with double outlet right ventricle, pulmonary stenosis or atresia and total anomalous pulmonary venous drainage. As there is no left atrium, the pulmonary venous drainage is always anomalous in this setting. However, in about half the cases, the pulmonary venous confluence drains directly to the atrial mass and do not cause a problem. On the other hand, if the veins drain to a supra- or infracardiac site, they are almost always obstructed to some extent, which is associated with a high neonatal mortality even if early surgery takes place. In contrast to left isomerism, the affected fetus with right atrial isomerism usually survives intrauterine life, but only palliation with a one ventricle repair is feasible in this condition. There is a high incidence of neonatal death, or death in childhood, despite surgical treatment.

Outcome data

There were 614 cases of a common atrioventricular junction in our series, 16% of the total and therefore one of the most common cardiac malformations identified prenatally. Cases were diagnosed between 11 and 39 weeks, at a mean gestation of 22.4 weeks in the early series and 18.6 in the later series. At least 141 (23%) had a heterotaxy syndrome, although the situs was not always documented in the early part of the series. There were 87 cases of left isomerism, 48 with complete heart block. There were 54 cases of right isomerism, most having double outlet right ventricle with pulmonary stenosis or pulmonary atresia in association. In the remaining cases with normal atrial situs, 49 had coarctation, 36 had double outlet right ventricle, 10 had tetralogy of Fallot, 9 aortic atresia, 3 a common arterial trunk and 7 a left superior caval vein as associated lesions. In addition, 15 were unbalanced, 9 with left ventricular, and 6 with right ventricular hypoplasia. Atrioventricular valve regurgitation was common when the diagnosis of a common valve was made before 14 weeks of gestation, especially in the group with trisomy 21, although uncommon in later pregnancy.

In the early series of 375 cases, the karyotype was documented in only 150 cases of which 87 had trisomy

21, 10 had trisomy 18, 3 had trisomy 13, 6 other chromosome anomalies, and 44 were normal. In the later series of 239 cases, the karyotype was documented in 206 cases. Of these, 116 had trisomy 21, 18 had trisomy 18, 6 had trisomy 13, 9 had other chromosomal anomalies, and 57 were normal. Associated structural extracardiac malformations, diaphragmatic hernia or exomphalos, for example, were common even in the absence of a chromosomal defect.

Of the total group, termination of pregnancy took place in 375 cases, there were 45 intrauterine deaths, 41 neonatal deaths and 14 deaths, in infancy or childhood. There were 126 children alive at short-term follow-up. Twelve patients were lost to follow-up. This represents a 55% mortality in the continuing pregnancies, emphasizing the complex nature of malformation in the isomerism group and the high mortality in the group with chromosomal defects. There has been a higher rate of termination in the later set of data because of the higher incidence of chromosomal anomalies, but a lower neonatal death rate.

Discordant AV junction

This is a relatively uncommon but complex abnormality, where the morphological left atrium connects to the right ventricle and the right atrium to the morphological left ventricle. There is nearly always a discordant ventriculo-arterial connection, thus "correcting" the path of blood flow. If there are no additional heart malformations, there may be no symptoms until middle adult life when the right ventricle (which is here the systemic pump) starts to fail. However, complete heart block is a common complication, the incidence of which increases with age, and often there is associated disease such a ventricular septal defect, Ebstein's malformation and pulmonary stenosis, which may require intervention in childhood. Chromosomal anomalies have to my knowledge never been described in association.

When atrioventricular discordance is associated with tricuspid atresia, a one-ventricle repair is the only option, albeit with some additional complications, such as obstruction to systemic outflow at the ventricular septal defect and a high incidence of heart block.

Outcome data

There were 26 cases in the total series, 5 with absent left connection (essentially tricuspid atresia on the left side), 5 with Ebstein's anomaly, 5 with a ventricular septal defect and pulmonary stenosis or atresia, 2 with aortic atresia, and 7 with just a ventricular septal defect in association. There was one fetus in the series with a microdeletion of chromosome 22, but extracardiac malformations are rare AV discordance. There were 12 terminations, 2 neonatal deaths, and 12 live births.

Double inlet AV junction

This is an uncommon condition where both atrioventricular valves connect to a dominant ventricle. Double inlet left ventricle is much more common than double inlet right. Chromosomal anomalies are not a recognized association. In double inlet left ventricle the great arteries are almost always transposed and there may be associated pulmonary stenosis, pulmonary atresia, or coarctation of the aorta. Double inlet right ventricle is associated with a double outlet connection. It has only rarely been possible to septate a double inlet ventricle and achieve a biventricular repair and a one ventricle repair is the usual treatment, with additional lesions providing added complications. If the single pump is a left ventricle, it is likely to have a better result than a single right ventricle.

Outcome data

There were 54 cases of double inlet ventricle in the series, 42 with double inlet left ventricle, 6 unspecified, and 6 double inlet right ventricle, diagnosed between 14 and 31 weeks of gestation. Fifteen had associated pulmonary stenosis or atresia and 7 coarctation. The great artery connection was discordant or double outlet right ventricle in all except one case with concordant great arteries. There was one case of trisomy 21, one deletion, and one microdeletion of chromosome 22. Extracardiac anomalies are uncommon in double inlet ventricle. Termination of pregnancy took place in 33 cases, there was one intrauterine death, 2 neonatal deaths, and 19 short-term survivors.

Ventricular septal defect

This is probably the most common form of heart abnormality, occurring in almost 20% of normal newborns if meticulously looked for with color flow echocardiography. The natural history of ventricular septal defects is to close spontaneously, especially if they are in the muscular septum and are small, which is common. As a result, most ventricular septal defects are not detected and are of no significance. However, the defects detected in fetal life are quite a different spectrum of disease, as they tend to be large in order to reach the attention of the fetal cardiologist and can be situated in any part of the ventricular septum. In our fetal series, therefore, there is a high association with chromosomal defects and malformations in extracardiac organs. A malaligned outlet defect without pulmonary stenosis is typical of trisomy 18, especially when there is associated polyvalvar dysplasia. The type of ventricular septal defect seen in fetal life will often require surgical repair, which is usually undertaken between 2 and 8 months of age. An inlet, perimembranous, or outlet defect can usually be repaired at low mortality and with good success. Large apical muscular defects may be very inaccessible to surgical repair and therefore difficult to manage but nowadays can be considered for a catheter approach for device closure. Associated extracardiac defects, however, may be more important in dictating the outcome than the ventricular septal defect itself.

Outcome data

There were 344 examples of ventricular septal defects seen in the total series, diagnosed between 12 and 40 weeks, with a further 28 cases where there was a suspicion of a VSD seen. Twenty-six/344 were described as malaligned. There was an associated possible coarctation in 33, a right aortic arch in 6, pulmonary stenosis in 2, and left atrial isomerism in 6. Chromosomal anomalies were found in 129 cases (37%) illustrating the unusual bias of the fetal series in comparison with postnatal life. The most common karyotype anomaly was trisomy 18, affecting 75 fetuses, 28 had trisomy 21, 12 trisomy 13, and 14 other various chromosome defects. In the group of suspected VSDs, there were 7 karyotype anomalies of 28 cases. Termination of pregnancy occurred in 132 cases. There were 30 spontaneous intrauterine deaths, 35 neonatal deaths, 2 infant deaths, and there were 136 short-term survivors. There were 9 cases lost to follow-up. Of the 28 suspected cases, there were 12 terminations, one intrauterine death, and the remainder were either lost to follow-up (4) or live born. No terminations took place in our series as a result of the diagnosis of a simple ventricular septal defect. With the improvement in image quality in recent ultrasound equipment, small muscular ventricular septal defects are increasingly seen during routine scanning, some of which are clearly documented to close prenatally or soon after birth. The detection of such defects in the fetus always raises the concern as to the possibility of a chromosomal anomaly but, in our experience, in the absence of extracardiac markers or any other high-risk feature, isolated small muscular VSDs should not be considered a risk factor for chromosomal anomalies or an indication for amniocentesis.

Left superior vena cava

This is a common normal variant occurring in about 1 in 300 normal people and has no functional significance in terms of venous return to the heart as the persistent vein still drains to the right side of the heart via the coronary sinus. It does, however, have an increased association with heart malformations, and with trisomy 13. It has been implicated as a "cause" of left heart hypoplasia and coarctation in the fetus, as a result of dilatation of the coronary sinus, which has been suggested to partially obstruct mitral valve flow, but this is very speculative. It is more likely that coarctation is simply a commonly associated finding. A left superior vena cava in the absence of associated heart or extracardiac malformations does not require intervention or follow-up.

Outcome

A left superior caval vein was frequently seen with other cardiac malformations, particularly with coarctation of the aorta. It has only been recorded in our most recent series, where it has been seen in 21 cases as an isolated cardiac finding, although there were two chromosomal anomalies in the group, trisomy 13 and a complex deletion.

Chiari network

This is a rare lesion. It consists of a network of redundant tissue related to the Eustachian valve, which is a ridge of tissue present in the right atrium of a normal heart. It rarely requires any intervention, although if the superfluous tissue obstructs the tricuspid valve, causing symptoms, it may require surgical removal. It has been seen in less than five cases in our series in the last 30 years and has not required intervention in any of our cases.

Tumor

The most common tumor seen in the fetus is the rhabdomyoma and these are usually multiple. Rhabdomyomas have a strong association with tuberous sclerosis, which can be associated with seizures and developmental delay, often profound. Tuberous

sclerosis is found in 95% of patients with multiple rhabdomyomas and in about 50% of single tumors. Cranial magnetic resonance imaging in the last trimester of pregnancy may help parents to decide about late termination of pregnancy, as multiple intracerebral tumors often indicate severe future handicap. If the cardiac tumors are not obstructive, no treatment is necessary in the neonate, as the natural history is for spontaneous involution after birth. Obstructive tumors occasionally require surgical removal or radiofrequency ablation. Fibromas or teratomas, which are much less common tumors, may cause hydrops and intrauterine fetal death. If they survive to delivery, they usually require surgical removal. Even though histologically benign and not associated with extracardiac malformations, if they are large, the prognosis for successful surgical excision is poor with a fibroma, although better in a teratoma.

Outcome data

There have been 42 cardiac tumors in our series. Of these, 35 were rhabdomyomas, and 7 were teratomas. Of the rhabdomyomas, all but one were multiple masses. Only the case of the single tumor was not associated with tuberose sclerosis. There were 4 intrauterine deaths, 13 terminations, and one neonatal death. There are 17 survivors all affected to varying degrees by tuberose sclerosis. The remaining 7 tumors were teratomas. Of this group, there were three intrauterine deaths, one neonatal death and two terminations because of increasing size of the mass and hydrops, developing at too early a stage of pregnancy for delivery to be a safe option. On the other hand, we have one perfect survivor, who did not develop prenatal compromise despite a large tumor (illustrated in Chapter 2) and who had successful postnatal removal.

Echogenic focus

An ecogenic focus in the heart has no relevance as far as the heart is concerned even when not small, single, and in the typical position in the papillary muscle of the mitral valve but multiple, septal, or larger than usual. Histologically, in cases were the pregnancy has been terminated for other reasons, echogenic foci are found to be calcium deposits in the myocardium. However, in the continuing pregnancy even where foci are multiple, they do not grow with the heart and therefore become smaller as pregnancy advances and do not impair cardiac function. An echogenic focus may be a "soft marker" for chromosomal anomalies, so other features of chromosomal disease should be looked for and a karyotype offered if appropriate. An echogenic focus is distinct from a tumor by its charcteristic brightness and typical position and from its tendency to become smaller rather than larger as gestation advances. It is also distinct from the linear calcification in the papillary muscles of the mitral or tricuspid valves which can occur in aortic or pulmonary atresia, respectively. As long as the function of both ventricles is unimpaired, excess echogenicity in the heart is not necessarily pathological and should be sequentially observed.

Ectopia cordis

This is a rare lesion but, when the whole heart lies outside the fetal thorax, the diagnosis is readily made, even as early as the nuchal scan. The outcome of surgical repair is extremely poor if the pregnancy continues. The chest cavity is too small to contain the heart, which cannot be compressed, so a cage has to be built outside the chest to protect the heart.

Outcome data

There have been five cases of complete ectopia cordis in our series, one diagnosed at 14 weeks after the nuchal scan, two with associated tetralogy of Fallot. In all cases the pregnancy was interrupted. There have been, in addition, five cases of pentalogy of Cantrell, which is a less extreme form of ectopia where the apex is partially outside the thorax, at least in early pregnancy, in addition to exomphalos, a sternal and diaphragmatic defect. Of the five, two had tetralogy of Fallot, one a ventricular septal defect. One pregnancy was terminated. Four cases survived although multiple surgeries and some degree of long-term disability was involved for all the survivors.

Ventricular aneurysm

These are uncommon lesions but, despite our paucity of data (we have only seen three cases in 30 years) and its often frightening appearance, the majority of cases seem to have a good outcome, usually without requiring intervention as has been the case in two of our cases. In one case, drainage of an associated pericardial effusion was the only intervention necessary prenatally, with successful surgical excision of the defect after birth. In the literature, some cases have had surgical treatment with a good result in the short term.

Criss-cross, upstairs/downstairs connections

These are rare complex forms of intracardiac malformation. Surgical options have to be tailored to the individual case but often are limited to a one ventricle repair. We have seen four cases, two of which were terminated. There was one death at 3 years at surgery and there is one survivor with a one-ventricle repair.

Straddling AV valve

This is a rare associated finding, seen in the four-chamber view, in transposition with a ventricular septal defect or double outlet right ventricle. It may have profound implications on the surgical management, rendering a biventricular repair difficult or impossible. We have seen two cases, both of whom have required a one-ventricle repair.

Cardiomyopathy

This is an umbrella term for a rag-bag of different underlying conditions, united in the finding of decreased cardiac function usually causing hydrops and equally affecting both ventricles. It can be secondary to viral infection, such as parvovirus or coxsackie, part of a twin-to-twin transfusion syndrome, or to unusual genetic conditions such as mitochondrial disease, storage diseases and other rarities. Of 66 cases, there has been a high rate of intrauterine death, termination of pregnancy and neonatal death with only a handful of short-term survivors. There is no evidence that treatment with drugs, such as digoxin prenatally, has any beneficial effect. There were a further nine cases where the dysfunction appeared to only affect the right ventricle. In one of the five survivors of this group, left ventricular dysfunction developed after birth necessitating transplant, which was not available, and the infant died.

Aortic atresia

This is complete obstruction of the aortic valve and is usually associated with mitral stenosis or atresia in the hypoplastic left heart syndrome, although rarely it can occur with two normal sized ventricles and a ventricular septal defect. Chromosomal anomalies occur in about 2%–4% of cases of the hypoplastic left heart syndrome but about 10% have extracardiac malformations, which add to the risk of surgical management.

Postnatal treatment of the hypoplastic left heart syndrome entails three stages of major cardiac surgery in the first years of life, resulting in a one-ventricle repair with the right ventricle as the pump. There is a significant mortality to the surgeries of at least 30% at the present time with considerable uncertainty about survival after 20–30 years. In addition, some degree of neurological impairment is frequent in the survivors.

Outcome data

There were 460 cases of aortic atresia, two with a ventricular septal defect and therefore a normal-sized left ventricle, but the rest being typical hypoplastic left heart syndromes. This condition represents 12% of the total series of CHD and is one of the commonest cardiac abnormalities recognized in the fetus. In the earlier part of the series, the gestational age at diagnosis ranged between 15 and 42 weeks but in the later series, 30% of the cases were diagnosed at 14 weeks or earlier. As there was no surgical treatment available for a large proportion of the early series, the karyotype was rarely tested. Of about 10/351 tested, trisomy 18 and Turner's syndrome predominated. In the later series, 76/109 cases were karyotyped, of which there were 48 normal, 3 trisomy 13, 3 trisomy 18, one triploidy and one XYY, and 20 cases of Turner's syndrome.

Termination of pregnancy took place in 286/460 cases, there were 24 intrauterine deaths, 81 neonatal deaths, and 9 deaths recorded in later childhood. There were 54 neonates alive at last follow-up. Six cases were lost to follow-up.

Aortic stenosis

This is a fairly uncommon condition. It is partial obstruction to the aortic valve, and varies in severity from a mild obstruction to critical stenosis. There is often associated mitral valve stenosis and/or incompetence. Chromosomal and extracardiac anomalies are rare. Mild or moderate degrees of aortic stenosis can be treated fairly conservatively with balloon valvoplasty or the Ross operation, which replaces the aortic valve with the native pulmonary valve and uses a homograft in the pulmonary position. Alternatively, valve replacement is avoided if possible until the child is fully grown, when an artificial valve can be used to replace the diseased aortic valve, although this commits the patient to life-long anticoagulant treatment. The most severe cases of aortic stenosis, particularly those with a restrictive atrial septum, can result in intrauterine or early postnatal death. Severe cases of aortic stenosis, who survive to postnatal life, may need to be treated as the hypoplastic left heart syndrome, if the left ventricle is small or dysfunctional, and the patient subjected to staged surgery to a one-ventricle repair.

Outcome data

There have been 85 cases in total, diagnosed between 14 and 40 weeks. There have been two documented chromosomal anomalies, one trisomy 18 and one isodicentric chromosome 9. Two cases in our series have survived prenatal balloon valvoplasty of 5 where it was attempted. There have been 4 intrauterine deaths, 41 terminations, 21 neonatal deaths, one infant death and there were 15 alive at last follow-up. There have been 3 cases lost to follow-up.

Aortic dysplasia

This is rare and mainly occurs in the setting of polyvalvar dysplasia in trisomy 18.

Aorto-left ventricular tunnel

This is a very rare entity where there is a tunnel-like connection between the aorta and the left ventricle around the cusp of the aortic valve. It results in severe aortic regurgitation, producing left ventricular dilatation. It can be successfully repaired surgically but, as the aortic valve is often stenotic and left ventricular function damaged, the results are mixed.

There were five cases in our early series but we have seen none latterly. There is only one survivor from that early series, one died as an infant and there were three terminations.

Pulmonary atresia

This is complete obstruction to the pulmonary valve. It can occur with an intact ventricular septum or with a ventricular septal defect, the latter being an extreme form of the tetralogy of Fallot. Alternatively, it can occur in the setting of complex heart disease such as double outlet right ventricle. When it occurs with an intact septum, the right ventricle is small and the tricuspid valve may also be stenotic. In the most severe cases, there are right ventricular to coronary artery fistulas, which can result in coronary artery damage. If the right ventricle is of adequate size, which occurs in about one-third of cases, radiofrequency puncture of the pulmonary valve followed by balloon dilatation may render a biventricular repair possible postnatally. More commonly however, only a one-ventricle repair is possible, with an arterial shunt placed as the first of successive procedures. The worst cases, with the smallest ventricles and those cases with fistulas have a high mortality in early childhood, whereas those who achieve a biventricular repair do fairly well into at least young adult life. In an attempt to improve the proportion of biventricular repairs, prenatal balloon valvoplasty of the atretic pulmonary valve has been attempted with some success. Tetralogy of Fallot or double outlet right ventricle with pulmonary atresia are discussed under these headings.

Outcome data

There have been 103 cases seen in our series, diagnosed between 12 and 37 weeks of gestation. There have been two cases of trisomy 18, and two unbalanced translocations. There have been 61 terminations of pregnancy, 7 intrauterine deaths, 8 neonatal deaths and 2 infant deaths. There were 23 patients alive at last follow-up. Two patients were lost to follow-up.

Pulmonary stenosis

Mild or moderate pulmonary valve obstruction is common in postnatal life. It is not, however, a common diagnosis in isolation in fetal life, although it can occur. The only finding in the fetus may be mild to moderate acceleration of flow across the right ventricular outflow tract, often coupled with mild hypoplasia of the pulmonary artery. The condition can be readily treated postnatally with balloon valvoplasty, with good results. Pulmonary stenosis is a common component of more complex heart disease and is usually indicated by hypoplasia of the pulmonary artery relative to the aorta.

Outcome data

There have been 35 isolated cases in our series, diagnosed between 16 and 33 weeks of gestation. There has been one case of triploidy and one unbalanced translocation. There have been eight cases associated with twin-to-twin transfusion syndrome and one with Noonan's syndrome. There have been ten terminations, one intrauterine death, two neonatal deaths, two infant deaths, and 20 live births.

Pulmonary valve dysplasia

This is uncommon. It can occur in tetralogy of Fallot and is known as the absent pulmonary valve syndrome in this setting. Alternatively, it can occur with dysplasia of other cardiac valves in trisomy 18. The absent pulmonary valve syndrome tends to have a very poor

prognosis when it is recognized in fetal life, as the most severe cases, with gross dilatation of the branch pulmonary arteries are preferentially diagnosed.

Outcome data

There have been 26 cases of absent pulmonary valve syndrome, diagnosed between 17 and 40 weeks of gestation. Twenty-one cases were associated with tetralogy of Fallot, 5 had a ventricular septal defect in a different site (not in the outlet septum as in tetralogy). There was one case of trisomy 18 in the early series, although few were tested. There were two cases of microdeletion of chromosome 22 of six tested in the later series. Termination of pregnancy occurred in 12 cases, intrauterine death in 4, neonatal death in 4, infant death in 2 and there were 3 survivors at last follow-up. One case was lost to follow-up.

Arterial valve override

Tetralogy of Fallot with pulmonary stenosis or atresia

Tetralogy of Fallot is a common condition in postnatal life, making up about 6%–10% of major heart disease in children. Although this is not the common understanding of it in postnatal life, in the fetus, it is commonly associated with extracardiac malformations and chromosomal anomalies. The extracardiac findings often lead the patient to the fetal cardiologist and in turn to the cardiac diagnosis. Associated chromosome anomalies can be trisomy 21, 18 or 13, more complex translocations/deletions or a microdeletion of 22q11. Particular associations with extracardiac malformations include exomphalos and diaphragmatic hernia, but neurological or renal anomalies can also occur.

A classic case of tetralogy of Fallot, with a main and branch pulmonary arteries of good size and without extracardiac malformations, should have a good prognosis for surgical repair at low risk (<2% mortality). Repair usually can be undertaken between 3–9 months of age with good long-term results into adult life. However, at the other end of the severity scale, cases with complete pulmonary atresia with discontinuous or very hypoplastic branch pulmonary arteries can have an extremely poor result in terms of exercise capacity after surgery or can even be inoperable. Intermediate cases, who require a shunt procedure in infancy or early repair, tend to fare reasonably well but with a more complicated course in terms of repeated intervention. Both the cardiac and extracardiac anatomical details therefore are essential to define in the fetus because of their important bearing on prognosis.

Outcome data

There were 231 cases of tetralogy of Fallot in our series, excluding the cases of the absent pulmonary valve syndrome described above. The diagnosis was made as early as 12 weeks' gestation to as late as 36. There was pulmonary atresia in 71 cases and an associated AVSD in 14. In the later series of 121 cases, the arch was noted to be right-sided in 10 and there was a left superior caval vein in 4.

Chromosomal anomalies and miscellaneous extracardiac malformations, such as the VACTERL syndrome and exomphalos, for example, were common but less completely ascertained in the early series. There were 7 cases of trisomy 13, 17 of trisomy 18, 26 of trisomy 21, including 11/14 cases of AVSD with tetralogy, 17 with microdeletion of 22q11 and 6 with other chromosomal anomalies. Thus, there was at least an incidence of 24% of chromosomal anomalies in our series. This, of course, has a profound influence in the outcome of this condition, which is usually considered to be relatively benign to the cardiologist or surgeon who only deals with postnatal life.

There were 96 terminations of pregnancy, 16 intrauterine deaths, 17 neonatal deaths, 9 deaths in later infancy or childhood, and there are 87 short-term survivors. Six patients were lost to follow-up.

Common arterial trunk

A common trunk is a relatively uncommon condition. It can be associated with extracardiac and chromosomal anomalies, particularly 22q11 deletion, but this is less common than in tetralogy of Fallot. If the truncal valve is "good," that is, neither stenotic nor incompetent, the surgical repair can be accomplished at a mortality risk of around 10% in the first weeks of life, using a homograft to connect the right ventricle with the pulmonary artery. The homograft will need to be replaced with growth, probably twice before adult size is reached, which means the child will of necessity require repeated interventions, which carry an intrinsic risk. If, on the other hand, the single arterial valve is severely stenotic or incompetent, this increases the risk of the initial repair and will necessitate repair of the neo-aortic valve or even replacement. Valve replacement is not ideal management for a child as it subjects him or her to the complications of life-long anticoagulant therapy.

Outcome data

There were 41 cases in the series, diagnosed between 13 and 33 weeks of gestation. There were 8 chromosomal anomalies, 4 of 11 tested in the later series. There were 3 cases of microdeletion of chromosome 22, 2 of trisomy 21, one each of trisomies 18, 21 and 9. There were 19 terminations of pregnancy, 8 neonatal deaths, 5 deaths in later childhood and 9 short-term survivors.

Pulmonary override in double outlet right ventricle or transposition

This condition is either part of double outlet right ventricle, if the pulmonary arises mainly (>50%) from the right ventricle, or part of transposition, if the pulmonary arises mainly (>50%) from the left ventricle, and is dealt with under these headings.

Transposition of the great arteries

With AV concordance

This is a relatively common condition in pediatric cardiology, constituting nearly 10% of infants with congenital heart disease, although it is less commonly diagnosed in the fetus. This is because transposition can usually only be diagnosed on great artery views and is not commonly associated with extracardiac malformations. Chromosomal anomalies are not a recognized association. Most commonly, transposition is "simple," that is, there are no associated cardiac defects, but transposition can also occur with ventricular septal defects, pulmonary stenosis and coarctation of the aorta. Transposition occurs in about 20% of cases of tricuspid atresia and in the majority of cases of double inlet left ventricle, but these are very different entities, the outlook for which is described under these headings.

Simple transposition can be satisfactorily treated by the arterial switch operation in the first week of life, with good results and low mortality (<5%), even if there are complicating lesions, such as a ventricular septal defect or coarctation, which will also need to be repaired. Coronary artery transfer is the most difficult aspect of the surgery and, if they arise from the aorta in an unusual pattern, can increase the perioperative mortality. About 10%–20% of cases of transposition are urgent within hours after birth, because they have an inadequate size of patent atrial communication, which is essential in this condition for "mixing" and for survival. Balloon atrial septostomy, or tearing the atrial septum to enlarge the atrial communication, may be necessary to stabilize the neonate until surgery can be performed. This is a procedure that may be performed in the intensive care unit under echocardiographic control but requires the skills and surgical back-up associated with a specialist cardiac center. Prenatal diagnosis of this condition is therefore highly advantageous for the affected newborn, as delivery can be arranged when and where emergency intervention can be easily undertaken if indicated. Current results suggest that these children have a good result until well into adult life although truly long-term results are still not available.

Cases of transposition, which are complicated by pulmonary stenosis together with a ventricular septal defect, constitute about 10%–20% of all transposition and are not suitable for switch surgery. They need to undergo the more difficult Rastelli repair, where the aorta is connected to the left ventricle by patch repair of the ventricular septal defect and a conduit is placed between the right ventricle and the pulmonary artery. These cases do not usually require urgent treatment, because there is mixing at the ventricular septal defect, and surgery can be delayed until the heart is a little bigger, after 6 months or even a year. Surgical mortality lies between 5% and 10% and repeated intervention to replace the conduit with growth adds to the morbidity.

Outcome data

There have been 95 cases in our series, diagnosed between 12 and 35 weeks of gestation. Note that detection of tetralogy, despite it being a diagnosis of similar frequency in children, has been more than twice as common as transposition in the fetus, although both require correct evaluation of the great artery views. This is because tetralogy is frequently associated with extracardiac malformations which bring the fetus to detailed attention, whereas transposition is not.

There have been 31 cases of transposition with a ventricular septal defect, 6 with pulmonary stenosis, 5 with coarctation, one with a left superior caval vein, one with left isomerism and one with mitral valve straddling. There were no chromosomal anomalies in our series. As our data extends to the 1980s when the prognosis for surgical treatment was not so good as it is now, 20 cases resulted in termination of pregnancy. There were 5 neonatal deaths, 3 deaths in infancy and there are 66 survivors. Note that our mortality in continuing pregnancies in our more recent series was still 8%, occurring for a variety of reasons in the "uncomplicated" cases of transposition, despite prenatal diagnosis and optimum perinatal management. This is higher than most surgeons would quote for the arterial switch procedure. This illustrates the general point that prenatal counseling, even in a condition which is considered low risk for postnatal treatment, must be a little more cautious than the results which are quoted in the literature. The one case with a straddling mitral valve was only suitable for a one-ventricle repair and all six cases with pulmonary stenosis had a Rastelli repair.

With AV discordance (corrected transposition)

This is a relatively uncommon condition, but one which must not be mistaken for simple transposition, as it has very different implications. It is very rarely associated with extracardiac or chromosomal lesions. If isolated, it may be completely asymptomatic and require no intervention until middle adult life. On the other hand, if there are associated intracardiac lesions, such as ventricular septal defects, pulmonary stenosis or Ebstein's anomaly, which occur in the majority of cases, surgery may be necessary in childhood. Complete heart block is also a common complication. The risk of heart block developing increases with age or with surgical intervention, and patients will usually require pacemaker placement in time, with its attendant complications.

Outcome data

These have been detailed above under discordant atrioventricular junction.

Double outlet right ventricle

This is relatively uncommon but because of the high incidence of extracardiac malformations is preferentially diagnosed prenatally. There is always a ventricular septal defect in association but the position of the defect relative to the great arteries dictate the difficulty of surgical repair. If the anatomy is "tetralogy-like," that is, with a subaortic ventricular septal defect, the surgical repair is similar to a tetralogy repair with a low mortality (<5%) and good long-term outcome. On the other hand, if the anatomy is "transposition-like," with a subpulmonary ventricular septal defect, the approach is more like a Rastelli repair, with a slightly higher mortality and morbidity. In the rare cases where the ventricular septal defect is not related to either great artery, a biventricular repair may be impossible

239

and a Fontan repair necessary, which would entail a still higher mortality and morbidity, with a less good long-term outlook.

Outcome data

There were 114 cases diagnosed between 12 and 35 weeks' gestation. Additional cardiac malformations to the central diagnosis of double outlet right ventricle were common. There was associated pulmonary stenosis in 28 cases, pulmonary atresia in 14, mitral stenosis in 2, coarctation in 3, interrupted aortic arch in one, heart block in 2, an isomerism syndrome in 4, left superior caval vein in 3, right aortic arch in one, left heart hypoplasia in 6 and dextrocardia in 4.

Because of the high rate of extracardiac malformations, karyotyping was obtained in the majority of the later series of 52 cases. There was a chromosome anomaly in 35% of those tested in this group. In the whole series, there were 10 cases of trisomy 18, 5 of trisomy 13, one trisomy 21 and 6 other chromosomal anomalies.

Termination of pregnancy took place in 67 cases, there were 8 intrauterine deaths, 7 neonatal deaths, and 3 deaths in later infancy. There were 28 short-term survivors and one patient was lost to follow-up.

Arch anomalies

Coarctation

This is a common condition in the neonate occurring in over 10% of infants with congenital heart disease. If there is a good standard of obstetric screening, the most severe cases can be detected during routine scanning and referred for fetal echocardiography. Milder cases, on the other hand, can be missed in the fetal period. Cases can also come to attention because of quite a high association with extracardiac malformations and chromosomal defects. Down's syndrome is a less common association but Turner's syndrome and trisomy 18 are not uncommon. Turner's syndrome and coarctation, presenting with a markedly increased nuchal measurement at the 11–14-week window, has a high rate of spontaneous intrauterine death.

If coarctation is isolated, an arch repair can be accomplished in the neonatal period with a low mortality and a good prognosis at least in the intermediate term. Sometimes the arch re-stenoses, but nowadays this can be successfully treated at low risk, by dilation with a balloon catheter or stent placement. A

ventricular septal defect, a commonly associated lesion, will complicate the repair and add a little to the mortality. Occasionally, a coarctation is associated with multiple levels of left heart disease, so-called Schone's syndrome, where there is mitral stenosis and subaortic or aortic stenosis in addition. This combination often necessitates repeated surgery with a poor outlook for survival or for a good quality of life after surgery. Sometimes, the left ventricle grows poorly as gestation advances and the patient needs to be treated as a hypoplastic left heart syndrome with a first stage Norwood operation in the neonatal period. If the left ventricle is already small in mid-gestation, this possibility may need to be included in the counselling.

Coarctation is one of the few conditions which can be falsely diagnosed prenatally. A fetal diagnosis of coarctation is often a provisional one, to be confirmed or refuted after birth. The neonate needs serial echocardiography and to be carefully observed for symptoms and signs until after the duct closes. In a few cases where coarctation was suspected in utero and apparently excluded in the neonatal period, the child has been found to have coarctation weeks or months later, so follow-up is essential.

Outcome data

There were 471 cases in our series, representing 12% of our cases, therefore one of the most commonly recognized (or suspected) defects in the fetus. However, it should be noted that a significant proportion of our cases (up to 30%) were suspected cases, which were not confirmed postnatally. Some cases were suspected from as early as 11 weeks of gestation. An associated ventricular septal defect was documented in 54 cases, mitral stenosis in 2, aortic or subaortic stenosis in 5. A left superior caval vein was quite a common association but not documented until recently. Tricuspid regurgitation was a common associated feature of the cases diagnosed at the nuchal scan.

There were 66 cases of Turner's syndrome, 21 of trisomy 13, 31 of trisomy 18, 22 of trisomy 21, 3 microdeletions of chromosome 22 and 14 other miscellaneous chromosome anomalies. Of the 227 cases tested in the recent series of 281 cases, 50% had a chromosome anomaly.

There were 29 intrauterine deaths, 214 terminations of pregnancy, 34 neonatal deaths, 7 deaths in infancy or later childhood and there were 181 short-term survivors. Six patients were lost to follow-up.

Interruption of the aorta

This is a relatively rare condition. The most common form of interrupted aorta is the so-called type B, where the interruption occurs between the left common carotid artery and the left subclavian artery. This has a high association with 22q11 chromosomal microdeletion. In the even less common type A, the arch is interrupted after the left subclavian artery. This has no, or a much less common, association with 22q11 deletion. Type B is relatively easily diagnosed as there is a very small aorta and no transverse arch, whereas type A will show the same signs as coarctation and can be difficult to differentiate from it. Surgical repair takes place in the neonatal period and is more difficult than repair of coarctation. Mobilization and reconstruction of the arch is required as well as closure of the usually large ventricular septal defect. Subaortic stenosis coexists or develops later in up to one-third of cases.

Outcome data

We have seen 12 cases of type B interrupted aortic arch in our series. Interestingly, all were diagnosed at or after 20 weeks of gestation, although there is no reason to suppose that diagnosis cannot be made earlier. There was one case of associated trisomy 18. Obviously, the early cases were not tested with the more modern methods for a microdeletion of chromosome 22, but there were no microdeletions in the last six cases, which is perhaps rather surprising. There were three terminations of pregnancy, one intrauterine death, four neonatal deaths and four successful surgical repairs, all in the more recent data.

Right aortic arch

This occurs as an isolated condition or with additional intracardiac lesions, particularly tetralogy of Fallot (in about 30%) and common arterial trunk (about 10%). The detection of it during routine fetal scanning as an isolated defect is increasing as the skills in routine scanning improve, suggesting that it may be more common in the normal population than previously thought. It can be associated with chromosomal or other extracardiac anomalies, particularly if there are associated intracardiac defects. The most common chromosomal defect is 22q11 deletion but other chromosomal defects can occur, such as trisomy 21 or 18. In its isolated form, it is asymptomatic and requires no treatment or intervention. It is important to differentiate it from a double aortic arch but this can be difficult, even on the postnatal echocardiogram. Magnetic resonance imaging may be necessary to clarify the arch anatomy, although, as this requires a general anesthetic in the infant, it is generally not used unless there are symptoms.

Outcome data

A right aortic arch has only been diagnosed in the recent series. It is recognized with other forms of CHD such as tetralogy of Fallot. These cases have been enumerated in the appropriate sections. There have been 28 cases of isolated right aortic arch, 2 diagnosed at the nuchal scan. Two cases have been documented to have a microdeletion of chromosome 22 and one a complex translocation. There were 2 terminations of pregnancy, 2 intrauterine deaths and 22 were normal live-births. Two cases were lost to follow-up.

Double aortic arch

A double aortic arch is where both limbs of the embryonic arch persist. Usually the left sided arch is smaller than the right. It has the potential for compressing the trachea which can lead to stridor in the infant and in some cases tracheomalacia or permanent damage to the trachea. It can be difficult to differentiate echocardiographically from a simple right sided aortic arch, which usually does not lead to symptoms. A double aortic arch can be readily corrected surgically at low risk and, except in those few cases where tracheal damage has occurred, the long-term outcome is good. We have seen two cases in our most recent series, both of whom have had successful surgical repair.

Aberrant right subclavian artery

An aberrant right subclavian artery describes the situation where instead of arising from the arch as a common origin with the right common carotid, the right subclavian arises as the most distal (fourth) branch of the arch, coursing behind the trachea to reach the right arm. It is not associated with postnatal symptoms. It may occur as an isolated variant, in association with heart defects. It occurs in about 1.5% of normal fetuses but in up to 20% of Down syndrome fetuses. It therefore increases the risk of trisomy 21 by 10 or more times. We have seen 11 cases where it was an isolated finding, one of which had trisomy 21. One of our cases, where the karyotype was unknown, had a spontaneous intrauterine death for no obvious reason, but the others are all normal survivors.

Aorto-pulmonary window

This is a rare defect and one which is very difficult to diagnose in the fetus. We have only diagnosed one case prenatally, who had successful surgical repair. To our knowledge we have not overlooked a case. There is a defect in the wall between the aorta and pulmonary artery, just above the valve rings. It is usually isolated but can occur with aortic arch lesions or with tetralogy of Fallot. There is a high mortality in those cases with other cardiac defects, but as an isolated lesion, it can be readily repaired surgically at low risk. The patient typically presents in the first month or two of life with symptoms suggestive of a large ventricular septal defect but none is found echocardiographically. This should lead to a search for a shunt at another site.

Abnormalities of the arterial duct

A small or even completely closed duct appears to be well tolerated in the late fetus, although some case reports suggest right heart failure in this context, which completely resolves after delivery. I find this rather dubious as I have never seen it, but it may be a real entity. Certainly, a tortuous or kinked duct is common in late gestation with no apparent consequences. The size of the duct is relevant in transposition of the great arteries, where it may result in severe early cyanosis, if it occurs in association with a restrictive atrial septum. A small duct may also be associated with poor development of the lung vasculature in the setting of tetralogy of Fallot.

A constricted duct is one where there is acceleration of flow across the duct. It is usually a response to maternal ingestion of non-steroidal anti-inflammatory medication. It is more likely to occur in response to these drugs after 30–32 weeks' gestation than in earlier pregnancy. It can lead to tricuspid regurgitation. It is usually reversible if the drugs are stopped, although pulmonary hypertension after birth is a theoretical complication. We have no experience of ductal constriction in our series.

Absence of the arterial duct has been described as a benign incidental finding, but it must be very rare as an isolated finding.

An "aneurysm" of the duct appears to be common as a mild dilation in late pregnancy, although less common as a more marked dilatation. We have seen three cases of the latter. Both types appear to be benign asymptomatic findings, which do not require treatment.

Arrhythmias

There are only data available for the last 9 years, during which time we have seen five cases of complete heart block, one of 2 to 1 block and one fetus with a prolonged P–R interval. Presentation ranged between 16 (2 to 1 block) and 31 weeks of gestation. One fetus was treated with salbutamol prenatally. One case was lost to follow-up but the remaining six were live births. A pacemaker has been necessary in two of six cases. The fetus with first-degree heart block, whose mother had systemic lupus erythematosis, remains well and asymptomatic at 6 months of age having received no treatment.

There were 27 cases of a tachycardia, 6 with atrial flutter and 21 with a supraventricular tachycardia. Gestation at presentation ranged from 21 to 40 weeks. There was hydrops at presentation in 8/27 cases. Three cases were not treated prenatally, two because of presentation at term and one because the tachycardia was intermittent. Fourteen cases were treated successfully with digoxin alone, administered transplacentally in 13 and to the umbilical vein in one. There were three cases treated with flecainide alone and one with sotalol alone. Four cases were treated with a combination of digoxin and flecainide and two with digoxin and sotalol. All, except one case of atrial flutter, achieved conversion to sinus rhythm prenatally. There are four cases lost to follow-up and the rest were live births. All are well at follow-up and most are not receiving any anti-arrhythmic drugs.

Summary

We have tried to indicate the results of current management of the cardiac malformations which we have seen in fetal life. For a variety of reasons, this is somewhat different from the results in the literature for postnatal treatment. The prognosis for many children in terms of mortality has improved dramatically over the 30-year period which I have been involved in this field and will continue to do so in the future. However, quality of life in terms of on-going physical disability, neurological damage and long-term outcome must always be kept under scrutiny, so that the parents can be realistically counseled during pregnancy.

Bibliography

Outcome

Allan LD, Apfel HD, Printz BF. Outcome after prenatal diagnosis of the hypoplastic left heart syndrome. *Heart* 1998; **79**: 371–374.

Allan LD, Sharland G. Prognosis in fetal tetralogy of Fallot. *Pediatr Cardiol* 1992; **13**: 1–4.

Allan LD, Sharland G, Tynan MJ. The natural history of the hypoplastic left heart syndrome. *Int J Cardiol* 1989; **25**: 341–343.

Andrews RE, Simpson JM, Sharland GK, Sullivan ID, Yates RW. Outcome after preterm delivery of infants antenatally diagnosed with congenital heart disease. *J Pediatr* 2006; **148**: 213–216.

Berg C, Kamil D, Geipel A, *et al*. Absence of ductus venosus – importance of umbilical venous drainage site. *Ultrasound Obstet Gynecol* 2006; **28**: 275–281.

Bernasconi A, Azancot A, Simpson JM, Jones A, Sharland GK. Fetal dextrocardia: diagnosis and outcome in two tertiary centres. *Heart* 2005; **91**: 1590–1594.

Bonnet D, Coltri A, Butera G *et al*. Detection of transposition of the great arteries in fetuses reduces neonatal morbidity and mortality. *Circulation* 1999; **99**: 916–918.

Brenner JI. Prevalence and outcome of congenital heart disease in infancy: a 10 year population based experience. In: *Progress in Obstetric and Gynecological Sonography Series. Ultrasound and the Fetal Heart*. Eds. Wladimiroff JW and Pilu G. New York, London: Parthenon Press, 1996: 107–115.

Celermajer DS, Bull C, Till JA *et al*. Ebstein's anomaly: presentation and outcome from fetus to adult. *J Am Coll Cardiol* 1994; **23**: 170–176.

Chang AC, Huhta JC, Yoon GY *et al*. Diagnosis, transport and outcome in fetuses with left ventricular outflow obstruction. *J Thorac Cardiovasc Surg* 1991; **102**: 841–846.

Chiappa E, Micheletti A, Sciarrone A, Botta G, Abbruzzese P. The prenatal diagnosis of, and short-term outcome for, patients with congenitally corrected transposition. *Cardiol Young* 2004; **14**: 265–276.

Daubeney PE, Sharland GK, Cook AC, Keeton BR, Anderson RH, Webber SA. Pulmonary atresia with intact ventricular septum: impact of fetal echocardiography on incidence at birth and postnatal outcome. *Circulation* 1998; **98**: 562–566.

Duke C, Sharland GK, Jones AM, Simpson JM. Echocardiographic features and outcome of truncus arteriosus diagnosed during fetal life. *Am J Cardiol* 2001; **88**: 1379–1384.

Fuchs IB, Müller H, Abdul-Khaliq H, Harder T, Dudenhausen JW, Henrich W. Immediate and long-term outcomes in children with prenatal diagnosis of selected isolated congenital heart defects. *Ultrasound Obstet Gynecol* 2007; **29**: 38–43.

Gardiner HM, Belmar C, Tulzer G *et al*. Morphologic and functional predictors of eventual circulation in the fetus with pulmonary atresia or critical pulmonary stenosis with intact septum. *J Am Coll Cardiol* 2008; **51**: 1299–1308.

Groves AM, Fagg NLK, Cook AC, Allan LD. Cardiac tumours in intrauterine life. *Arch Dis Child* 1992; **67**: 1189–1192.

Head CE, Jowett VC, Sharland GK, Simpson JM. Timing of presentation and postnatal outcome of infants suspected of having coarctation of the aorta during fetal life. *Heart* 2005; **91**: 1070–1074.

Holley DG, Martin GR, Brenner JI *et al*. Diagnosis and management of fetal cardiac tumors: a multicenter experience and review of published reports. *J Am Coll Cardiol* 1995; **26**: 516–520.

Hornberger LK, Sahn DJ, Kleinman CS, Copel JA, Reed KL. Tricuspid valve disease with significant tricuspid insufficiency in the fetus: diagnosis and outcome. *J Am Coll Cardiol* 1991; **17**: 167–173.

Hornberger LK, Sahn DJ, Kleinman C, Copel J, Silverman N. Antenatal diagnosis of coarctation of the aorta. A multicenter experience. *J Am Coll Cardiol* 1994; **23**: 417–423.

Huggon IC, Cook AC, Smeeton NC, Magee AG, Sharland GK. Atrioventricular septal defects diagnosed in fetal life: associated cardiac and extra-cardiac abnormalities and outcome. *J Am Coll Cardiol* 2000; **36**: 593–601.

Jaeggi ET, Fouron JC, Hornberger LK *et al*. A genesis of the ductus venosus that is associated with extrahepatic umbilical vein drainage: prenatal features and clinical outcome. *Am J Obstet Gynecol* 2002; **187**: 1031–1037.

Jaeggi ET, Sholler GF, Jones OD, Cooper SG. Comparative analysis of pattern, management and outcome of pre- versus postnatally diagnosed major congenital heart disease: a population-based study. *Ultrasound Obstet Gynecol* 2001; **17**: 380–385.

Jouannic JM, Gavard L, Fermont L *et al.* Sensitivity and specificity of prenatal features of physiological shunts to predict neonatal clinical status in transposition of the great arteries. *Circulation* 2004; **110**: 1743–1746.

McElhinney DB, Salvin JW, Colan SD *et al.* Improving outcomes in fetuses and neonates with congenital displacement (Ebstein's malformation) or dysplasia of the tricuspid valve. *Am J Cardiol* 2005; **96**: 582–586.

Menon SC, O'Leary PW, Wright GB, Rios R, MacLellan-Tobert SG, Cabalka AK. Fetal and neonatal presentation of noncompacted ventricular myocardium: expanding the clinical spectrum. *J Am Soc Echocardiogr* 2007; **20**: 1344–1350.

Moon-Grady AJ, Tacy TA, Brook MM, Hanley FL, Silverman NH. Value of clinical and echocardiographic features in predicting outcome in the fetus, infant, and child with tetralogy of Fallot with absent pulmonary valve complex. *Am J Cardiol* 2002; **89**: 1280–1285.

Pascal CJ, Huggon I, Sharland GK, Simpson JM. An echocardiographic study of diagnostic accuracy, prediction of surgical approach, and outcome for fetuses diagnosed with discordant ventriculo-arterial connections. *Cardiol Young* 2007; **17**: 528–534.

Pedra SR, Smallhorn JF, Ryan G *et al.* Fetal cardiomyopathies: pathogenic mechanisms, hemodynamic findings, and clinical outcome. *Circulation* 2002; **106**: 585–591.

Roman KS, Fouron JC, Nii M, Smallhorn JF, Chaturvedi R, Jaeggi ET. Determinants of outcome in fetal pulmonary valve stenosis or atresia with intact ventricular septum. *Am J Cardiol* 2007; **99**: 699–703.

Salvin JW, McElhinney DB, Colan SD *et al.* Fetal tricuspid valve size and growth as predictors of outcome in pulmonary atresia with intact ventricular septum. *Pediatrics* 2006; **118**: 415–420.

Simpson JM, Sharland GK. Natural history and outcome of aortic stenosis diagnosed prenatally. *Heart* 1997; **77**: 205–210.

Sivasankaran S, Sharland GK, Simpson JM. Dilated cardiomyopathy presenting during fetal life. *Cardiol Young* 2005; **15**: 409–416.

Taketazu M, Lougheed J, Yoo SJ, Lim JS, Hornberger LK. Spectrum of cardiovascular disease, accuracy of diagnosis, and outcome in fetal heterotaxy syndrome. *Am J Cardiol* 2006; **97**: 720–724.

Tworetzky W, McElhinney DB, Reddy VM, Brook MM, Hanley FL, Silverman NH. Improved surgical outcome after fetal diagnosis of hypoplastic left heart syndrome. *Circulation* 2001; **103**: 1269–1273.

Vesel S, Rollings S, Jones A, Callaghan N, Simpson J, Sharland GK. Prenatally diagnosed pulmonary atresia with ventricular septal defect: echocardiography, genetics, associated anomalies and outcome. *Heart* 2006; **92**: 1501–1505.

Vida VL, Bacha EA, Larrazabal A *et al.* Hypoplastic left heart syndrome with intact or highly restrictive atrial septum: surgical experience from a single center. *Ann Thorac Surg* 2007; **84**: 581–585.

Wald RM, Tham EB, McCrindle BW *et al.* Outcome after prenatal diagnosis of tricuspid atresia: a multicenter experience. *Am Heart J* 2007; **153**: 772–778.

Yagel S, Weissman A, Rotstein Z *et al.* Congenital heart defects. Natural course and in utero development. *Circulation* 1997; **96**: 550–555.

General references

Allan LD, Chita SK, Anderson RH, Fagg N, Crawford DC, Tynan MJ. Coarctation of the aorta in prenatal life: an echocardiographic, anatomical, and functional study. *Br Heart J* 1988; **59**: 356.

Allan LD, Crawford DC, Chita SK, Tynan MJ. Prenatal screening for congenital heart disease. *Br Med J* 1986; **292**: 1717–1719.

Allan LD, Crawford DC, Tynan M. Evolution of coarctation of the aorta in intrauterine life. *Br Heart J* 1984; **52**: 471–473.

Allan LD, Crawford DC, Tynan MJ. Pulmonary atresia in prenatal life. *J Am Coll Cardiol* 1986; **8**: 1131–1136.

Allan LD, Joseph MD, Boyd EGCA, Campbell S, Tynan MJ. M-Mode echocardiography in the developing human fetus. *Br Heart J* 1982; **47**: 573–584.

Allan LD, Sharland GK. The echocardiographic diagnosis of totally anomalous pulmonary venous connection in the fetus. *Heart* 2001; **85**: 433–437.

Allan LD, Sharland GK, Milburn A *et al.* Prospective diagnosis of 1006 consecutive cases of congenital heart disease in the fetus. *J Am Coll Cardiol* 1994; **23**: 1452–1458.

Allan LD, Tynan M, Campbell S, Wilkinson JL, Andersen RH. Echocardiographic and anatomical correlates in the fetus. *Br Heart J* 1980; **44**: 444–451.

Axt-Fleidner R, Schwarze A, Smrcek J, Germer U, Krapp M, Gembruch U. Isolated ventricular septal defects detected by color Doppler imaging: evolution during fetal and first year of postnatal life. *Ultrasound Obstet Gynecol* 2006; **27**: 266–273.

Berg C, Bender F, Soukup M *et al.* Right aortic arch detected in fetal life. *Ultrasound Obstet Gynecol* 2006; **28**: 882–889.

Berg C, Geipel A, Smrcek J *et al.* Prenatal diagnosis of cardiosplenic syndromes: a 10-year experience. *Ultrasound Obstet Gynecol* 2003; **22**: 451–459.

Berg C, Kremer C, Geipel A, Kohl T, Germer U, Gembruch U. Ductus venosus blood flow alterations in fetuses with obstructive lesions of the right heart. *Ultrasound Obstet Gynecol* 2006; **28**: 137–142.

Chaoui R, Heling KS, Kalache KD. Caliber of the coronary sinus in fetuses with cardiac defects with and without left persistent superior vena cava and in growth-restricted fetuses with heart-sparing effect. *Prenat Diagn* 2003; **23**: 552–557.

Chaoui R, Heling KS, Sarioglu N, Schwabe M, Dankof A, Bollmann R. Aberrant right subclavian artery as a new cardiac sign in second- and third-trimester fetuses with Down syndrome. *Am J Obstet Gynecol* 2005; **192**: 257–263.

Chaoui R, Hoffmann J, Heling KS. Three-dimensional (3D) and 4D color Doppler fetal echocardiography using spatio-temporal image correlation (STIC). *Ultrasound Obstet Gynecol* 2004; **23**: 535–545.

Chaoui R, Kalache KD, Heling KS, Tennstedt C, Bommer C, Körner H. Absent or hypoplastic thymus on ultrasound: a marker for deletion 22q11.2 in fetal cardiac defects. *Ultrasound Obstet Gynecol* 2002; **20**: 546–552.

Chaoui R, McEwing R. Three cross-sectional planes for fetal color Doppler echocardiography. *Ultrasound Obstet Gynecol* 2003; **21**: 81–93. Review.

Contratti G, Banzi C, Ghi T, Perolo A, Pilu G, Visentin A. Absence of the ductus venosus: report of 10 new cases and review of the literature. *Ultrasound Obstet Gynecol* 2001; **18**: 605–609.

Cook AC, Fagg NL, Ho SY *et al.* Echocardiographic-anatomical correlations in aorto-left ventricular tunnel. *Br Heart J* 1995; **74**: 443–448.

Cordes TM, O'Leary PW, Seward JB, Hagler DJ. Distinguishing right from left: a standardized technique for fetal echocardiography. *J Am Soc Echocardiogr* 1994; **7**: 47–53.

DeVore GR, Falkensammer P, Sklansky MS, Platt LD. Spatio-temporal image correlation (STIC): new technology for evaluation of the fetal heart. *Ultrasound Obstet Gynecol* 2003; **22**: 380–387.

Dyamenahalli U, Smallhorn JF, Geva T *et al.* Isolated ductus arteriosus aneurysm in the fetus and infant: a multi-institutional experience. *J Am Coll Cardiol* 2000; **36**: 262–269.

Espinoza J, Gonçalves LF, Lee W, Mazor M, Romero R. A novel method to improve prenatal diagnosis of abnormal systemic venous connections using three- and four-dimensional ultrasonography and "inversion mode". *Ultrasound Obstet Gynecol* 2005; **25**: 428–434.

Ettedgui JA, Sharland GK, Chita SK, Cook A, Fagg N, Allan LD. Absent pulmonary valve syndrome with ventricular septal defect: role of the arterial duct. *Am J Cardiol* 1990; **66**: 233–234.

Ferencz C, Boughman JA, Neill CA, Brenner JI, Perry LW. Congenital cardiovascular malformations: questions on inheritance. *J Am Coll Cardiol* 1989; **14**: 756–763.

Ferencz C, Rubin JD, Loffredo CA, Magee CA. Perspectives in Pediatric Cardiology, vol. 4. *Congenital Heart Disease – The Baltimore Washington Infant Study 1981–1989.* New York: Futura, 1993.

Ferencz C, Rubin JD, McCarter RJ *et al.* Congenital heart disease: prevalence at livebirth. The Baltimore–Washington Infant Study. *Am J Epidemiol* 1985; **121**: 31–36.

Fishman NH, Hof RB, Rudolph AM, Heymann MA. Models of congenital heart disease in fetal lambs. *Circulation* 1978; **58**: 354–364.

Fouron JC, Skoll A, Sonesson SE, Pfizenmaier M, Jaeggi E, Lessard M. Relationship between flow through the fetal aortic isthmus and cerebral oxygenation during acute placental circulatory insufficiency in ovine fetuses. *Am J Obstet Gynecol* 1999; **181**: 1102–1107.

Fyler DC, Buckley LP, Hellenbrand WE, Cohn HE. Report of the New England Regional Infant Cardiac Care Program. *Pediatrics* 1980; **65**(suppl): 376–461.

Garne E, Stoll C, Clementi M; Euroscan Group. Evaluation of prenatal diagnosis of congenital heart diseases by ultrasound: experience from 20 European registries. *Ultrasound Obstet Gynecol* 2001; **17**: 386–391.

Gembruch U, Smrcek JM. The prevalence and clinical significance of tricuspid valve regurgitation in normally grown fetuses and those with intrauterine growth retardation. *Ultrasound Obstet Gynecol* 1997; **9**: 374–382.

Gill HK, Splitt M, Sharland GK, Simpson JM. Patterns of recurrence of congenital heart disease: an analysis of 6,640 consecutive pregnancies evaluated by detailed fetal echocardiography. *J Am Coll Cardiol* 2003; **42**: 923–929.

Goldmuntz E, Clark BJ, Mitchell LE *et al.* Frequency of 22q11 deletions in patients with conotruncal defects. *J Am Coll Cardiol* 1998; **32**: 499–501.

Gonçalves LF, Espinoza J, Romero R *et al.* Four-dimensional ultrasonography of the fetal heart using a novel Tomographic Ultrasound Imaging display. *J Perinatal Med* 2006; **34**: 39–55.

Gonçalves LF, Lee W, Chaiworapongsa T *et al.* Four-dimensional ultrasonography of the fetal heart with spatiotemporal image correlation. *Am J Obstet Gynecol* 2003; **189**: 1792–1802.

Hornberger LK, Sanders SP, Rein AJ, Spevak PJ, Parness IA, Colan SD. Left heart obstructive lesions and left ventricular growth in the midtrimester fetus. A longitudinal study. *Circulation* 1995; **92**: 1531–1538.

Hornberger LK, Sanders SP, Sahn DJ *et al.* In utero pulmonary artery and aortic growth and potential for progression of pulmonary outflow tract obstruction in tetralogy of Fallot. *J Am Coll Cardiol* 1995; **25**: 739–745.

Humpl T, Huggan P, Hornberger LK, McCrindle BW. Presentation and outcomes of ectopia cordis. *Can J Cardiol.* 1999; **15**: 1353–1357.

Karatza AA, Wolfenden JL, Taylor MJ, Wee L, Fisk NM, Gardiner HM. Influence of twin-twin transfusion syndrome on fetal cardiovascular structure and function: prospective case-control study of 136 monochorionic twin pregnancies. *Heart* 2002; **88**: 271–277.

Kiserud T, Rasmussen S. Ultrasound assessment of the fetal foramen ovale. *Ultrasound Obstet Gynecol* 2001; **17**: 119–124.

Kleinman CS, Hobbins JC, Jaffee CC, Lynch DC, Talner NS. Echocardiographic studies of the human fetus: prenatal diagnosis of congenital heart disease and cardiac dysrhythmias. *Pediatrics* 1980; **65**: 1059–1067.

Lang D, Oberhoffer R, Cook A *et al.* The pathologic spectrum of malformations of the tricuspid valve in prenatal and neonatal life. *J Am Coll Cardiol* 1991; **17**: 1161–1167.

Lange LW, Sahn DJ, Allen HD, Goldberg SJ, Anderson C, Giles H. Qualitative real-time cross-sectional echocardiographic imaging of the unborn human fetus during the second half of pregnancy. *Circulation* 1980; **62**: 799–806.

Lougheed J, Sinclair BG, Fung Kee Fung K et al. Acquired right ventricular outflow tract obstruction in the recipient twin in twin-twin transfusion syndrome. *J Am Coll Cardiol* 2001; **38**: 1533–1538.

Luchese S, Mânica JL, Zielinsky P. Intrauterine ductus arteriosus constriction: analysis of a historic cohort of 20 cases. *Arq Bras Cardiol* 2003; **81**: 405–10, 399–404.

Machado MV, Crawford DC, Anderson RH, Allan LD. Atrioventricular septal defect in prenatal life. *Br Heart J* 1988; **59**: 352–355.

Maeno YV, Boutin C, Hornberger LK et al. Prenatal diagnosis of right ventricular outflow tract obstruction with intact ventricular septum, and detection of ventriculocoronary connections. *Heart* 1999; **81**: 661–668.

Maeno YV, Kamenir SA, Sinclair B, van der Velde ME, Smallhorn JF, Hornberger LK. Prenatal features of ductus arteriosus constriction and restrictive foramen ovale in d-transposition of the great arteries. *Circulation* 1999; **99**: 1209–1214.

Mäkikallio K, McElhinney DB, Levine JC et al. Fetal aortic valve stenosis and the evolution of hypoplastic left heart syndrome: patient selection for fetal intervention. *Circulation* 2006; **113**: 1401–1405.

Mäkikallio K, Vuolteenaho O, Jouppila P, Räsänen J. Ultrasonographic and biochemical markers of human fetal cardiac dysfunction in placental insufficiency. *Circulation* 2002; **105**: 2058–2063.

Makrydimas G, Sotiriadis A, Huggon IC et al. Nuchal translucency and fetal cardiac defects: a pooled analysis of major fetal echocardiography centers. *Am J Obstet Gynecol* 2005; **192**: 89–95.

Marino B, Digilio MC, Toscano A et al. Anatomic patterns of conotruncal defects associated with deletion 22q11. *Genet Med* 2001; **3**: 45–48.

Marshall AC, van der Velde ME, Tworetzky W et al. Creation of an atrial septal defect in utero for fetuses with hypoplastic left heart syndrome and intact or highly restrictive atrial septum. *Circulation* 2004; **110**: 253–258.

Mavrides E, Cobian-Sanchez F, Tekay A, Moscoso G, Campbell S, Thilaganathan B, Carvalho JS. Limitations of using first-trimester nuchal translucency measurement in routine screening for major congenital heart defects. *Ultrasound Obstet Gynecol* 2001; **17**: 106–110.

Maxwell D, Allan LD, Tynan MJ. Balloon dilatation of the aortic valve in the fetus: a report of two cases. *Br Heart J* 1991; **65**: 256–258.

McEwing RL, Chaoui R. Congenitally corrected transposition of the great arteries: clues for prenatal diagnosis. *Ultrasound Obstet Gynecol* 2004; **23**: 68–72.

Michailidis GD, Economides DL. Nuchal translucency measurement and pregnancy outcome in karyotypically normal fetuses. *Ultrasound Obstet Gynecol* 2001; **17**: 102–105.

Michailidis GD, Simpson JM, Tulloh RM, Economides DL. Retrospective prenatal diagnosis of scimitar syndrome aided by three-dimensional power Doppler imaging. *Ultrasound Obstet Gynecol* 2001; **17**: 449–452.

Michelfelder E, Gomez C, Border W, Gottliebson W, Franklin C. Predictive value of fetal pulmonary venous flow patterns in identifying the need for atrial septoplasty in the newborn with hypoplastic left ventricle. *Circulation* 2005; **112**: 2974.

Mielke G, Benda N. Reference ranges for two-dimensional echocardiographic examination of the fetal ductus arteriosus. *Ultrasound Obstet Gynecol* 2000; **15**: 219–225.

Nikkilä A, Björkhem G, Källén B. Prenatal diagnosis of congenital heart defects – a population based study. *Acta Paediatr* 2007; **96**: 49–52.

Park JK, Taylor DK, Skeels M, Towner DR. Dilated coronary sinus in the fetus: misinterpretation as an atrioventricular canal defect. *Ultrasound Obstet Gynecol* 1997; **10**: 126–129.

Pasquini L, Mellander M, Seale A et al. Z-scores of the fetal aortic isthmus and duct: an aid to assessing arch hypoplasia. *Ultrasound Obstet Gynecol* 2007; **29**: 628–633.

Pepas LP, Savis A, Jones A, Sharland GK, Tulloh RM, Simpson JM. An echocardiographic study of tetralogy of Fallot in the fetus and infant. *Cardiol Young* 2003; **13**: 240–247.

Phillipos EZ, Robertson MA, Still KD. The echocardiographic assessment of the human fetal foramen ovale. *J Am Soc Echocardiogr* 1994; **7**: 257–263.

Pitkänen OM, Hornberger LK, Miner SE et al. Borderline left ventricles in prenatally diagnosed atrioventricular septal defect or double outlet right ventricle: echocardiographic predictors of biventricular repair. *Am Heart J* 2006; **152**: 163–167.

Raboisson MJ, Fouron JC, Lamoureux J et al. Early intertwin differences in myocardial performance during the twin-to-twin transfusion syndrome. *Circulation* 2004; **110**: 3043–3048.

Respondek M, Kammermeier M, Ludomirsky A, Weil SR, Huhta JC. The prevalence and clinical significance of fetal tricuspid valve regurgitation with normal heart anatomy. *Am J Obstet Gynecol* 1994; **171**: 1265–1270.

Rudolph AM. Distribution and regulation of blood flow in the fetal and neonatal lamb. *Circ Res* 1985; **57**: 811–820.

Sahn DJ, Lange LW, Allen HD et al. Quantitative real-time cross-sectional echocardiography in the development of normal human fetus and newborn. *Circulation* 1980; **62**: 588–595.

Sandor GG, Cook AC, Sharland GK, Ho SY, Potts JE, Anderson RH. Coronary arterial abnormalities in pulmonary atresia with intact ventricular septum diagnosed during fetal life. *Cardiol Young* 2002; **12**: 436–444.

Sau A, Sharland G, Simpson J. Agenesis of the ductus venosus associated with direct umbilical venous return into the heart–case series and review of literature. *Prenat Diagn* 2004; **24**: 418–423.

Schneider C, McCrindle BW, Carvalho JS, Hornberger LK, McCarthy KP, Daubeney PL. Development of Z-scores for fetal cardiac dimensions from echocardiography. *Ultrasound Obstet Gynecol* 2005; **26**: 599–605.

Sharland GK, Allan LD. Normal fetal cardiac measurements derived by cross-sectional echocardiography. *Ultrasound Obstet Gynecol* 1992; **2**: 175–181.

Sharland GK, Allan LD. Screening for congenital heart disease prenatally. Results of a 2 1/2 year study in the South East Thames Region. *Br J Obstet Gynaecol* 1992; **99**: 220–225.

Sharland GK, Chan K–Y, Allan LD. Coarctation of the aorta: difficulties in prenatal diagnosis. *Br Heart J* 1994; **71**: 70–75.

Sharland GK, Chita SK, Allan LD. The use of colour Doppler in fetal echocardiography. *Int J Cardiol* 1990; **28**: 229–236.

Sharland GK, Chita SK, Allan LD. Tricuspid valve dysplasia or displacement in intrauterine life. *J Am Coll Cardiol* 1991; **17**: 944–949.

Shipp TD, Bromley B, Hornberger LK, Nadel A, Benacerraf BR. Levorotation of the fetal cardiac axis: a clue for the presence of congenital heart disease. *Obstet Gynecol* 1995; **85**: 97–102.

Simpson JM, Cook A. Repeatability of echocardiographic measurements in the human fetus. *Ultrasound Obstet Gynecol* 2002; **20**: 332–339.

Smith RS, Comstock CH, Kirk JS, Lee W. Ultrasonographic left cardiac axis deviation: a marker for fetal anomalies. *Obstet Gynecol* 1995; **85**: 187–191.

Smrcek JM, Germer U, Gembruch U. Functional pulmonary valve regurgitation in the fetus. *Ultrasound Obstet Gynecol* 1998; **12**: 254–259.

Taketazu M, Lougheed J, Yoo SJ, Lim JS, Hornberger LK. Spectrum of cardiovascular disease, accuracy of diagnosis, and outcome in fetal heterotaxy syndrome. *Am J Cardiol* 2006; **97**: 720–724.

Tan J, Silverman NH, Hoffman JIE, Villegas M, Schmidt KG. Cardiac dimensions determined by cross-sectional echocardiography in the normal human fetus from 18 weeks to term. *Am J Cardiol* 1992; **70**: 1459–1467.

Tegnander E, Eik-Nes SH, Johansen OJ, Linker DT. Prenatal detection of heart defects at the routine fetal examination at 18 weeks in a non-selected population. *Ultrasound Obstet Gynecol* 1995; **5**: 372–380.

Tegnander E, Williams W, Johansen OJ, Blaas HG, Eik-Nes SH. Prenatal detection of heart defects in a non-selected population of 30,149 fetuses – detection rates and outcome. *Ultrasound Obstet Gynecol* 2006; **27**: 252–265.

Tometzki AJ, Suda K, Kohl T, Kovalchin JP, Silverman NH. Accuracy of prenatal echocardiographic diagnosis and prognosis of fetuses with conotruncal anomalies. *J Am Coll Cardiol* 1999; **33**: 1696–1701.

Tulzer G, Arzt W, Franklin RC, Loughna PV, Mair R, Gardiner HM. Fetal pulmonary valvuloplasty for critical pulmonary stenosis or atresia with intact septum. *Lancet* 2002; **360**: 1567–1568.

Tworetzky W, McElhinney DB, Margossian R *et al.* Association between cardiac tumors and tuberous sclerosis in the fetus and neonate. *Am J Cardiol* 2003; **92**: 487–489.

Tworetzky W, Wilkins-Haug L, Jennings RW *et al.* Balloon dilation of severe aortic stenosis in the fetus: potential for prevention of hypoplastic left heart syndrome: candidate selection, technique, and results of successful intervention. *Circulation* 2004; **110**: 2125–2131.

Valsangiacomo ER, Hornberger LK, Barrea C, Smallhorn JF, Yoo SJ. Partial and total anomalous pulmonary venous connection in the fetus: two-dimensional and Doppler echocardiographic findings. *Ultrasound Obstet Gynecol* 2003; **22**: 257–263.

Viñals F, Poblete P, Giuliano A. Spatio-temporal image correlation (STIC): a new tool for the prenatal screening of congenital heart defects. *Ultrasound Obstet Gynecol* 2003; **22**: 388–394.

Wladimiroff JW, McGhie JS. M-mode ultrasonic assessment of fetal cardiovascular dynamics. *Br J Obstet Gynaecol* 1981; **88**: 1241–1245.

Yagel S, Arbel R, Anteby EY, Raveh D, Achiron R. The three vessels and trachea view (3VT) in fetal cardiac scanning. *Ultrasound Obstet Gynecol* 2002; **20**: 340–345.

Yagel S, Benachi A, Bonnet D *et al.* Rendering in fetal cardiac scanning: the intracardiac septa and the coronal atrioventricular valve planes. *Ultrasound Obstet Gynecol* 2006; **28**: 266–274.

Yeager SB, Parness IA, Spevak PJ, Hornberger LK, Sanders SP. Prenatal echocardiographic diagnosis of pulmonary and systemic venous anomalies. *Am Heart J* 1994; **128**: 397–405.

Yoo SJ, Lee YH, Kim ES *et al.* Three-vessel view of the fetal upper mediastinum: an easy means of detecting abnormalities of the ventricular outflow tracts and great arteries during obstetric screening. *Ultrasound Obstet Gynecol* 1997; **9**: 173–182.

Yoo SJ, Min JY, Lee YH. Normal pericardial fluid in the fetus: color and spectral Doppler analysis. *Ultrasound Obstet Gynecol* 2001; **18**: 248–52.

Zidere V, Tsapakis EG, Huggon IC, Allan LD. Right aortic arch in the fetus. *Ultrasound Obstet Gynecol* 2006; **28**: 876–881.

Zosmer N, Bajoria R, Weiner E, Rigby M, Vaughan J, Fisk NM. Clinical and echographic features of in utero cardiac dysfunction in the recipient twin in twin–twin transfusion syndrome. *Br Heart J* 1994; **72**: 74–79.

Doppler

Al-Ghazali W, Chapman MG, Allan LD. Doppler assessment of the cardiac and uteroplacental circulations in normal and abnormal fetuses. *Br J Obstet Gynaecol* 1988; **95**: 575–580.

Allan LD, Chita SK, Al-Ghazali W, Crawford DC, Tynan MJ. Doppler echocardiographic evaluation of the normal human fetal heart. *Br Heart J* 1987; **57**: 528–533.

Axt-Fliedner R, Wiegank U, Fetsch C et al. Reference values of fetal ductus venosus, inferior vena cava and hepatic vein blood flow velocities and waveform indices during the second and third trimester of pregnancy. *Arch Gynecol Obstet* 2004; **270**: 46–55.

Berg C, Kremer C, Geipel A, Kohl T, Germer U, Gembruch U. Ductus venosus blood flow alterations in fetuses with obstructive lesions of the right heart. *Ultrasound Obstet Gynecol* 2006; **28**: 137–142.

Better DJ, Apfel HD, Zidere V, Allan LD. Pattern of pulmonary venous blood flow in the hypoplastic left heart syndrome in the fetus. *Heart* 1999; **81**: 646–649.

Better DJ, Kaufman S, Allan LD. The normal pattern of pulmonary venous flow on pulsed Doppler examination of the human fetus. *J Am Soc Echocardiogr* 1996; **9**: 281–285.

Carceller-Blanchard A, Fouron JC. Determinants of the Doppler flow velocity profile through the mitral valve of the human fetus. *Br Heart J* 1995; **70**: 457–460.

Chaoui R, Taddei F, Rizzo G, Bast C, Lenz F, Bollman R. Doppler echocardiography of the main stems of the pulmonary arteries in the normal human fetus. *Ultrasound Obstet Gynecol* 1998; **11**: 167–172.

Chiba Y, Kanzaki T, Kobayashi H, Murakami M, Yutani C. Evaluation of fetal structural heart disease using color flow mapping. *Ultrasound Med Biol* 1990; **16**: 221–229.

Chintala K, Tian Z, Du W, Donaghue D, Rychik J. Fetal Pulmonary venous Doppler patterns in hypoplastic left heart syndrome: relationship to atrial septal restriction. *Heart* Oct 8 2007 (Epub).

Crowe DA, Allan LD. Patterns of pulmonary venous flow in the fetus with disease of the left heart. *Cardiol Young* 2000; **11**: 369–374.

De Smedt MCH, Visser GHA, Meijboom EJ. Fetal cardiac output estimated by Doppler echocardiography during mid- and late gestation. *Am J Cardiol* 1987; **60**: 338–342.

DeVore GR, Horenstein J, Siassi B, Platt LD. Fetal echocardiography, VII. Doppler color flow mapping: a new technique for the diagnosis of congenital heart disease. *Am J Obstet Gynecol* 1987; **156**: 1054–1064.

Feller Printz B, Allan LD. Abnormal pulmonary venous return diagnosed prenatally by pulsed Doppler flow imaging. *Ultrasound Obstet Gynecol* 1997; **9**: 347–349.

Fouron JC, Gosselin J, Amiel-Tison C et al. Correlation between prenatal velocity waveforms in the aortic isthmus and neurodevelopmental outcome between the ages of 2 and 4 years. *Am J Obstet Gynecol* 2001; **184**: 630–636.

Fouron JC, Zarelli M, Drblik SP, Lessard M. Normal flow velocity profile of the fetal aortic isthmus through normal gestation. *Am J Cardiol* 1994; **74**: 483–486.

Friedman D, Buyon J, Kim M, Glickstein JS Fetal cardiac function assessed by Doppler myocardial performance index (Tei Index). *Ultrasound Obstet Gynecol* 2003; **21**: 33–36.

Gembruch U, Chatterjee MS, Bald R, Redel DA, Hansmann M. Color Doppler flow mapping of fetal heart. *J Perinatal Med* 1991; **19**: 27–32.

Gembruch U, Hansmann M, Redel DA, Bald R. Fetal two-dimensional Doppler echocardiography (colour flow mapping) and its place in prenatal diagnosis. *Prenat Diagn* 1989; **9**: 535–547.

Gudmundsson S, Tulzer G, Hutha JC, Marsal K. Venous Doppler in the fetus with absent end diastolic flow in umbilical artery. *Ultrasound Obstet Gynecol* 1996; **7**: 262–267.

Hecher K, Ville Y, Nicolaides KH. Fetal arterial Doppler studies in twin–twin transfusion syndrome. *J Ultrasound Med* 1995; **14**: 101–110.

Huhta JC, Moise KJ, Fisher DJ et al. Detection and quantitation of constriction of the fetal ductus arteriosus by Doppler echocardiography. *Circulation* 1987; **75**: 406–412.

Johnson P, Maxwell DJ, Tynan MJ, Allan LD. Intracardiac pressures in the human fetus. *Heart* 2000; **84**: 59–63.

Kenny JF, Plappert T, Doubilet P et al. Changes in intracardiac blood flow velocities and right and left ventricular stroke volumes with gestational age in the normal human fetus; a prospective Doppler echocardiographic study. *Circulation* 1986; **74**: 1208–1216.

Kessler J, Rasmussen S, Hanson M, Kiserud T. Longitudinal reference ranges for ductus venosus flow velocities and waveform indices. *Ultrasound Obstet Gynecol* 2006; **28**: 890–898.

Kiserud T, Eik-Nes SH, Hellevik LR, Blaas HG. Ductus venosus – a longitudinal Doppler velocimetric study of the human fetus. *J Matern Fetal Invest* 1992; **2**: 5–11.

Kiserud T, Rasmussen S, Skulstad S. Blood flow and the degree of shunting through the ductus venosus in the human fetus. *Am J Obstet Gynecol* 2000; **182**: 147–153.

Koyanagi T, Hara K, Satoh S, Yoshizato T, Nakano H. Relationship between heart rate and rhythm and cardiac performance assessed in the human fetus in utero. *Int J Cardiol* 1990; **28**: 163–171.

Laudy JAM, Huisman TWA, De Ridder MAJ, Wladimirrof JW. Normal fetal pulmonary blood flow velocity. *Ultrasound Obstet Gynecol* 1995; **6**: 277–281.

Machado MVL, Chita SK, Allan LD. Acceleration time in the aorta and pulmonary artery measured by Doppler echocardiography in the mid-trimester normal fetus. *Br Heart J* 1987; **58**: 15–18.

Maulik D, Nanda NC, Hsiung MC, Youngblood JP. Doppler color flow mapping of the fetal heart. *Angiology* 1986; **37**: 628–632.

Mielke G, Benda N. Cardiac output and central distribution of blood flow in the human fetus. *Circulation* 2001; **103**: 1662–1668.

Mitchell JM, Roberts AB, Lee A. Doppler waveforms from the pulmonary arterial system in normal fetuses and those with pulmonary hypoplasia. *Ultrasound Obstet Gynecol* 1998; **11**: 167–172.

Mori Y, Rice MJ, McDonald RW *et al*. Evaluation of systolic and diastolic ventricular performance of the right ventricle in fetuses with ductal constriction using the Doppler Tei index. *Am J Cardiol* 2001; **88**: 1173–1178.

Paladini D, Palmieri S, Celentano E *et al*. Pulmonary venous blood flow in the human fetus. *Ultrasound Obstet Gynecol* 1997; **10**: 27–31.

Prefumo F, Risso D, Venturini PL, De Biasio P. Reference values for ductus venosus Doppler flow measurements at 10–14 weeks of gestation. *Ultrasound Obstet Gynecol* 2002; **20**: 42–46.

Rasenen J, Huhta JC, Weiner S, Wood DC, Ludomirski A. Fetal branch pulmonary arterial vascular impedance during the second half of pregnancy. *Am J Obstet Gynecol* 1996; **174**: 1441–1449.

Rasanen J, Wood DC, Weiner S, Ludomirski A, Huhta JC. Role of the pulmonary circulation in the distribution of human fetal cardiac output during the second half of pregnancy. *Circulation* 1996; **94**: 1068–1073.

Reed KL, Meijboom EJ, Sahn DJ *et al*. Cardiac Doppler flow velocities in human fetuses. *Circulation* 1986; **73**: 41–56.

Reed KL, Sahn DJ, Scagnelli S, Anderson CF, Shenker L. Doppler echocardiographic studies of diastolic function in the human fetal heart: changes during gestation. *J Am Coll Cardiol* 1986; **8**: 391–395.

Schmidt KG, Di Tommaso M, Silverman NH, Rudolph AM. Doppler echocardiographic assessment of fetal descending aortic and umbilical blood flows. Validation studies in lambs. *Circulation* 1991; **83**: 1731–1737.

Schmidt KG, Silverman NH, Rudolph AM. Assessment of flow events at the ductus venosus–inferior vena cava junction and at the foramen ovale in fetal sheep by use of multimodal ultrasound. *Circulation* 1996; **93**: 826–833.

Sharland GK, Chita SK, Allan LD. The use of colour Doppler in fetal echocardiography. *Int J Cardiol* 1990; **28**: 229–236.

Sonesson SE, Fouron JC. Doppler velocimetry of the aortic isthmus in human fetuses with abnormal velocity waveforms in the umbilical artery. *Ultrasound Obstet Gynecol* 1997; **10**: 107–111.

St John Sutton MG, Gewitz MH, Shah B *et al*. Quantitative assessment of growth and function of the cardiac chambers in the normal human fetus: a prospective longitudinal echocardiographic study. *Circulation* 1984; **69**: 645–654.

St John Sutton M, Gill T, Plappert T, Saltzman DH, Doubilet P. Assessment of right and left ventricular function in terms of force development with gestational age in the normal human fetus. *Br Heart J* 1991; **66**: 285–289.

St John Sutton M, Groves A, MacNeil A, Sharland G, Allan L. Assessment of changes in blood flow through the lungs and foramen ovale in the normal human fetus with gestational age: a prospective Doppler echocardiographic study. *Br Heart J* 1994; **71**: 232–237.

van der Mooren K, Barendregt LG, Wladimiroff JW. Fetal atrioventricular and outflow tract flow velocity waveforms during normal second half of pregnancy. *Am J Obstet Gynecol* 1991; **165**: 668–674.

van der Mooren K, Barendregt LG, Wladimiroff JW. Flow velocity wave forms in the human fetal ductus arteriosus during the normal second half of pregnancy. *Pediatr Res* 1991; **30**: 387–490.

van der Mooren K, Wladimiroff JW, Stunen T. Effect of fetal breathing movements on fetal cardiac hemodynamics. *Ultrasound Med Biol* 1991; **17**: 787–790.

van Eyck T, Stewart PA, Wladimiroff JW. Human fetal foramen ovale flow velocity waveforms relative to behavioral states in normal term pregnancy. *Am J Obstet Gynecol* 1990; **163**: 1239–1242.

Wladimiroff JW, McGhie JS. M-mode ultrasonic assessment of fetal cardiovascular dynamics. *Br J Obstet Gynaecol* 1981; **88**: 1241–1245.

Wladimiroff JW, Stewart PA, Burghouwt MT, Stijnen T. Normal fetal cardiac flow velocity waveforms between 11 and 16 weeks of gestation. *Am J Obstet Gynecol* 1992; **167**: 736–773.

The early fetus

Achiron R, Weissman A, Rotstein Z *et al*. Transvaginal echocardiographic examination of the fetal heart between 13 and 15 weeks' gestation in a low-risk population. *J Ultrasound Med* 1994; **13**: 783.

Allan LD, Santos R, Pexieder T. Anatomical and echocardiographic correlates of normal cardiac morphology in the late first trimester fetus. *Heart* 1997; **77**: 68–72.

Borenstein M, Cavoretto P, Allan L, Huggon I, Nicolaides KH. Aberrant right subclavian artery at 11 + 0 to 13 + 6 weeks of gestation in chromosomally normal and abnormal fetuses. *Ultrasound Obstet Gynecol* 2008; **31**: 20–24.

Bronshtein M, Zimmer EZ. Sonographic diagnosis of fetal coarctation of the aorta at 14–16 weeks of gestation. *Ultrasound Obstet Gynecol* 1998; **11**: 254–257.

Huggon IC, Turan O, Allan LD. Doppler assessment of cardiac function at 11–14 weeks' gestation in fetuses with normal and increased nuchal translucency. *Ultrasound Obstet Gynecol* 2004; **24**: 390–398.

Hyett J, Moscoso G, Pappanagiotou G, Perdu M, Nicholaides KH. Abnormalities of the heart and great arteries in chromosomally normal fetuses with increased nuchal translucency thickness at 11–13 weeks gestation. *Ultrasound* 1996; **7**: 245–250.

Hyett JA, Perdu M, Sharland GK, Snijders RS, Nicolaides KH. Increased nuchal translucency at 10–14 weeks of gestation as a marker for major cardiac defects. *Ultrasound Obstet Gynecol* 1997; **10**: 242–246.

Lombardi CM, Bellotti M, Fesslova V, Cappellini A. Fetal echocardiography at the time of the nuchal translucency scan. *Ultrasound Obstet Gynecol* 2007; **29**: 249–257.

Mäkikallio K, Jouppila P, Räsänen J. Human fetal cardiac function during the first trimester of pregnancy. *Heart* 2005; **91**: 334–338.

Nicolaides KH, Azar G, Burn D, Mansur C, Marks K. Fetal nuchal translucency; ultrasound screening for chromosomal defects in the first trimester of pregnancy. *Br Med J* 1992; **304**: 867–869.

Simpson JM, Jones A, Callaghan N, Sharland GK. Accuracy and limitations of transabdominal fetal echocardiography at 12–15 weeks of gestation in a population at high risk for congenital heart disease. *Br J Obstet Gynaecol* 2000; **107**: 1492–1497.

Souka AP, Snijders RJM, Novakov A, Soares W, Nicolaides KH. Defects and syndromes in chromosomally normal fetuses with increased nuchal translucency thickness at 10–14 weeks gestation. *Ultrasound Obstet Gynecol* 1998; **11**: 391–401.

Arrhythmias

Allan LD, Anderson RH, Sullivan ID, Campbell S, Holt DW, Tynan MJ. Evaluation of fetal arrhythmias by echocardiography. *Br Heart J* 1983; **50**: 240–245.

Allan LD, Chita SK, Sharland GK, Maxwell D, Priestley K. Flecainide in the treatment of fetal tachycardias. *Br Heart J* 1991; **65**: 46–48.

Azancot-Benisty A, Jacqz-Aigrain E, Guirgis NM, Decrepy A, Oury JF, Blot P. Clinical and pharmacologic study of fetal supraventricular tachyarrhythmias. *J Pediatr* 1992; **121**: 608–613.

Beinder E, Grancay T, Menéndez T, Singer H, Hofbeck M. Fetal sinus bradycardia and the long QT syndrome. *Am J Obstet Gynecol* 2001; **185**: 743–747.

Berg C, Geipel A, Kohl T et al. Atrioventricular block detected in fetal life: associated anomalies and potential prognostic markers. *Ultrasound Obstet Gynecol* 2005; **26**: 4–15.

Breur JM, Gooskens RH, Kapusta L et al. Neurological outcome in isolated congenital heart block and hydrops fetalis *Fetal Diagn Ther* 2007; **22**: 457–461.

Buyon JP, Heibert R, Copel J et al. Autoimmune-associated congenital heart block: demographics, mortality, morbidity and recurrence rates obtained from a national neonatal lupus registry. *J Am Coll Cardiol* 1998; **31**: 1658–1666.

Buyon JP, Waltuck J, Kleinman C, Copel J. In utero identification and therapy of congenital heart block. *Lupus* 1995; **4**: 116–121.

Fouron JC, Proulx F, Miró J, Gosselin J. Doppler and M-mode ultrasonography to time fetal atrial and ventricular contractions. *Obstet Gynecol* 2000; **96**: 732–736.

Friedman DM, Kim MY, Copel JA et al. for the PRIDE Investigators. Utility of cardiac monitoring in fetuses at risk for congenital heart block. The PR Interval and Dexamethasone Evaluation (PRIDE) Prospective Study. *Circulation* 2008; **117**: 485–493.

Gardiner HM, Belmar C, Pasquini L et al. Fetal ECG: a novel predictor of atrioventricular block in anti-Ro positive pregnancies. *Heart* 2007; **93**: 1454–1460.

Groves AM, Allan LD, Rosenthal E. Outcome of isolated congenital complete heart block diagnosed in utero. *Heart* 1996; **75**: 190–194.

Groves AMM, Allan LD, Rosenthal E. Therapeutic trial of sympathomimetics in three cases of complete heart block in the fetus. *Circulation* 1995; **92**: 3394–3396.

Hofbeck M, Ulmer H, Beinder E, Sieber E, Singer H. Prenatal findings in patients with prolonged QT interval in the neonatal period. *Heart* 1997; **77**: 198–204.

Jaeggi E, Fouron JC, Fournier A et al. Ventriculo-atrial time interval measured on M-mode echocardiography: a determining element in diagnosis treatment and prognosis of fetal supraventricular tachycardia. *Heart* 1998; **79**: 582–587.

Jaeggi ET, Fouron JC, Silverman ED, Ryan G, Smallhorn J, Hornberger LK. Transplacental fetal treatment improves the outcome of prenatally diagnosed complete atrioventricular block without structural heart disease. *Circulation* 2004; **110**: 1542–1548.

Jaeggi ET, Hamilton RM, Silverman ED, Zamora SA, Hornberger LK. Outcome of children with fetal, neonatal or childhood diagnosis of isolated congenital atrioventricular block. A single institution's experience of 30 years. *J Am Coll Cardiol* 2002; **39**: 130–137.

Jaeggi ET, Hornberger LK, Smallhorn JF, Fouron JC. Prenatal diagnosis of complete atrioventricular block associated with structural heart disease: combined experience of two tertiary care centers and review of the literature. *Ultrasound Obstet Gynecol* 2005; **26**: 16–21.

Kleinman C, Donnerstein R, Jaffe C, DeVore G et al. Fetal echocardiography. A tool for evaluation of in utero cardiac arrhythmias and monitoring of in utero therapy: analysis of 71 patients. *Am J Cardiol* 1983; **51**: 237–243.

Krapp M, Kohl T, Simpson JM, Sharland GK, Katalinic A, Gembruch U. Review of diagnosis, treatment, and outcome of fetal atrial flutter compared with supraventricular tachycardia. *Heart* 2003; **89**: 913–917.

Machado MLV, Tynan MJ, Curry PVL, Allan LD. Fetal complete heart block. *Br Heart J* 1988; **60**: 512–515.

Maxwell D, Crawford D, Curry P, Tynan M, Allan L. Obstetric importance, diagnosis, and management of fetal tachycardias. *Br Med J* 1988; **297**: 107–110.

Naheed ZJ, Strasburger JF, Deal BJ, Woodrow Benson Jr DW, Gidding SS. Fetal tachycardias: mechanisms and predictors of hydrops fetalis. *J Am Coll Cardiol* 1996; **27**: 1736–1740.

Nield LE, Silverman ED, Taylor GP *et al.* Maternal anti-Ro and anti-La antibody-associated endocardial fibroelastosis. *Circulation* 2002; **105**: 843–848.

Rein AJ, O'Donnell C, Geva T *et al.* Use of tissue velocity imaging in the diagnosis of fetal cardiac arrhythmias. *Circulation* 2002; **106**: 1827–1833.

Robinson BV, Ettedgui JA, Sherman FS. Use of terbutaline in the treatment of complete heart block in the fetus. *Cardiol Young* 2001; **11**: 683–686.

Schmidt KG, Ulmer HE, Silverman NH, Kleinman CS, Copel JA. Perinatal outcome of fetal complete atrioventricular block: a multicenter experience. *J Am Coll Cardiol* 1991; **91**: 1360–1366.

Simpson JM, Sharland GK. Fetal tachycardias: management and outcome of 127 consecutive cases. *Heart* 1998; **79**: 576–581.

Simpson JM, Yates RW, Sharland GK. Irregular heart rate in the fetus – not always benign. *Cardiol Young* 1996; **6**: 28–31.

Sonnesson ES, Fouron JC, Wesslen-Eriksson E, Jaeggi E, Winberg P. Fetal supraventricular tachycardia treated with sotalol. *Acta Paediatr* 1998; **87**: 584–587.

Sonesson SE, Salomonsson S, Jacobsson LA, Bremme K, Wahren-Herlenius M. Signs of first-degree heart block occur in one-third of fetuses of pregnant women with anti-SSA/Ro 52-kd antibodies. *Arthritis Rheum* 2004; **50**: 1253–1261.

Strasburger JF, Huhta JC, Carpenter RJ, Garson Jr A, McNamara DG. Doppler echocardiography in the diagnosis and management of persistent fetal arrhythmias. *J Am Coll Cardiol* 1986; **7**: **1386**–1391.

Van Engelen AD, Weijtens O, Brenner JI *et al.* Management, outcome and follow-up of fetal tachycardia. *J Am Coll Cardiol* 1994; **24**: 1371–1375.

Ward RM. Pharmacological treatment of the fetus. *Clin Pharmacokinet* 1995; **28**: 343–350.

Zhao H, Cuneo BF, Strasburger JF, Huhta JC, Gotteiner NL, Wakai RT. Electrophysiological characteristics of fetal atrioventricular block. *J Am Coll Cardiol* 2008; **51**: 77–84.

Index